OXFORD MEDICAL PUBLICATIONS

Oxford Handbook of
Rheumatology

Published and forthcoming Oxford Handbooks

Oxford Handbook of
Rheumatology

Second Edition

Alan J. Hakim

Consultant Physician and Rheumatologist,
Whipps Cross University Hospital,
London, UK

and

Honorary Consultant Rheumatologist,
University College London Hospital,
London, UK

Gavin P.R. Clunie

Consultant Rheumatologist,
The Ipswich Hospital NHS Trust,
Ipswich, Suffolk, UK

Inam Haq

Senior Lecturer in Medical Education and Rheumatology,
Brighton and Sussex Medical School,
Mayfield House,
University of Brighton,
Falmer, Essex, UK

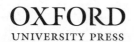

OXFORD
UNIVERSITY PRESS

OXFORD
UNIVERSITY PRESS

Great Clarendon Street, Oxford OX2 6DP

Oxford University Press is a department of the University of Oxford.
It furthers the University's objective of excellence in research, scholarship,
and education by publishing worldwide in

Oxford New York

Auckland Cape Town Dar es Salaam Hong Kong Karachi
Kuala Lumpur Madrid Melbourne Mexico City Nairobi
New Delhi Shanghai Taipei Toronto

With offices in

Argentina Austria Brazil Chile Czech Republic France Greece
Guatemala Hungary Italy Japan Poland Portugal Singapore
South Korea Switzerland Thailand Turkey Ukraine Vietnam

Oxford is a registered trade mark of Oxford University Press
in the UK and in certain other countries

Published in the United States
by Oxford University Press Inc., New York

British Library Cataloguing in Publication Data
Data available

Library of Congress Cataloging in Publication Data
Hakim, Alan.
   Oxford handbook of rheumatology / Alan J. Hakim, Gavin P.R. Clunie.
      p. ; cm.—(Oxford medical publications)
   Includes bibliographical references and index.
1. Rheumatology—Handbooks, manuals, etc.   I. Clunie, Gavin P. R.   II. Title.
III. Title: Handbook of rheumatology.   IV. Series.
   [DNLM: 1. Rheumatic Diseases—Handbooks. WE 39 H155o 2006]
   RC927.O952 2006
   616.7'23—dc22   2006009451

Typeset by Newgen Imaging Systems (P) Ltd., Chennai, India
Printed in China
on acid-free paper by Asia Pacific Offset

ISBN 978–0–19–857135–3 (Flexicover: alk paper)

10 9 8 7 6 5 4 3 2

Foreword

Rheumatic or musculoskeletal disorders can present in a number of familiar ways but sometimes are atypical and occasionally bewildering. They may appear insidiously or acutely and their impact ranges from a temporary nuisance, to a condition that is persistent and increasingly disabling, and sometimes a severe, even life-threatening illness.

Not only are they common, and increasingly so in an ageing population, they are often compounded by other disorders associated with ageing. But they affect people of all ages and especially those of working age in whom they are a major cause of sickness absence and curtailment of normal working life. Most do not call for specialist rheumatological care provided the General Practitioner and General Practitioner with a Special Interest are practiced in their diagnosis and treatment, and long-term care. Specialist referral is sought when the diagnosis is uncertain, the treatment ineffective, or a patient is acutely ill, which in some instances will lead to tertiarly referral.

This small book is up-to-date, based soundly on evidence and good clinical practice. It provides a compact but remarkably comprehensive vade mecum both for clinicians in training and trained clinicians who encounter patients with rheumatologic conditions in any guise, and specialists too. Notably, this new edition includes an important chapter on emergencies in rheumatology.

It is a book that I should have been glad to have by me from the beginning of my own career in rheumatology, and I commend it to clinicians today.

Carol Black
Professor Dame Carol Black, President,
Royal College of Physicians, and Professor of Rheumatology,
Royal Free & University College Medical School,
London.

Preface

Rheumatic conditions are common both in general and hospital practice. Musculoskeletal symptoms are a primary feature of many multisystem illnesses, not only in the autoimmune joint and connective tissue diseases, but also metabolic, endocrine, neoplastic, and infectious conditions. Symptoms are also common in the context of injury, age-related change, and psychological distress. Many conditions in rheumatology are a major source of morbidity and mortality.

We have kept to the format of the first edition of this book, focusing first on history and physical signs in the differential diagnosis of rheumatic disease. The reader is then encouraged to consider diseases in more detail. There have been major advances in rheumatology, not least the introduction of biologic therapy. The second edition reflects this in being up-to-date with assessment, guidelines, and treatment options in 2006. We have also introduced several new chapters in Part 2 including one on rheumatological emergencies.

Part 1 offers a practical guide to arriving at an appropriate differential diagnosis given the realistic presentation of rheumatic disease; for example, how to assess someone complaining of a pain in the elbow, knee pain, or of difficulty moving the shoulder, etc. The book suggests appropriate lines of enquiry for patients who present with characteristic patterns of abnormality such as widespread joint or muscle pain, or joint pains in association with a rash. The aim is to provide a guide for obtaining diagnostic information but also for discriminating good from bad information—where to lay emphasis in eliciting a history and examination signs. In most chapters in Part 1, text is laid out under the headings of Taking a history, Examination, and Investigations, with the subheadings indicating important considerations and areas of enquiry.

Part 2 lists a number of rheumatic conditions encountered in rheumatology and general practice. There is a focus on clinical features, specific findings of relevant investigations, and management. There is reference to childhood and adolescent rheumatic disease throughout. The aim is to provide a comprehensive, clinically orientated text. Some reference is made to disease epidemiology and pathophysiology. However, for more detail on the basic sciences the reader is referred to *The Oxford Textbook of Rheumatology*.

Acknowledgements

We would like to thank the editors of *The Oxford Textbook of Rheumatology* third edition and Dr Richard Watts, Dr Mark Lillicrap, and Dr Rachel Jeffery who reviewed the second edition, and the staff at Oxford University Press for their support and encouragement during the preparation of this book.

Contents

Part 1: The presentation of rheumatic disease

**Part 2: The clinical features and management
of rheumatic diseases**

Detailed Contents

Editorial Advisers

Professor David A. Isenberg,
Bloomsbury Rheumatology Unit,
University College London, UK

Professor Peter J. Maddison,
Department of Rheumatology,
Ysbyty Gwynedd, Bangor, North Wales, UK

Professor Patricia Woo,
Centre of Paediatric and Adolescent Rheumatology,
Windeyer Institute,
London, UK

Professor David Glass,
Division of Rheumatology,
Childrens' Hospital Medical Center,
Cincinnati, Ohio, USA

Symbols and abbreviations

⚠	alert/warning
1°	primary
2°	secondary
↑	increase/raise
↓	decrease/reduce
♂	male(s)
♀	female(s)
±	plus or minus
α	alpha
β	beta
ACA	Anticentromere antibody
AC(J)	Acromioclavicular (joint)
ACR	American College of Rheumatology
ADM	Abductor digiti minimi
ALP	Alkaline phosphatase
ALT	Alanine transaminase
ANA	Anti-nuclear antibody
ANCA	Antineutrophil cytoplasmic antibody
AP	Anteroposterior
APB	Abductor pollicis brevis
APL	Abductor pollicis longus
APS	Antiphospholipid (antibody) syndrome
ARA	American Rheumatism Association
AS	Ankylosing spondylitis
AST	Aspartate transaminase
ASOT	Antistreptolysin O titre
ASU	Avocado/soybean unsaponifiable
AZA	Azathioprine
BCP	Basic calcium phosphate (crystals)
bd	Twice daily
BJHS	Benign joint hypermobility syndrome
BMC	Bone mineral content
BMD	Bone mineral density
BSR	British Society of Rheumatology
C	Cervical (e.g. C6 is the sixth cervical vertebra)
CA	Coracoacromial

CINCA	Chronic, infantile, neurological, cutaneous, and articular syndrome
CK	Creatine phosphokinase
CMC(J)	Carpometacarpal (joint)
CMV	Cytomegalovirus
CPPD	Calcium pyrophosphate deposition (arthritis)
CREST	Calcinosis, Raynaud's, Oesophageal dysmotility, Sclerodactyly, Telangiectasia (syndrome)
CRP	C reactive protein
CS	Congenital scoliosis
CSS	Churg–Strauss syndrome
CT	Computed tomography
CTS	Carpal tunnel syndrome
CXR	Chest radiograph
dcSScl	Diffuse cutaneous systemic sclerosis
DEXA/DXA	Dual-energy X-ray absorptiometry
DIP(J)	Distal interphalangeal (joint)
DISH	Diffuse idiopathic skeletal hyperostosis
DLCO	Diffusion capacity for carbon monoxide
DM	Dermatomyositis
DMARD	Disease-modifying antirheumatic drug
DVT	Deep vein thrombosis
EA	Enteropathic arthritis
EBV	Epstein–Barr virus
ECG (EKG)	Electrocardiograph
ECM	Erythema chronicum migrans
ECRB	Extensor carpi radialis brevis
ECRL	Extensor carpi radialis longus
ECU	Extensor carpi ulnaris
ED	Extensor digitorum
EDL	Extensor digitorum longus
EDM	Extensor digiti minimi
EDS	Ehlers–Danlos syndrome
EHL	Extensor hallucis longus
EI	Extensor indicis
ELMS	Eaton–Lambert myasthenic syndrome
EMG	Electromyography
EN	Eythema nodosum
ENA(S)	Extractable nuclear antigen(s)
EPB	Extensor pollicis brevis
EPL	Extensor pollicis longus
ERA	Enthesitis-related arthritis

ESR	Erythrocyte sedimentation rate
ESSG	European Spondylarthropathy Study Group
EULAR	European League Against Rheumatism
FBC (CBC)	Full blood count
FCR	Flexor carpi radialis
FCU	Flexor carpi ulnaris
FDP	Flexor digitorum profundus
FDS	Flexor digitorum superficialis
FHB	Flexor hallucis brevis
FM	Fibromyalgia
FMF	Familial Mediterranean fever
FPL	Flexor pollicis longus
FR	Flexor retinaculum
GARA	Gut associated reactive arthritis
GBS	Guillain Barre syndrome
GCA	Giant cell arteritis
GFR	Glomerular filtration rate
GI	Gastrointestinal
GOA	Generalized osteoarthritis
HA	Hydroxyapatite
HIV	Human immunodeficiency virus
HLA	Human leucocyte antigen
HO	Hypertrophic osteoarthropathy
HSP	Henoch–Schönlein purpura
HTLV	Human T-cell leukaemia virus
IL	Interleukin
ILAR	International League of Associations for Rheumatology
IM	Intramuscular(ly)
INR	International normalized ratio
ITB	Iliotibial band
ITP	Idiopathic thrombocytopenic purpura
JCA	Juvenile chronic arthritis
JIA	Juvenile idiopathic arthritis
JIO	Juvenile idiopathic osteoporosis
KD	Kawasaki disease
L	Lumbar (e.g. L5 is the fifth lumbar vertebra)
LCL	Lateral collateral ligament
LDH	Lactate dehydrogenase
LFTS	Liver function tests
lcSScl	Limited cutaneous systemic sclerosis
MCP(J)	Metacarpophalangeal (joint)
MCL	Medial collateral ligament

MCTD	Mixed connective tissue disease
MG	Myasthenia gravis
MND	Motor neuron disease
MPA	Microscopic polyangiitis
MR	Magnetic resonance
MTP(J)	Metatarsophalangeal (joint)
MTX	Methotrexate
NMS	Neuromuscular scoliosis
nocte	Every night
NSAID	Non-steroidal anti-inflammatory drug
OA	Osteoarthritis
OI	Osteogenesis imperfecta
PAN	Polyarteritis nodosa
PBC	Primary biliary cirrhosis
PCR	Polymerase chain reaction
PIN	Posterior interosseous nerve
PIP(J)	Proximal interphalangeal (joint)
PL	Palmaris longus
PLM	Polarized light microscopy
PM	Polymyositis
PMN	Polymorphonuclear neutrophil
PMR	Polymyalgia rheumatica
PSA	Psoriatic arthritis
PSA	Prostatic specific antigen
PTH	Parathyroid hormone
PV	Plasma viscosity
PVNS	Pigmented villonodular synovitis
qds	Four times daily
RA	Rheumatoid arthritis
RF	Rheumatoid factor
RNP	Ribonuclear protein
RP	Raynaud's phenomenon
REA	Reactive arthritis
RSD	Reflex sympathetic dystrophy (algo/osteodystrophy)
RSI	Repetitive strain injury
RS_3PE	Remitting seronegative symmetrical synovitis with pitting oedema
RTA	Renal tubular acidosis
sACE	Serum angiotensin converting enzyme
SAI	Subacromial impingement
SAPHO	Synovitis, acne, palmoplantar pustolosis, hyperostosis, aseptic osteomyelitis (syndrome)
SARA	Sexually transmitted reactive arthritis

s/c	Subcutaneous(ly)
SC(J)	Sternoclavicular (joint)
SI(J)	Sacroiliac (joint)
SLE	Systemic lupus erythematosus
SS	Sjögren's syndrome
SScl/Scl	Systemic sclerosis/Scleroderma
T	Thoracic (e.g. T5 is the fifth thoracic vertebra)
TB	Tuberculosis
tds	Three times daily
TENS	Transcutaneous electrical nerve stimulation
TFTs	Thyroid function tests
TIA	Transient ischaemic attack
TM(J)	Temperomandibular (joint)
TNF(α)	Tumour necrosis factor (alpha)
TPMT	Thiopurine S-methyltransferase
TRAPs	Tumour necrosis factor-associated periodic syndrome
TSH	Thyroid stimulating hormone
UC	Ulcerative colitis
U&E	Urea and electrolytes
US	Ultrasound
UV	Ultraviolet
WG	Wegener's granulomatosis
WHO	World Health Organization

Part I

The presentation of rheumatic disease

Evaluating musculoskeletal pain

Introduction

Pain is the most common musculoskeletal symptom. It is defined by its subjective description, which may vary depending on its physical/biological cause, the patient's understanding of it, its impact on function, and the emotional and behavioural response it invokes. Pain is also often 'coloured' by cultural, linguistic, and religious differences. Therefore pain is not merely an unpleasant sensation; it is in effect an 'emotional change'. The experience is different for every individual.

In children and adolescents the evaluation of pain is sometimes complicated further by the interacting influences of the experience of pain within the family, school, and peer group.

Localization of pain and pain patterns

- Adults usually accurately localize joint or muscle pain, although there are some situations worth noting in rheumatic disease where pain can be poorly localized (see Table 1.1).
- Pain may be well localized but caused by a distant lesion, e.g. interscapular pain caused by postural/mechanical problems in the cervical spine.
- Pain caused by neurological abnormalities, ischaemic pain, and pain referred from viscera is less easy for the patient to visualize or express and the history may be given with varied interpretations.
- Bone pain is generally constant despite movement or change in posture—in comparison with muscular, synovial, ligament, or tendon pain—and often disturbs sleep. Fracture, tumour, and metabolic bone disease are all possible causes. Such constant, local, sleep-disturbing pain should always be considered sinister and investigated.
- Patterns of pain distribution are associated with certain musculoskeletal conditions, e.g. shoulder girdle muscle pain in poly-myalgia rheumatica (PMR) and symmetrical/peripheral joint pain in rheumatoid arthritis (RA). The patterns describe a typical case but are not invariable.
- Patterns of pain distribution may overlap, especially in the elderly where common diseases coexist, e.g. hip and/or knee osteoarthritis (OA), peripheral vascular disease, degenerative lumbar spine.

The quality of pain

Some individuals find it hard to describe pain or use descriptors of severity. A description of the quality of pain can often help to discriminate the cause. Certain pain descriptors are associated with non-organic pain syndromes (see Table 1.2):

- Burning pain, hyperpathia, and allodynia suggest a neurological cause.
- A change in the description of pain in a patient with a long-standing condition is worth noting as it may denote the presence of a second condition, e.g. a fracture or septic arthritis in a patient with established RA.

Repeated, embellished, or elaborate description may suggest non-organic pain, but be aware that such a presentation may be cultural for example.

Table 1.1 Clinical pointers in conditions where pain is poorly localized

Diagnosis	Clinical pointer
Periarticular shoulder pain	Referred to deltoid insertion
Carpal tunnel syndrome	Nocturnal parasthesiae and/or pain, often diffuse
Trochanteric bursitis	Nocturnal pain lying on affected side
Hip Synovitis	Groin/outer thigh pain radiating to the knee

Table 1.2 Terms from the McGill pain scale that help distinguish between organic and non-organic pain syndromes

Organic	Non-organic
Pounding	Flickering
Jumping	Shooting
Pricking	Lancinating
Sharp	Lacerating
Pinching	Crushing
Hot	Searing
Tender	Splitting
Nagging	Torturing
Spreading	Piercing
Annoying	Unbearable
Tiring	Exhausting
Fearful	Terrifying
Tight	Tearing

Eliciting changes in pain by the use of examination techniques

Eliciting changes in pain by the use of different examination techniques may be used to provide clues to the diagnosis:

- Palpation and specific resisted and passive movements can be used to reproduce pain, localizing pathology. For validity, however, a good knowledge of anatomy and a practiced technique are required.
- Given the context in which the examination is done and the effects of suggestibility, manoeuvres should always be interpreted carefully and many experienced clinicians would agree that in certain clinical settings there continues to be a high degree of interobserver variation in diagnosis. Diagnostic examination criteria continue to develop, and many are now validated for research purposes.
- Palpation and passive movement of structures are performed whilst the patient is static. The concept of 'passive' movement is the assumption that muscles and tendons around the joint are removed as potential sources of pain, i.e. one is left just eliciting limitation of movement at the articular surface. This assumption has its own limitations, not least because passive movements of the joint will still cause movement of the soft tissues. In some cases, e.g. shoulder rotator cuff disease, the joint may be painful to move passively because of subluxation or impingement 2° to a musculotendinous lesion.
- The clinician should be aware of myofascial pain when palpating musculotendinous structures, especially around the neck and shoulder regions. Myofascial pain is said to occur when there is activation of a trigger point that elicits pain in a zone stereotypical for the individual muscle. It is often aching in nature.
- Trigger points are associated with palpable tender bands. It is not clear whether trigger points are the same as the tender points characteristic of fibromyalgia.
- Local anaesthetic infiltration at the site of a painful structure is sometimes used to help localize pathology, e.g. injection under the acromion followed by a repeat of an 'impingement test' gauging change from a previously positive test. However, the technique is only reliable if precise localization of injected anaesthetic can be guaranteed. Few, if any, rigorously controlled trials have shown it to give specific results for any condition.

The assessment of pain in young children

The assessment of pain in young children is often difficult:

- Young children often localize pain poorly. Careful identification of the painful area is necessary through observation and palpation.
- A child may not admit to pain but will withdraw the limb or appear anxious when the painful area is examined.
- Observing a child's facial expression during an examination is very important, as is the parent's response.
- Quantification of pain often requires non-verbal clues such as the child's behaviour. Pain rating scales are often helpful (see Fig. 1.1).

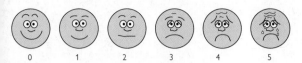

Fig. 1.1 Pain assessment in children—the faces rating scale.

Regional musculoskeletal conditions: making a working diagnosis

Introduction

This chapter aims to provide a guide to constructing an appropriate differential diagnosis in the patient who presents with regional musculoskeletal symptoms. It does not make reference to all possible diagnoses, only the most common. The section is divided into discussion of the neck, upper limb (shoulder, elbow, wrist), hand, thoracolumbar spine, lower limb (pelvis, groin, thigh, knee), and foot.

General consideratons

- Findings from conventional clinical examination and imaging of the musculoskeletal system usually reflect a static situation. Examination in the context of function (i.e. carrying, lifting, walking, bending, etc.) is not easy, though it is arguably more appropriate. Therefore a thorough history utilizing a good depth of knowledge of functional anatomy is the best alternative and an invaluable way of obtaining good information about abnormal function and its causes.

- Time spent obtaining a detailed account of the onset of symptoms is often helpful whether or not the symptoms are of recent onset or chronic or obviously associated with trauma. Patients usually have a clearer concept of injury-induced disease and may try to rationalize the appearance of non-trauma-related symptoms by association with an event or injury.

- Weakness (as a symptom) may be due to a neuropathic or myopathic condition or it may be perceived according to the impact of other symptoms such as pain.

- With children it is important to obtain a history from both the carer (parent, nanny, or other adult) and the child. Second-hand information, even if provided by the mother, may be less reliable than direct information from the carer.

- Regional musculoskeletal lesions may be a presenting feature of a systemic disorder such as an autoimmune rheumatic disease, malignancy or infection. Clinical suspicion should trigger a common 'screen' of investigations.

- Screening for disseminated malignancy, lymphoma, myeloma, and infection should at least include an FBC, immunoglobulins, ESR, CRP and bone biochemistry. Thereafter tests should be directed specifically towards the clinical scenario.

Corticosteroid injections and rehabilitation, as part of regional pain treatment, are discussed in general terms at appropriate points in the text. The practical approach to these therapies is presented at the end of this chapter.

Neck pain

Background epidemiology

- About 10% of the adult population has neck pain at any one time, although many people do not seek medical help.
- About 1% of adult patients with neck pain develop neurological deficit, but overall levels of disability are lower than for patients with low back pain.
- Isolated neck pain in children and adolescents is unusual. More commonly it accompanies thoracic spine pain or pathology.
- A continuum of radiological appearances exists in relation to age: intervertebral disc narrowing, marginal end-plate osteophytes, and facet joint changes. The appearances are often termed 'degenerative'; however, their correlation with the presence and severity of pain is poor.

Table 2.1 lists the major causes of neck pain in adults.

Functional anatomy

- The neck is the most mobile (37 separate articulations) but least stable part of the spine. There are seven vertebrae (C1–C7) and five intervertebral discs (C2/3–C6/7). The C7/T1 disc is most often associated with radicular symptoms and 'degenerative' disease is common between C5 and T1. If it occurs, cord compression is most likely in this region, though atlantoaxial subluxation may produce the same picture.
- Minor congenital abnormalities are not infrequent and increase the risk of degenerative changes.
- Nerve roots C2 and C3 cover sensation over the back of the head, the lower jaw line, and the neck.
- Nerve roots (C4–T1) leave the spine in dural root sleeves, traverse the intervertebral foramina and form the brachial plexus.
- Cervical nerves have a dermatomal representation (Fig. 2.1) and supply upper limb musculature in a predictable way.

Taking a history

The site, radiation, and description of pain

- Nerve root (radicular) pain is usually sharp and reasonably well-localized in the arms. It is often 'burning' and associated with parasthesiae and numbness. Nerve root irritation and compression by an intervertebral disc are common causes of radicular pain. However, in older adults and those who suffer recurrent bouts of pain it is usually due to encroachment of vertebral end-plate or facet joint osteophytes, or thickened soft tissue/fibrosis on the nerve leading to stenosis of the exit foramen.

Table 2.1 The major causes of neck pain in adults

Soft tissue lesions (posture, psychogenic issues, and overuse as modifiers)	Neck strain
	Torticollis
	Myofascial pain
	Trauma (e.g. acute flexion—extension injury ('whiplash'))
	Cervicothoracic interspinous bursitis
Degenerative and mechanical lesions	Spondylosis
	Disc prolapse
	Thoracic outlet syndrome
	Diffuse idiopathic skeletal hyperostosis (DISH)
Inflammatory conditions	Rheumatoid arthritis (RA)
	Spondylarthropathy (associated with fracture and inflammatory discitis) (Chapter 8)
	Juvenile idiopathic arthritis (Chapter 7)
	Polymyalgia rheumatica (PMR) (Chapter 14)
	Myelitis
Bone lesions	Traumatic fracture
	Osteomyelitis (e.g. TB)
	Osteoporosis (fragility fracture) (Chapter 16)
	Osteomalacia (bone disease or muscle pain)
	Paget's disease
Non-osseous infections	General systemic infection (general/cervical myalgia)
	Meningitis
	Discitis
Malignancy	Primary (rare) or 2° tumours (and pathological fracture)
	Myeloma, lymphoma, leukaemias
Brachial plexus lesions	Trauma
	Thoracic outlet syndromes (e.g. cervical rib)
Referred pain from	Acromioclavicular or temporomandibular joint
	Heart and major arteries (e.g. angina, thoracic aorta dissection)
	Pharynx (e.g. infection, tumour)
	Lung and diaphragm (e.g. Pancoast tumour, subphrenic abscess)
	Abdomen (e.g. gallbladder, stomach, oesophageal, or pancreatic disease)
	Shoulder (e.g. adhesive capsulitis) (Chapter 2 and 19)

- Pain from deep cervical structures is common. It often localizes poorly across the upper back. It can be referred to the upper arms, is typically described as 'heavy' or 'aching' and is more diffuse than nerve root pain.
- Muscle spasm often accompanies various lesions. It can be very painful.
- Pain from the upper cervical spine (C1–C3) can be referred to the temperomandibular joint (TMJ) or retro-orbital regions. Conversely, pain from both TMJ disorders and as a result of dental malocclusion can be referred to the neck.
- Pain from the lower neck may be referred to the interscapula and anterior thoracic wall regions. The latter may mimic cardiac ischaemic pain.
- Florid descriptions of the pain and of its extent and severity are associated with prominent psychological modulators of pain.
- Evaluation of the shoulder joint is often necessary as pathology there often coexists and symptoms around the shoulder often complicate neck evaluation.
- Occipital headache is a common manifestation.

Acute neck pain with trauma

⚠ Acute neck pain with trauma requires urgent assessment even if there are no obvious neurological symptoms:

- Acute trauma requires urgent evaluation and consideration of fracture, spinal cord damage, and vertebral instability. About 80% of serious injuries occur from an accelerating head hitting a stationary object.
- An abrupt flexion injury may fracture the odontoid (this occurs less commonly with extension); however, < one in five injuries at C1/C2 produce neurological deficit because of the wide canal at this level.
- If not traumatic or osteoporotic (the latter being relatively rare in the cervical spine), fractures may occur in bone invaded by malignancy.

New and/or associated symptoms

Ask about associated leg weakness and new bladder or bowel symptoms. New onset acute neck pain with neurological features needs urgent evaluation. Neurological symptoms may also accompany chronic neck pain:

- Spinal osteomyelitis, meningitis, discitis (infection or inflammation), myelitis and fracture may all present with acute or subacute neck pain. All may cause cord compression. Myelopathy due to spondylosis typically presents with a slowly progressive disability over weeks/months, although it can be acute, particularly if associated with central disc prolapse.
- Subacute pain, flaccid paralysis and profound distal neurological signs may suggest myelitis, a condition caused mainly by infections and autoimmune diseases.
- Tinnitus, gait disturbance, blurring of vision and diplopia associated with neck pain are all ascribed to irritation of the cervical sympathetic nerves.

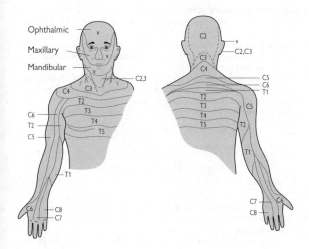

Fig. 2.1 Dermatomal distribution of the cervical and upper thoracic nerves reflecting the radicular pattern of nerve root lesions.

- The vertebral arteries pass close to the facet joints just anterior to emerging nerve roots. Dogma invokes disruption of vertebral blood flow as a cause of dizziness in severe cases of neck spondylosis.

Previous trauma

Ask about previous trauma—it often precedes and influences chronic pain:
- Acute and occupational (chronic overuse) trauma is a common antecedent of chronic neck pain.
- Unresolved litigation associated with trauma is a recognized correlate of the persistence of neck pain and reported disability.
- Cervical dystonia (torticollis) can occur 1 to 4 days after acute trauma, it responds poorly to treatment and can be long-standing. It may also complicate arthropathy such as in RA or Parkinson's disease.
- Whiplash injury is associated with chronic myofascial pain.
- In some patients with chronic pain following, sometimes trivial, trauma there may be dissatisfaction with the quality of care received at the time of the injury.

Occupational and leisure activities

Some occupations and sports/activities are associated with recurrent neck pain:

- Neck pain (and early spondylosis) is prevalent in people whose occupations require persistent awkward head and neck postures, e.g. professional dancers.
- Though biomechanical factors may be an important influence in initiating and aggravating neck pain, there may also be an underlying genetic predisposition to OA and/or hypermobility.

Other points

Establish whether the pain started or varies with any non-musculoskeletal symptoms:

- Cardiac ischaemia, dyspepsia, or abdominal pain can result in referred pain to the neck (see Table 2.9).

Examination

The neck is part of the functional upper limb and symptoms in the arms and legs may be relevant. Neurological examination of the arms is important.

- Inspection from front and back may reveal specific muscle wasting or spasm and poor posture.
- Observing active movements reveals little if the patient has severe pain or muscle spasm. Inability to move the neck even small distances is characteristic in advanced ankylosing spondylitis (AS) (Chapter 8).
- Tenderness often localizes poorly in degenerative disease. Exquisite tenderness raises the possibility of a disc lesion, osteomyelitis, or malignancy (the latter two are rare).
- There may be 'trigger points' in neck stabilizer and extensor muscles. Activation of a trigger point elicits myofascial pain in a zone that is stereotypical for the individual muscle.
- Tender points (localized, non-radiating pain elicited on thumb pad pressure), notably at the occipital origin of the trapezius, the medial scapular border and the mid-belly of the trapezius, are features of fibromyalgia (FM) (Chapter 18). It is not clear whether tender and trigger points are the same.
- Examination of passive mobility may be helpful primarily if it reveals gross asymmetry. The normal range of movement varies depending on age, sex, and ethnicity. Generally, at least 45° of lateral flexion and 70° of rotation should be achieved in a middle-aged adult. Global loss of passive mobility is non-specific and occurs with increasing age. The range of movement that might indicate hypermobility has not been established.
- Care should be taken if neck instability is a possibility (e.g. fracture, RA). Vigorous passive examination of forward flexion may exacerbate disc lesions.
- Examination of the shoulder is important to evaluate any referred pain or associated articular lesion (e.g. adhesive capsulitis) (Chapter 19).
- Neurological examination of upper and lower limbs is important in all cases where pain is referred to the arms and/or the legs if cord compression is a possibility: look for ↑ tone, clonus, pyramidal weakness and extensor plantar response. Check for a cervicothoracic sensory level.

Investigations
Radiographs
Radiographs should be requested with specific objectives in mind:
- A lateral neck film may demonstrate soft tissue thickening in infection or synovium in RA (Chapter 5), will document spondylitis (syndesmophytes, discitis and periosteal apposition (in posterior elements associated with psoriasis)), and the severity of spondylosis.
- Oblique views centred on the suspected level may show nerve root foramen stenosis from bony encroachment in patients with radiculopathy. There may be underlying OA (Chapter 6).
- High cervical flexion and extension views and a 'through-the-mouth' view are useful to demonstrate odontoid pathology.
- In a patient with RA, if the distance between the anterior arch of the atlas and odontoid process is > 3 mm on a lateral film taken in flexion, there is likely to be C1/C2 AP subluxation.
- On a lateral film superior odontoid subluxation in RA can be judged from a reduced distance from the anteroinferior surface of C2 to a line drawn between the hard palate and base of the occiput (McGregor's line). The distance should be >34 mm in men and >29 mm in women. Lateral odontoid subluxation is best demonstrated with magnetic resonance (MR) imaging.
- Stepwise vertebral subluxation throughout the cervical spine demonstrated on a lateral film is characteristic of (advanced) RA.
- There may be only a few but important signs of spinal infection such as a soft tissue mass or isolated loss of joint space.

Magnetic resonance (MR) and computed tomography (CT)
- MR has largely superceded CT, arthrography, and CT-arthrography in assessing cervical spine/nerve, dural, vertebral, disc, and other soft tissue lesions in the neck.
- In many cases the relevance of some MR 'abnormalities' is still being established—patterns of signal abnormality do occur in asymptomatic people. The frequency of these effects increases with age.
- MR is the technique of choice for imaging disc prolapse, myelopathy (Plate 1), myelitis and for excluding infection or tumours. MR is used to help evaluate the need for, and plan, neurosurgical intervention in high cervical instability in RA patients.
- MR may show soft-tissue swelling around the odontoid in CPPD disease (Chapter 15) but the diagnosis is best made with CT which shows calcification around the odontoid and of adjacent ligaments ('crowned dens syndrome').
- In patients with the combination of unexplained radiographic signs and generalized symptoms MR is an important investigation. Cases of spinal infection such as TB or brucellosis and lymphoma and can be picked up (Chapter 17).

Scintigraphy
- Scintigraphy has little role in diagnosing neck lesions.
- Despite improved image quality and tomographic images, on an isotope bone scan the neck remains one of the most poorly imaged regions of the skeleton and it is non-specific.

Treatment

Table 2.2 shows the principles of treating mechanical cervical syndromes and the timing of MR scanning.

- Remember to review the diagnosis if pain is persistent depite treatment and symptoms seem disproportionate to the results or reports of imaging. In our experience inflammatory psoriatic-related neck pains are often mistaken for 'cervical spondylosis'. This may be because the clinician too readily assumes the latter diagnosis and/or radiologists misreport radiographs.

Table 2.2 The principles of treating mechanical neck syndromes and the timing of mr scanning

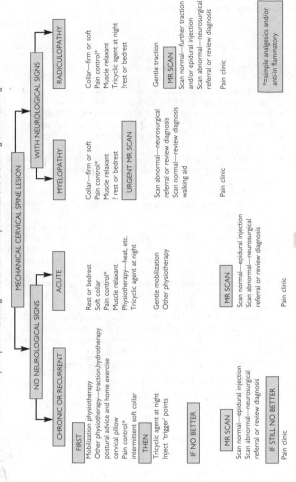

MECHANICAL CERVICAL SPINE LESION

NO NEUROLOGICAL SIGNS

CHRONIC OR RECURRENT

FIRST
Mobilization physiotherapy
Other physiotherapy—traction,hydrotherapy
postural advice and home exercise
cervical pillow
Pain control*
intermittent soft collar

THEN
Tricyclic agent at night
Inject 'trigger' points

IF NO BETTER

MR SCAN
Scan normal—epidural injection
Scan abnormal—neurosurgical
referral or review diagnosis

IF STILL NO BETTER

Pain clinic

ACUTE

Rest or bedrest
Soft collar
Pain control*
Muscle relaxant
Physiotherapy—heat, etc.
Tricyclic agent at night

Gentle mobilization
Other physiotherapy

MR SCAN
Scan normal—epidural injection
Scan abnormal—neurosurgical
referral or review diagnosis

Pain clinic

WITH NEUROLOGICAL SIGNS

MYELOPATHY

Collar—firm or soft
Pain control*
Muscle relaxant
? rest or bedrest

URGENT MR SCAN

Scan abnormal—neurosurgical
referral or review diagnosis
Scan normal—review diagnosis
walking aid

Pain clinic

RADICULOPATHY

Collar—firm or soft
Pain control*
Muscle relaxant
Tricyclic agent at night
?rest or bedrest

Gentle traction

MR SCAN
Scan normal—further traction
and/or epidural injection
Scan abnormal—neurosurgical
referral or review diagnosis

Pain clinic

*=simple analgesics and/or
anti-inflammatory

Shoulder pain

Anatomy of the shoulder (see Fig. 2.2)

- The glenohumeral joint is a ball and socket joint. The shallow glenoid cavity permits a wide range of movement. The circular fibrocartilagenous labrum sits on the glenoid and increases the articular surface area and acts as a static joint stabilizer.
- Normal glenohumeral movements include depression then glide and rotation of the humeral head under the coracoacromial (CA) arch to enable elevation of the arm. As the arm elevates there is smooth rotation and elevation of the scapula on the thoracic wall.
- Shoulder movements are a synthesis of four joints: glenohumeral, acromioclavicular (AC), sternoclavicular (SC), and scapulothoracic.
- Movements at AC and SC joints enable slight clavicular rotation, shoulder elevation/depression, and protraction/retraction.
- The rigid CA arch protects the glenohumeral joint from trauma and it, and the overlying deltoid, are separated from the capsule by the subacromial (subdeltoid) bursa.
- A cuff of muscles surrounds the glenohumeral joint capsule. These 'rotator cuff ' muscles are supraspinatus, infraspinatus, teres minor, and subscapularis.
- Supraspinatus initiates abduction by depressing the humeral head then elevating the arm alone for the first 10° of movement. The more powerful deltoid then takes over abduction. Infraspinatus/ teres minor and subscapularis externally and internally rotate the arm in the anatomical position respectively (see Fig. 2.3).
- Production of powerful shoulder movements requires some degree of arm elevation as the larger muscles such as deltoid, latissimus dorsi (extensor), and teres major (adductor) work inefficiently with the arm in the anatomical position. The rotator cuff muscles act synchronously as joint stabilizers throughout the range of shoulder movement.
- The long head of biceps tendon originates above the glenoid usually attached to the labrum and runs within the glenohumeral joint capsule anteromedially in a bony groove.

Pain and shoulder lesions (see Chapter 19)

- Shoulder pain is common and may have its origin in articular or periarticular structures or may be referred from the cervical or thoracic spine, thoracic outlet or subdiaphragmatic structures (Table 2.3).
- Shoulder lesions often produce pain referred to the humeral deltoid insertion (patient points to upper arm).
- Periarticular disorders, mainly subacromial impingement (SAI) disorders, are the commonest cause of shoulder pain in adults (> 90% of cases).

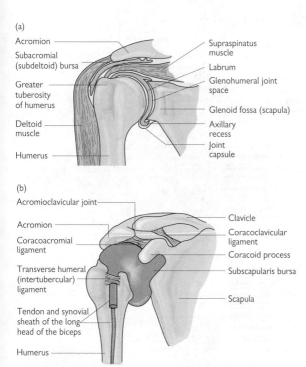

Fig. 2.2 (a) Major shoulder structures. (b) The relationship of the joint capsule to its bony surround and the coracoacromial arch

- Traumatic or inflammatory lesions of many different shoulder structures and conditions that result in neuromuscular weakness of the rotator cuff or scapular stabilizers may result in impingement pain.
- Impingement pain is thought to be generated by the 'squashing' of subacromial structures between the greater tuberosity of the humeral head and the CA arch during rotation/elevation of the humeral head.

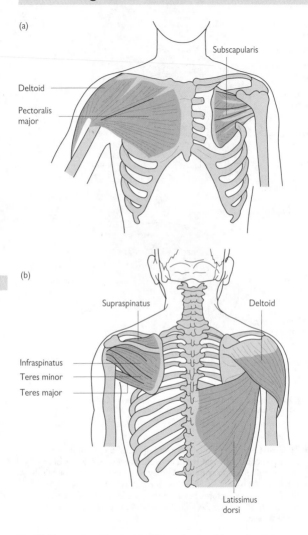

Fig. 2.3 The muscles of the shoulder: (a) anterior view; (b) posterior view

Table 2.3 The commonest causes of shoulder pain

Periarticular lesions (often manifest as subacromial impingement pain)	Rotator cuff tendonitis/tears (very common age 40y+)
	Calcific tendonitis
	Bicipital tendonitis
	Subacromial bursitis
	Milwaukee shoulder (basic calcium phosphate crystal periarthritis)
	Periarticular muscle weakness
Articular lesions	Synovitis (glenohumeral or AC)
	OA (glenohumeral or AC)
	Glenohumeral instability (e.g. labral tears)
	Adhesive capsulitis ('frozen shoulder')
Neurological	Cervical nerve root and radicular referred pain
	Neuralgic amyotrophy
	Spinal cord lesions: tumours, syringomyelia
Neurovascular	Algodystrophy (see Chapter 18)
Thoracic conditions (referred pain)	Mediastinal tumours
	Angina
Systemic and diffuse conditions	Polymyalgia rheumatica (see Chapter 14)
	Myositis (see Chapter 13)
	Chronic pain disorders (see Chapter 18)
	Polyarticular synovitis
Bone disorders	Tumours
	Osteonecrosis (see Chapter 16)
	Paget's disease (see Chapter 16)
Subdiaphragmatic (referred pain)	Gallbladder disease
	Subphrenic abscess

Taking a history

When did the pain start? Injury?

Injurious conditions are common and are both acute and chronic (overuse).

- Rotator cuff lesions (inflammation, degenerative weakness, or tear) are often associated with activities and occupations that involve straining the arm in abduction or forward flexion. A history of an acute 'injury', however, is not always obtained. Subsequent calcification in the tendon following a supraspinatus injury can be asymptomatic or present with acute pain.
- Manual labour (e.g. seamstress) is a risk for rotator cuff lesions. There is typically no acute injury but a history of recurrent provocative movements over years.
- Athletes employed in throwing and racket sports are at risk of rotator cuff tendonopathy and labral tears. Rugby players are at risk of clavicle fracture, shoulder dislocation (and long-term instability), and disruption of the acromioclavicular joint (ACJ).
- Pain from degenerative glenohumeral or ACJ arthritis might be a long-term sequelae of a bone or joint injury.
- The shoulder girdle is one of the commonest sites for a chronic pain syndrome.
- Myofascial pain of the shoulder girdle is common and may mimic the symptoms of cervical radiculopathy and even reflux oesophagitis or ischaemic heart disease.
- Severe, persistent, sleep-disturbing pain of recent onset may be indicative of avascular necrosis, osteomyelitis, or of bony tumours. Though uncommon in the shoulder region these conditions should not be missed.

Where is the pain?

- Pain from the shoulder may be referred to the deltoid insertion.
- Well-localized pain may occur with ACJ arthritis (e.g. patient places a finger on the affected joint) though referred C4 nerve root pain and pain from bone lesions of the distal clavicle is maximal in the same area.
- Glenohumeral articular and capsulitis pain is not well localized (e.g. the patient covers their shoulder with their hand).
- Periscapular pain may be associated with SAI syndromes but may also be myofascial (typically) or referred from the cervicothoracic spine.
- Bilateral shoulder pain should increase suspicion of the presence of an inflammatory polyarthritis such as RA (see Chapter 5), juvenile idiopathic arthritis (JIA, Chapter 7), psoriatic arthritis (see Chapter 8) or CPPD arthritis (see Chapter 15)—these would be rare without other joint symptoms.
- Diffuse pain across shoulder girdle muscles in those over 55 years of age raises the possibility of PMR (see Chapter 14). This pain is often associated with immobility and stiffness.
- A deep aching pain associated with stiffness is characteristic of adhesive capsulitis (frozen shoulder). The use of the term frozen shoulder is popular, though often incorrectly applied. It is a condition that is rare in patients under 40 years of age. The condition is invariably

phasic: a painful phase, an adhesive ('frozen') phase, and a resolution phase. Phases often overlap and the duration varies but long-term limitation of shoulder movement remains in up to 15% of patients. It is associated with diabetes.

Does the pain vary?

Movement- or posture-related pain may be a clue to its cause:

- Rotator cuff lesions often present to rheumatologists with an SAI pattern of pain—that is, pain reproducibly aggravated by specific movements during each day such as reaching up with the arm. Articular, bone, and adhesive capsulitis pain is more likely to be persistent.
- A history of recurrent bouts of shoulder pain in children and adolescents may suggest glenohumeral instability owing to hypermobility or previous trauma, e.g. a labral tear. In an unstable shoulder, pain may result from synovitis, subchondral bone damage, or a 2° SAI disorder. The frequency of recurrent anterior subluxation is inversely proportional to the age at which the initial dislocation occurs.

Are there spinal symptoms?

There is an association between neck conditions and shoulder pain. C4 nerve root pain is referred to the shoulder, adhesive capsulitis is associated with cervical nerve root symptoms (the nature of the link is unknown), and inflammatory neck lesions such as CPPD and psoriatic spondylitis forms can be associated with bilateral shoulder pain referral and can mimic PMR.

Examination

Visual inspection

Inspect the neck, shoulders, and arms from the front, side, and back with the patient standing.

- Abnormality of the contour of the cervicothoracic spine could indicate muscle imbalance/spasm or might be associated with a nerve root origin of pain.
- Scapular asymmetry at rest is especially relevant when examining children and may indicate a congenital bony deformity. Subtle degrees of asymmetry are common and are not usually due to specific pathology nor are they of consequence.
- Diffuse swelling of the whole shoulder may suggest a shoulder effusion/haemarthrosis or subacromial bursitis. In the elderly, possibly Milwaukee shoulder. Swelling of the ACJ occurs with joint diastasis, arthritis and distal clavicular bone lesions.
- Arm swelling and skin changes distally could indicate algodystrophy (see Chapter 18).

Elicit any tenderness

Eliciting tenderness of discrete shoulder structures is often unrewarding:

- Tenderness of the ACJ, humeral insertion of the supraspinatus tendon, and the long head of biceps tendon may be clues to pathology but palpation will not be specific for diagnosis.

- An appreciation of trigger points associated with myofascial pain and tender points in fibromyalgia (see Chapter 18) is important in the interpretation of regional soft tissue tenderness.

Document bilateral shoulder movements

This aids diagnosis but also gives an indication of the level of functional impairment and can help in monitoring changes over time (Table 2.4). The movements are first tested actively (the patient does the movement) and then passively (the clinician supports the limb). Muscle strength can also be assessed whilst testing active movement.

- Observe arm elevation in the scapular plane from behind, noting symmetry of scapular movement, the pattern of pain during elevation, and the range of elevation. Hunching of the shoulder at the outset of arm elevation often occurs with an impingement problem. A painful arc may suggest a rotator cuff lesion. Inability to lift the arm suggests a rotator cuff tear or weakness, capsulitis, or severe pain, e.g. acute calcific supraspinatus tendonitis.
- Observe and compare internal rotation of shoulders judged by how far up the back the hand can reach. Poor performance may be due to weakness of cuff or scapular stabilizing muscles or pain, usually as a result of subacromial impingement. This manoeuvre assumes normal elbow function.
- Observe the range of external rotation of the humerus from the front. Ask the patient to flex their elbows as if they were holding a tray and rotate the arms outwards. Minor degrees of restriction caused by pain are not specific but severe restriction is characteristic of adhesive capsulitis.

Test for subacromial impingement

- Always compare the affected with the non-symptomatic side and make conservative judgments about muscle weakness if there is pain impeding voluntary effort.
- Most tests rely on their ability to narrow the distance between the humeral head and the CA arch, by driving the greater tuberosity under the CA arch as the humerus rotates (see Fig. 2.4).
- Whether the tests are specific for lesions of the subacromial structures or for the site of impingement is unknown.

Movement of the glenohumeral joint

Move the glenohumeral joint passively in all directions by moving the upper arm with one hand and placing the other over the shoulder to feel for clunks, crepitus, and resistance to movement:

- If the humeral head can be slid anteriorly (often with a 'clunk') clearly without rotation in the glenoid it suggests instability.
- Grossly reduced passive shoulder movement (notably external rotation, with or without pain) is the hallmark of adhesive capsulitis.
- Pull down on both (hanging) arms. If the humeral head moves inferiorly (sulcus sign) there may be glenohumeral instability.

Table 2.4 Isolated muscle testing of shoulder girdle muscles

Muscle: nerve root, peripheral nerve supply and muscle action	Muscle position	Isolated muscle test	Common pathology affecting muscle strength/bulk
Supraspinatus: C5/C6. Suprascapular nerve. Initial humeral abduction and stability of raised upper arm	From behind, seen and felt above the scapular spine at rest and when activated	Abduct arm from neutral against resistance	Tear or disuse following damage, e.g. after a fall, chronic overuse stress, or in athletes (throwing arm)
Infraspinatus: C5/C6. Suprascapular nerve. External rotation and stability of humeral head	From behind, seen and felt arising from medial scapular border passing laterally (below the scapular spine)	External rotation of arm in neutral, elbow supported and flexed at 90°	Tear or disuse following chronic damage
Serratus anterior: C5–C7. Long-thoracic nerve. Pulls the scapula forward on the thoracic wall (extends forward reach of arm)	Appreciated from behind when patient is pushing against a wall with arms outstretched in front, in that scapula remains fixed	Test by pushing wall with an outstretched arm or push-up. If paralysed there will be lifting and lateral excursion of the scapula	Damage to long-thoracic nerve from trauma. Patient may also have SAI
Deltoid: C5/C6. Axillary nerve. Flexion, extension but mainly abduction of humerus	Arises from the scapular spine and acromion, then swathes the shoulder inserting into the humerus laterally	Wasting may be obvious. Weakness in isometric strength of an arm abducted to 90°	Lesions of axillary nerve damaged by anterior shoulder dislocation (external rotation may also be weak from denervation of teres minor)

Stress the acromioclavicular joint

Stressing the ACJ may reproduce the pain. This is conventionally done by compression or shear tests:

- These tests should not normally be painful. Although painful tests have not proved to be specific for ACJ pathology (pain from SAI may also be present), a positive test may provide a clue that the ACJ is arthritic, dynamically unstable, or that impingement of structures in the subacromial space under the ACJ is occurring.
- Hold the patient's arm in forward flexion (90°) and draw it across the top of the patient's chest. The resulting compression of the ACJ may produce pain. ACJ pain can also be elicited by passively elevating the arm through 180° bringing the hand to the ceiling. Pain is experienced in the upper 10° or so of movement.

Shoulder examination with the patient supine

Examine the shoulders with the patient supine to test whether there is anterior cuff deficiency, glenohumeral joint laxity, or a labral tear: this is especially important in young adults and adolescents to identify an 'unstable shoulder'. Hold and support the upper arm held in slight abduction and external rotation (the elbow is flexed). Move the arm gently (cranially in the coronal plane) and apply gradual degrees of external rotation.

- Deficiency of anterior structures is suggested by patient apprehension that pain is imminent or that the shoulder will slip forward. With a labral tear there may be an audible/palpable 'clunk'.
- Pressure downward on the upper arm (taking the pressure off anterior shoulder structures by an anteriorly translocated humeral head) may relieve this apprehension or the pain associated with it (positive relocation test).
- An unstable shoulder identified with the above tests may denote previous traumatic injury (e.g. shoulder dislocation) or a hyper-mobility disorder.

Investigations

The optimum initial imaging for investigating undiagnosed shoulder pain is disputed. Some clinicians advocate management of shoulder problems based on history and examination alone. This is a practical approach to a common problem as, it is said, many problems get better in the short-term. The long-term sequelae of such management strategies, where a firm diagnosis has not been made, are unknown however. Studies of shoulder pain in Primary Care suggest that chronic shoulder problems are common, often despite initial improvement.

(a)

Painful arc
(active)

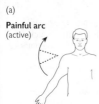

Action: Patient standing.
Slow arm abduction
(scapular plane).

Positive Pain onset (maximal)
test: at (variable) angular
range.

(b)

Neer test
(passive)

Action: Patient sitting/standing.
Passive forward flexion.
Scapula fixed.

Positive Pain at (variable) angle
test: of flexion.

(c)

Empty can
(active)

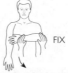

Action: Patient sitting/standing.
Active forward flexion
to 90° then internal
rotation—'can empties'.

Positive Pain with flexion or
test: rotation of arm.

(d)

Kennedy–Hawkins
(passive)

FIX

Action: Patient sitting/standing.
Passive forward flexion (90°).
Fix elbow with hand.
Passive internal rotation.

Positive Pain at some stage of
test: elevation or rotation.

Fig. 2.4 Tests useful for eliciting subacromial impingement

Radiographs

- The standard projection for screening purposes is anteroposterior (AP), though the AP axial–lateral view taken with the arm abducted may add information about the relationship of the glenoid and humeral head. Look for calcific deposits in soft-tissue (possible basic calcium/phosphate crystals: Milwaukee Shoulder—see Chapter 15).
- Supraspinatus outlet views are often used to assess acromial configuration and identify inferior acromial osteophytes in patients with SAI.
- If recurrent dislocation is suspected, associated humeral head defects may be identified by an AP with internal humeral rotation or a Stryker view. Bilateral films distinguish anomaly (invariably bilateral) from abnormality.
- Bilateral AP ACJ views with the patient holding weights may identify, and grade degrees of, ACJ diastasis. Distal clavicular erosion may be due to RA, hyperparathyroidism, myeloma, metastases, or post-traumatic osteolysis.
- Though characteristic patterns of abnormality are associated with SAI (see Plate 2), minor age-related radiographic abnormalities may normally exist.

Other imaging: ultrasound, arthrography, CT arthrography, MR, bone scintigraphy

- Ultrasound scoring systems for locating and grading rotator cuff tears now exist. The technique permits examination of the rotator cuff with the shoulder in different positions but is highly operator dependent.
- Patterns of rotator cuff abnormality and subacromial impingement are well recognized with both arthrography and MR. However, there is no consensus about which of ultrasound, MR, or arthrography is most accurate for detecting rotator cuff tears.
- Children, adolescents, and young adults with suspected unstable shoulders should have an MR examination as detailed views of the humeral head, glenoid labrum, periarticular glenohumeral soft tissues, and subacromial area are important.
- MR is the imaging of choice in young adults where instability is diagnosed. Rotator interval lesions and labral abnormalities are best assessed with MR. Enhancement with IV contrast may increase the chance of detecting a labral tear.
- No specific patterns of bone scan abnormality have been consistently recognized for isolated shoulder lesions, although a three-phase study may be diagnostic for algodystrophy in the upper limb.

Other investigations

- Local anaesthetic injection may help disclose the site of shoulder pain, although it is possible that by the time anaesthesia occurs the injected anaesthetic has spread to areas not intended as a target.
- Joint aspiration is essential if infection is possible. Fluid is usually aspirated easily from a grossly distended shoulder capsule. Haemarthroses can occur in degenerate shoulders (often in association with chondrocalcinosis), haemophilia, trauma, and pigmented villonodular synovitis.

- Electrophysiological tests may confirm muscle weakness and help establish the presence of neuromuscular disease, e.g. myositis or neuralgic amyotrophy.
- Blood tests are required if looking for infection, inflammatory disease, etc.
  - A normal creatine kinase (CK) will rule out myositis in the majority of cases.
  - Blood urea, electrolytes, creatinine, alkaline phosphatase (ALP), calcium, phosphate, thyroid function tests, and myeloma screen should be considered if metabolic bone or myopathic disease is considered.

Treatment (see Chapter 19)
- Physiotherapy should play a focal part in encouraging mobilization of the joint, and early assessment is recommended. The following principles are recommended:
  - know whether there is an additional neck/spinal generated pain component (physiotherapists are independent diagnosticians and many physiotherapists erroneously aim therapy at cervicothoracic segments for individual shoulder lesions).
  - do not refer to physiotherapy without knowledge of who will see the patient.
  - do not refer to physiotherapy without knowing the approach taken by the specific physiotherapist for instability and rotator cuff weakness.
- Simple analgesics are often necessary.
- Local steroid injections (see Plates 12 and 13) can be considered in the following situations:
  - tendonitis of the rotator cuff
  - adhesive capsulitis (see Plate 12)
  - ACJ pain
  - subacromial bursitis (see Plate 13).
- The principles of steroid injection and rehabilitation are dealt with in the last two sections of this chapter.
- There are several situations where local steroids should be avoided:
  - bicipital tendonitis (rest, analgesia, physiotherapy).
  - the first 6 weeks of an acute rotator cuff tear.
  - where symptoms have become chronic and conservative therapy has not helped for a presumptive clinical diagnosis (this requires reassessment, imaging and a diagnosis as surgery may be required).
- Surgical intervention may take the form of subacromial decompression arthroscopy, synovectomy of the SCJ and ACJ, or excision of the distal end of the clavicle.
  - subacromial decompression may be necessary for chronic rotator cuff tendonitis especially where imaging has shown inferior acromial osteophytes.
  - other interventions include repair of a rotator cuff or biceps tendon rupture and joint replacement (for pain relief rather than improvement in function mainly).
- Lithotripsy does not offer advantages over steroid injection and physiotherapy for calcific supraspinatus tendonitis.

Pain around the elbow

Functional anatomy

- The humeroulnar articulation is the prime (hinge) joint at the elbow, though the radius also articulates with the humerus and, to allow forearm and hand supination/pronation, with the ulna at the elbow (see Fig. 2.5).
- Normal extension results in a straight arm although some muscular people lack the last 5–10° of extension and some (especially women) have up to an extra 10° of extension (hyperextension).
- Normal flexion is to 150–160° and forearm supination/pronation range is about 180°.
- Due to obliquity of the trochlea, extension is associated with slight valgus that can be accentuated in women (up to 15°).
- Unilateral acute traumatic or chronic overuse lesions of the elbow are common. Bilateral symptoms may occur in these situations but be suspicious of referred pain from the neck or possibly an inflammatory articular condition involving both elbows.

Pain may also be referred from proximal neurological lesions in the arm, the shoulder or even from distal lesions such as carpal tunnel syndrome (CTS).

Taking a history

Is the pain exclusively located in the elbow or referred from elsewhere?

Establish whether the pain is associated with neck pain and whether it has neurogenic qualities or is associated with parasthesiae or numbness. There may be referral of pain from C6 or C7 nerve roots, shoulder lesions, or even from compression of the median nerve in the wrist.

Is there a history of acute or chronic (overuse) trauma?

- Pain at the lateral epicondyle 1–2 weeks after a weekend of 'home maintenance' might suggest lateral epicondylitis (tennis elbow) following excessive use of a screwdriver, for example.

Other common sites of pain, where characteristic conditions related to overuse are recognized, include medial humeral epicondyle (golfer's elbow) and olecranon bursa (repetitive pressure/friction). Although typically acute in onset, these conditions may develop insidiously.

- Fractures around the elbow and fractures/dislocations in the forearm are common. Dislocation of the radial head alone is rare and is usually associated with concurrent fracture of the ulna (radiographs may not easily identify the fracture). If not associated with fracture (and especially if recurrent) the condition may be associated with generalized hypermobility (see Chapter 16) or shortening of the ulna due to bone dysplasia.
- In children, a strong pull of the forearm or wrist (occurring primarily in pre-school children) can tear the radioulnar ligament surrounding the radial neck (nursemaid's elbow).

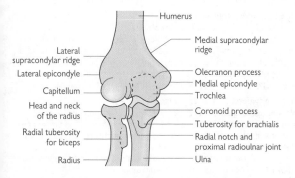

Fig. 2.5 Bony configuration at the (right) elbow (anterior view)

- In children, osteochondritis of the humeral capitellum can occur in mid to late childhood (Panner's disease) typically following repeated trauma.

Does the pain radiate distally?
- Forearm pain may be an additional clue to C6 or C7 radicular pain but may also be due to the spread of musculoskeletal pain along the extensor group of muscles from lateral epicondylitis or rarely from entrapment of the median nerve in the elbow region.
- Associated with occupational overuse, a condition termed peri-tendonitis crepitans is used to characterize symptoms of pain, tenderness, and swelling in the forearm. It is thought to be due to damage of the long wrist/hand flexors and extensors at the muscle–tendon junction.
- Diffuse pain in the forearm can occur as a result of overuse injury, particularly in musicians and typists, though there is overlap with regional pain syndromes.
- Pain around the forearm may also arise from inflammation at the wrist (see the next section) particularly in De Quervain's tenosynovitis.

Is there prominent stiffness with the pain?
- Stiffness is often non-specific but may denote inflammation such as synovitis of the joint or olecranon bursa and, therefore, raises the possibility of an autoimmune rheumatic or crystal deposition disease.
- In the middle aged and elderly, gout (see Chapter 15) of the olecranon bursa and surrounding soft tissues, particularly overlying the border of the ulna, is not uncommon and is often misdiagnosed as infection.

Ask about locking
Locking of the elbow either in flexion or supination/pronation may be due to loose intra-articular bodies. A single loose body is most commonly due to osteochondritis dissecans of the capitellum (e.g. in children with overuse throwing injury—'Little League elbow') and multiple loose bodies are associated with OA or synovial chondromatosis.

Is the pain unremitting and severe?

This type of pain suggests bony pathology:

- Although non-fracture bone pathology is rare in the elbow region, local bony pain might suggest osteochondritis or avascular necrosis, or, if part of a wider pattern of bony pain, metabolic bone disease.
- In the elderly and others at high risk for osteoporosis, supracondylar and other fractures may occur with surprisingly little trauma.

Are there symptoms in other joints?

Ask about other joints, low back (sacroiliac) pains and risks for gout:

- Elbow synovitis alone is an uncommon though recognized presenting feature of adult RA. Elbow synovitis occurs in children presenting with JIA (see Chapter 7) but is rare (3%).
- Peri-articular enthesitis is a recognized feature of spondylarthropathy (SpA) (see Chapter 8) and may mimic tennis elbow.
- The periarticular tissue around the elbow is a moderately common site for gout.

Examination

Look for abnormality then palpate with the thumb. Observe the active, passive, and resisted active range of joint and related tendon movements and consider examining for local nerve lesions. A complete assessment should include examination of the neck, shoulder, and wrist.

Visual inspection

Look for obvious deformity or asymmetry in the anatomical position:

- Up to 10° of extension from a straight arm is normal. More extension might suggest a hypermobility disorder.
- A child with an elbow lesion typically holds the extended arm close to the body, often in pronation.

Look for swelling or nodules:

- Swelling owing to joint synovitis is difficult to see in the antecubital fossa unless it is florid: it is most easily seen (and more easily felt) adjacent to the triceps tendon insertion.
- The olecranon bursa, which may be inflamed, overlies the olecranon and does not as a rule communicate with the joint. Overlying erythema, although non-specific, may be associated with infection or gout.
- Nodules over the extensor surface or ulna border may be associated with RA (see Chapter 5).
- Psoriatic plaques are commonly found at the elbow extensor surface.

Observe active flexion and supination/pronation with the elbows held in 90° of flexion:

- Although the range of movement may be affected by extra-articular pain, loss of range usually implies an intra-articular disorder.

Palpate the lateral epicondyle of the humerus

- In lateral epicondylitis (tennis elbow) there is tenderness, which may extend a little distally. Resisted wrist and finger extension with the elbow in extension or passively stretching the tendons (make fist, flex wrist, pronate forearm, then extend elbow) may reproduce the pain.
- Lateral epicondyle tenderness may be due to inflammation of the radiohumeral bursa that lies under the extensor tendon aponeurosis.
- Note that tenderness of lateral and sometimes medial epicondyles can occur in chronic pain syndromes. In these cases, however, the relevant extensor or flexor tendon provocation tests are likely to be negative.

Palpate the medial humeral epicondyle

- Tenderness suggests traumatic medial epicondylitis (golfer's elbow), a regional or chronic pain syndrome, or enthesitis. Confirm the site of the pain by stretching the wrist flexors—supinate the forearm then passively extend both the wrist and elbow simultaneously. Resisted palmar flexion of the wrist or forearm pronation with elbow extension may also cause pain. Tasks that rely on this repetitive movement are often the provoking cause.
- Consider osteochondritis of the medial humeral epicondyle as a cause of persistent pain following an injury. The 8–15-year-old age group is at particular risk as this is a site of 2° ossification.

Passively flex and extend the elbow joint

Passively flex and extend the joint and note the range of movement and 'end-feel' (the feel of resistance at the end of the range of passive joint movement):

- 'End-feel' may tell you whether there is a block to full flexion or extension from a bony spur or osteophyte (solid end-feel) or from soft tissue thickening/fibrosis (springy, often painful).
- Note any crepitus (often associated with intra-articular pathology) and locking (may have loose bodies in the joint).

Supinate and pronate the forearm

Passively supinate and pronate the forearm supporting the elbow in 90° of flexion with your thumb over the radioulnar articulation:

- There may be crepitus or instability/subluxation associated with pain. Instability might suggest a tear or damage to the annular ligament (due to trauma or chronic/aggressive intra-articular inflammation).

Test peripheral nerve function if there are distal arm symptoms

- Given its course around the lateral epicondyle, the integrity of the radial nerve should always be tested when a lateral elbow lesion is suspected.
- The median nerve runs in the antecubital fossa and may be affected in traumatic elbow lesions. It is particularly susceptible where it runs between the two heads of pronator teres (from medial epicondyle and the coronoid process of the ulna) and separates into anterior interosseous and terminal median nerve branches.
- The ulnar nerve lies in the groove behind the medial epicondyle. Bony or soft tissue abnormality in this area may affect nerve function and cause reduced sensation in the little finger and weakness in

(for example) the small muscles of the hand, flexor carpi ulnaris (FCU), extensor carpi ulnaris (ECU), and abductor digiti minimi (ADM). The median and ulnar nerves are dealt with in more detail in the later sections on wrist and hand disorders pp.42–59.

Investigations
Radiographs and other imaging
- Standard AP and lateral radiographs are the most straightforward way of imaging the elbow initially. CT or MR may then be needed if the diagnosis is still obscure and referred pain can be ruled out.
- Look for periosteal lesions and enthesophytes (new bone spurs at clear entheses like the triceps insertion). Periosteal apposition and enthesophytes are typical in psoriatic arthritis (see Chapter 8).
- A lateral radiograph may identify displacement of the anterior fat pad associated with a joint effusion (sail sign).
- Dislocations of the radial head and associated ulna fractures in children are easily missed. To make this diagnosis a high degree of suspicion and further imaging are often needed.

Needle arthrocentesis/olecranon bursocentesis
- Arthrocentesis/bursocentesis with fluid sent for microscopy and culture should always be done in suspected cases of sepsis. Fluid should be sent for polarized light microscopy in cases of bursitis that may be due to gout. Serum urate is worth requesting but may not be raised even in acute gout.
- Examination of fluid for crystals should always be considered in cases of monoarthritis in the elderly or patients on dialysis.

Electrophysiology
If nerve entrapment is suspected and there is some uncertainty after clinical examination then electrophysiological tests may provide useful information. Testing can help identify the degree and likely site of nerve damage and can help to discriminate between a peripheral and nerve root lesion.

Treatment
- The management of fractures is beyond the scope of this text.
- Epicondylitis is best managed early on with rest, splinting, analgesia, and local steroid injections. The efficacy of physical manipulation has not been proven, though there are theoretical reasons why ultrasound therapy could be of value (it passes through the myofascial planes and concentrates near bone). Resistant cases may benefit from surgery—a 'lateral release'.
- There is anecdotal evidence for the utility of lithotripsy, dry needling, and autologous blood injection for lateral epicondylitis but robust studies showing significant efficacy have not been reported.
- Steroid injections may be of value in the following situations:
  - lateral or medial epicondylitis (hydrocortisone)
  - inflammatory arthritis (usually long acting steroid)
  - olecranon bursitis
  - ulnar nerve entrapment.

The principles of steroid injection and rehabilitation are dealt with at the end of this chapter pp.148–55; also see Plates 12–15.

- Surgical procedures include excision of nodules and bursae, transposition of the ulnar nerve, synovectomy, excision of the head of the radius, and arthroplasty.
- Arthroplasty in inflammatory arthritis is best reserved for intractable pain and should be undertaken by an experienced surgeon. Lesser procedures such as proximal radial head excision can be effective to improve pain and function if forearm pronation and supination are poor.
- Radiation synovectomy of the elbow (Y-90 or Re-186) for inflammatory arthritis, PVNS, or synovial chondromatosis (see Chapter 18) requires ultrasound guidance (see EANM guidelines www.eanm.org).

Wrist pain

Functional anatomy of the wrist

- The wrist comprises radiocarpal (scaphoid and lunate) and intercarpal articulations. The ulna does not truly articulate with the lunate but is joined to it, the triquetrum, and the radius (ulnar side of distal aspect), by the triangular fibrocartilage complex.
- The intercarpal joints are joined by intercarpal ligaments and are most stable when the wrist is in full extension. Anterior carpal ligaments are stronger than posterior ones and are reinforced by the flexor retinaculum. Wrist and finger flexor tendons, the radial artery, and the median nerve enter the hand in a tunnel formed by the carpal bones and the flexor retinaculum (carpal tunnel).
- Flexion (70°), extension (70°), radial and ulnar deviation (about 20° and 30° from midline respectively) occur at the wrist but supination/pronation of the wrist and hand is due to radiohumeral movement at the elbow.
- Flexor carpi radialis (FCR) and ulnaris (FCU) are the main flexors of the wrist though palmaris longus (PL) also helps (see Fig. 2.6). All arise from the medial humeral epicondyle.
- All carpal extensors arise from the lateral humeral epicondyle (see Fig. 2.6).
- Radial deviation (abduction) occurs primarily when radial flexors and extensors act together. Ulnar deviation (adduction) occurs primarily when ulnar flexors and extensors act together.

Taking a history

Table 2.5 details the major diagnoses for painful conditions of the wrist and hand.

Determine the exact location of the pain

- Pain localizing only to the wrist is most likely to be from local tissue pathology. Cervical nerve root pain as a result of a C6, C7, or C8 lesion and pain from peripheral nerve lesions is likely to be located chiefly in the hand.
- Pain at the base of the thumb, aggravated by thumb movements, in middle and old age is typical of OA (see Chapter 6) of the trapezium—first metacarpal joint. Pain in this area might also be due to tenosynovitis of thumb tendons.

Trauma history

- Injury/post-injury conditions are common. A history of trauma is important.
- Common fractures in adults are: scaphoid and base of the first metacarpal (Bennett's), and head of the radius (Colles').
- Distal radioulnar physeal injuries may occur in children.
- Post-traumatic chronic wrist pain following injuries may be due to ligamentous injury and chronic carpal instability or osteonecrosis (lunate).

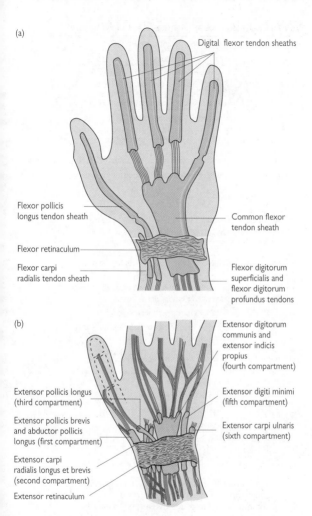

(a)

Digital flexor tendon sheaths

Flexor pollicis
longus tendon sheath

Common flexor
tendon sheath

Flexor retinaculum

Flexor carpi
radialis tendon sheath

Flexor digitorum
superficialis and
flexor digitorum
profundus tendons

(b)

Extensor digitorum
communis and
extensor indicis
proprius
(fourth compartment)

Extensor pollicis longus
(third compartment)

Extensor digiti minimi
(fifth compartment)

Extensor pollicis brevis
and abductor pollicis
longus (first compartment)

Extensor carpi ulnaris
(sixth compartment)

Extensor carpi
radialis longus et brevis
(second compartment)

Extensor retinaculum

Fig. 2.6 Flexor (a) and extensor (b) tendon sheaths crossing the wrist. Flexor carpi radialis (FCR) inserts into the second and third metacarpals. Flexor carpi ulnaris (FCU) inserts into the pisiform, hamate, and fifth metacarpal. Extensor carpi radialis longus (ECRL) inserts into the base of the second, extensor carpi radialis brevis (ECRB) into the third, and extensor carpi ulnaris (ECU) into the fifth metacarpal respectively

Table 2.5 Painful conditions of the wrist and hand: major diagnoses

Articular disorders	Inflammatory arthritis (e.g. RA, JIA)
	Degenerative arthritis*
	Crystal arthritis
	Ligamentous lesions*
	Carpal instability (e.g. lunate dislocation)
Periarticular disorders	De Quervain's tenosynovitis
	Tenosynovitis of common flexor/extensor tendon sheath
	Flexor pollicis tenosynovitis
	Distal flexor stenosing tenosynovitis (trigger finger or thumb)*
	Ganglia*, subcutaneous nodules, tophi
	Diabetic cheirarthropathy
	Dupuytren's contracture*
Bone pathology	Fracture*
	Neoplasia
	Infection
	Osteochondritis (lunate—Kienböck's; scaphoid—Prieser's) (see Chapter 16)
Neurological	Median nerve entrapment (carpal tunnel* or at pronator teres)
	Anterior interosseous nerve syndrome
	Ulnar nerve entrapment (cubital tunnel or in Guyon's canal in wrist)
	Posterior interosseous nerve entrapment
	Radial nerve palsy
	Brachial plexopathy
	Thoracic outlet syndrome
	Cervical nerve root irritation or entrapment*
	Algodystrophy (see Chapter 18)
	Spinal cord lesions, e.g. syringomyelia

*Common conditions.

- Unusual or florid pain descriptors suggest a regional pain syndrome (e.g. algodystrophy). Following trauma, regional pain syndromes are not uncommon in children, adolescents, or young adults.

Are there features to suggest synovitis?
- Pain due to wrist joint synovitis may be associated with 'stiffness' and be worse at night or in the early morning. Stiffness 'in the hand' may have various causes but these will include multiple tendon/small joint synovitis, diabetic cheirarthropathy, or even scleroderma (Scl) (see Chapter 12).

- Wrist synovitis occurs commonly in adult RA and in children with both systemic and rheumatoid factor positive JIA. It occurs in 5% of oligoarticular JIA cases (see Chapter 7).
- In the elderly, wrist synovitis may be due to calcium pyrophosphate dihydrate (CPPD) crystals (see Chapter 15).

The quality of the pain
- Although 1° bone pathology is rare, local bony pain (unremitting, severe, sleep disturbing) might suggest avascular necrosis in those at risk or, if part of a wider pattern of bony pain, metabolic bone disease (e.g. physeal pain in children with rickets).
- Radicular pain may be burning in quality and is typically associated with numbness and parasthesiae. Such neurogenic pain is commonly due to nerve root irritation or compression.

Other joint/musculoskeletal symptoms
- Wrist and extensor tendon sheath synovitis is a common presenting feature of adult RA. Other joints may be affected.
- CPPD arthritis commonly involves the wrist and can mimic RA in its joint distribution and presentation in the elderly.
- Wrist synovitis and enthesitis occurs in SpA. Pain may be considerable though swelling is minimal. There may be inflammatory-type symptoms of spinal pain and enthesitis elsewhere.

Ask specifically about job/leisure activities
- Repetitive lateral and medial wrist movements with thumb adducted can cause tenosynovitis of abductor pollicis longus (APL) or extensor pollicis brevis (EPB) commonly called De Quervain's tenosynovitis.
- If there is no obvious history of trauma, tendonitis may be a presenting feature of a systemic autoimmune rheumatic disease or even gonococcaemia in adolescents and young adults.
- Overuse pain syndromes may occur as a result of repetitive activity. The term 'repetitive strain injury' is controversial. Objective assessment of pain, location of swelling, etc. from the outset is invaluable in assessing the response to treatment. Lack of objective findings (if imaging subsequently normal) suggests a regional pain disorder.

Examination

Visual inspection
Inspect the dorsal surface of both wrists looking for swelling, deformity, or loss of muscle bulk.
- Diffuse swelling may be due to wrist or extensor tendon sheath synovitis.
- A prominent ulna styloid may result from subluxation at the distal radioulnar joint owing to synovitis or radioulnar ligament damage.
- Prominence ('squaring') of the trapezoid–first metacarpal joint commonly occurs in OA of this joint.
- Loss of muscle bulk in the forearm may be 2° to a chronic T1 nerve root lesion or disuse atrophy.

Flexion/extension range tests for major wrist lesions
- The normal range of both flexion and extension in Caucasian adults is about 70°. Synovitis invariably reduces this range.
- Where wrist synovitis is present, swelling on the dorsum of the wrist may become more apparent. Substantial common flexor or extensor tendon swelling will probably also block the full range of wrist movement (soft tissue approximation 'end-feel').
- There is normally an additional 20° of flexion and extension to the active range with passive movement.
- Elicited pain and crepitus are unlikely to be specific for any type of lesion but may draw your attention to the anatomical site of the lesion.

Examine the dorsum of the wrist in detail
- Note any abnormal excursion of the ulnar styloid associated with pain and/or crepitus suggesting synovitis.
- Post-traumatic carpal instability, particularly scapulolunate dissociation, is relatively common. The latter is demonstrated by eliciting dorsal subluxation of the proximal scaphoid pole by firm pressure on its distal pole as the wrist is deviated radially from a starting position with the forearm pronated and the wrist in ulnar deviation. Note any gap between scaphoid and lunate and any associated tenderness.
- Note any tenderness or thickening of the common extensor tendon sheath and tendon sheath of APL and EPB.
- Tenderness at the base of the thumb may be due to wrist synovitis, carpal or carpo–first metacarpal OA, tenosynovitis, a ganglion, or a ligament lesion.
- Finkelstein's test for De Quervain's tenosynovitis may be used to elicit APL/EPB tendon pain. With the thumb adducted and opposed, the fingers are curled to form a fist. Passive ulnar deviation at the wrist stretches the abnormal tendons and elicits pain. Although it is a sensitive test, it is not specific for tendon pain.
- In adults, protrusion of the thumb out of the fist on the ulnar side of the hand during the first part of this test is unusual and suggests thumb, and perhaps general, hypermobility.

Test the integrity of the tendons
Many muscles/tendons that move both the wrist and digits originate at the elbow; therefore, the quality of information gained from isolated tendon resistance tests (either for pain or strength) may be affected by pain elsewhere around the wrist, wrist deformity, or elbow lesions. Interpret findings cautiously. Useful information might be obtained by passive movement of a tendon rather than by resisted active movement, and also by feeling for thickening or crepitus of the tendons.

Investigation and treatment

The investigation and treatment of wrist conditions is covered in the following section on symptoms in the hand.

Symptoms in the hand

Symptoms in the hand are a common presenting feature of some systemic conditions, and localized neurological and musculoskeletal lesions are common, especially in adults. Detailed knowledge of anatomy is beyond the scope of this text. Functional anatomy is important and the more common abnormalities are summarized below.

Functional anatomy of the hand

The long tendons

- Digital power is provided primarily by flexor and extensor muscles arising in the forearm. Their action is supplemented and modified by small muscles in the hand. Precise movements of the hand are mainly due to small muscles.
- Powerful digital flexors (see Fig. 2.6): flexor digitorum superficialis (FDS), flexor digitorum profundus (FDP), and flexor pollicis longus (FPL).
- FDS flexes proximal interphalangeal joints (PIPJs) and, more weakly, metacarpophalangeal joints (MCPJs)/wrist.
- FDP flexes distal interphalangeal joints (DIPJs) and, increasingly weakly, PIPJs, MCPJs/wrist.
- FPL flexes (at 90° to other digits) mainly the PIPJ but also the whole thumb in a power grip (see below).
- Powerful digital extensors (see Fig. 2.6): extensor digitorum (ED) arises from the lateral epicondyle splitting at the wrist to insert into each digital dorsal expansion (digits two to five) that attaches to all three phalanges (see Fig. 2.7). The fifth digit has an additional tendon, extensor digiti minimi (EDM) that also arises at the lateral epicondyle.
- APL abducts the thumb at the MCPJ provided the wrist is stable.
- EPB and EPL extend the thumb.
- Extensor indicis (EI) arises from the ulna posterior border distal to EPL and joins the index finger ED tendon.
- The muscles of the thenar eminence (see Table 2.6) act synchronously. All except adductor pollicis (ulnar nerve, C8/T1) are supplied by the median nerve from C8/T1 nerve roots. All three muscles are supplied by the ulnar nerve (C8/T1).

The intrinsic muscles

- The longitudinal muscles of the palm (four dorsal and four palmar interossei and four lumbricals) all insert into digits.
- Palmar interossei, from metacarpals 1, 2, 4, and 5, insert into dorsal tendons.
- Each dorsal interosseous arises from origins on two adjacent metacarpals. The muscles abduct the second and fourth fingers and move the middle finger either medially or laterally.
- The four lumbricals (see Fig. 2.8, Table 2.7) arise from tendons of FDP in the palm passing to the lateral side of each MCPJ inserting into the dorsal expansions.
- The interossei combine with lumbricals to facilitate fine control of flexion and extension of MCPJs and PIPJs.

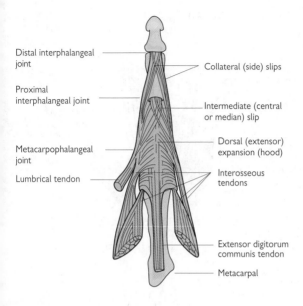

Fig. 2.7 Extensor expansion of a finger

Table 2.6 Muscles of the thenar eminence

Muscle	Origin	Insertion
Abductor pollicis brevis	Flexor retinaculum, scaphoid, and trapezium	Thumb proximal phalanx and dorsal expansion
Flexor pollicis brevis	Flexor retinaculum, trapezium, trapezoid, and capitate	Thumb proximal phalanx (base of radial side)
Opponens pollicis	Flexor retinaculum and tubercle of the trapezium	First metacarpal (lateral border)
Adductor pollicis	Capitate, bases of second/third metacarpals and distal third metacapal	Thumb proximal phalanx (medial side)

(a)

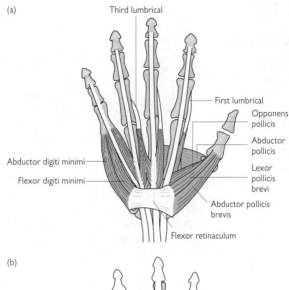

(b)

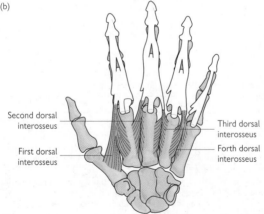

Fig. 2.8 (a) Lumbrical muscles and muscles of the thenar and hypothenar eminences. (b) Dorsal interossei

Table 2.7 Muscles of the hypothenar eminence

Muscle	Origin	Insertion
Abductor digiti minimi	Flexor retinaculum (FR), pisiform, and pisohamate Ligament	Base of the fifth proximal phalanx and dorsal expansion
Flexor digiti minimi brevis	Flexor retinaculum and hook of hamate	Base of the fifth proximal phalanx
Opponens digiti minimi	Flexor retinaculum and hook of hamate	Medial side of the fifth metacarpal

Grip

- For power, the wrist extends and adducts slightly and long digital flexors contract.
- A modified power grip, the hook grip, is used to carry heavy objects like a suitcase. The thumb is extended out of the way and extension at MCPJs accompanies flexion at PIPJs/DIPJs.
- More precision in the grip can be obtained using varying degrees of thumb adduction, abduction, and flexion. The thumb can be opposed with any of the four other digits depending on the shape of the object to be held and the type of manipulation required.

Taking a history

A history of acute or overuse trauma with subsequent localized symptoms requires a straightforward application of anatomical knowledge, precise examination, and judicious choice of imaging techniques for diagnosis. However, there are more subtle or less easily delineated patterns of symptoms in the hand, particularly where pain is diffuse or poorly localized.

Is the pain associated with immobility or stiffness?

- Stiffness may be associated with joint or tendon synovitis but is not specific. Prompting may provide more accurate localization of symptoms.
- If unilateral, especially on the dominant hand, be suspicious that diffuse hand pain may be due to a regional pain syndrome.

Is stiffness local or diffuse?

- Patterns of joint involvement in autoimmune rheumatic disease and polyarticular arthritides are summarized in Chapter 3.
- If localized in the palm there may be Dupuytren's contracture (associated with diabetes). If diffuse, there may be thickening of soft tissue from a systemic process, e.g. hypothyroidism, scleroderma, diabetic cheirarthropathy, or disorders of mucopolysaccharide metabolism (the latter especially in infants, although Fabry's syndrome can present in adulthood associated with acroparasthesiae and palmar telangiectasias).
- Stiffness due to an upper motor neuron lesion (an interpretation of ↑ tone) is unlikely to be confined to the hand and is likely to be associated with weakness. The pattern of symptoms over time should give a clue to its aetiology.

Are there neurological qualities to the pain or characteristics typical of a common nerve lesion?

- 'Burning' or 'deep' episodic pain varying with head, neck, and upper spinal position is typical of cervical nerve root pain. Ask about occupation and other activities that are associated with neck problems, e.g. adolescent ballerina, a seamstress, the relationship with sleep posture, and frequent headaches.
- Pain on the radial side of the hand waking the patient at night and often relieved, at least partially, by shaking the hand is typical of median nerve entrapment in the wrist. However, pain in this condition is often poorly localized at initial presentation. Remember other lesions that produce pain in the area around the thumb base: trapezoid–first metacarpal joint OA, tenosynovitis of APL/EPB (De Quervain's) or EPL, referred pain from a C6 nerve root lesion, and ligament lesions (e.g. ulnar collateral ligament of first MCPJ—'skier's thumb').

Tingling/pins and needles/numbness

Make sure both you and the patient understand what you each mean by these terms.

- Symptoms usually denote cervical nerve root or peripheral nerve irritation/compression though they can reflect underlying ischaemia.
- Tingling in the fingertips of both hands, however, is recognized to occur commonly in patients diagnosed with fibromyalgia.
- Symptoms associated primarily with specific positions of the whole arm may be 2° to thoracic outlet compression of neurovascular structures.

Pain arising from bone

Pain in the hands arising from bones may be difficult to discriminate. Radiographs will often lead to confirmation of the diagnosis.

- The commonest tumour in the hand is an enchondroma. It is usually painless. Once painful then suspect infarction or malignant change.
- Secondary metastases and 1° malignant bone tumours in the hand are rare but must be ruled out in children, adolescents, and young adults with persistent localized bone pain.
- Paget's disease of hand bones can occur but is relatively rare.
- Digital bone pain from osteomalacia/rickets occurs but is unusual at presentation.
- Digital pain may rarely be due to sarcoidosis, hyperparathyroid bone disease, thyroid acropachy, hypertrophic (pulmonary) osteoarthropathy (HO), or pachydermoperiostitis. Look for clubbing.

Ischaemic pain?

A history suggestive of ischaemic pain in the hands is rare in rheumatological practice. Persistent ischaemic digital pain is a medical emergency.

- Digital vasomotor instability (e.g. Raynaud's phenomenon (RP)) is episodic and triggered by cold and emotion, and characterized by digital colour changes: white/blue then red.
- Pain from vasculitis is likely to be persistent and associated with a purpuric rash, nail-fold infarcts, or splinter haemorrhages.
- Ischaemic pain associated with cervicothoracic posture or prolonged arm elevation manoeuvres may be due to a lesion of the thoracic outlet.

- Pain may be due to thromboembolism, e.g. antiphospholipid syndrome, infective endocarditis, or thromboarteritis obliterans (Buerger's disease).

'Swelling'
Examination is more reliable than a history.
- Apart from isolated lesions such as ganglia, patients' description of soft tissue or joint swelling may be unreliable and should be substantiated by examination. Nerve lesions can give the impression that swelling is present (think what a dentist's local anaesthetic does for your lip!).

'Weakness'
Ask about trauma, neck, and median nerve entrapment symptoms.
- Acute tendon injuries are common industrial accidents. Chronic occupational overuse may also lead to rupture.
- If weakness is profound and provided that there has been no obvious trauma, then the cause is likely to be neuromuscular.
- If not associated with pain then weakness is more likely to be neurological than musculoskeletal in origin.
- Weakness associated with pain may be due to a neurological or musculoskeletal lesion, the latter situation often due to an inability to use the hand (or part of it) because of pain or an alteration in biomechanical function as a result of deformity, which may only be slight.
- True weakness associated with stiffness is associated with myelopathy or even motor neuron disease. A detailed history of the progression of symptoms is important and neurological examination should be thorough.

'Catching' of a finger
This may denote stenosing tenosynovitis of a digital flexor tendon (trigger finger). Damage to the tendon and its sheath can result in a fibrous nodule attached to the tendon that moves and catches under the proximal annular ligament just distal to the MCPJ. It may not be painful. This most commonly affects middle and ring fingers and is prevalent amongst professional drivers, cyclists, and those in occupations requiring repeated use of hand-held heavy machinery.

Examination
The sequence below is comprehensive but should be considered if a general condition is suspected. Often an examination only needs to be more specifically directed.

Inspection of the nails and fingers
- Pits/ridges are associated with psoriatic arthritis (see Plate 3).
- Splinter haemorrhages may be traumatic but are associated with infective endocarditis or rheumatoid vasculitis.
- Obvious cuticle damage and punctate cuticle erythema (dilated capillary loops) are features of severe RP/Scl (see Plate 4).
- Periungual erythema is associated with a number of autoimmune rheumatic and connective tissue diseases.
- Multiple telangiectasias are associated with limited cutaneous Scl (lcScl) (see Chapter 12).

- Diffuse finger thickening (dactylitis) may be due to gross tendon thickening (e.g. SpA or sarcoid, see Plate 19), or connective tissue fibrosis/thickening (Scl, cheirarthropathy). Bony or soft-tissue DIPJ or PIPJ swelling should be discriminated.
- A shiny/waxy skin appearance, often pale, may indicate Scl.
- Scattered, tiny, non-blanching dark red punctate lesions are typical of cutaneous skin vasculitis.
- Erythematous or violacious scaly papules/plaques over MCPJs or PIPJs may suggest dermatomyositis.

Note any diffuse swelling of the hand
- Diffuse soft-tissue/skin swelling, may occur in association with RA, RS$_3$PE syndrome, JIA, algodystrophy (see Plate 5), and Scl.
- RS$_3$PE (remitting seronegative symmetrical synovitis with pitting oedema), which presents mainly in adults in their 70s, may be a distinct type of non-erosive polyarticular/tendon synovitis but may be associated with other, often haematological conditions.
- Swelling associated with algodystrophy may be localized or diffuse (see Plate 5). Skin may be shiny and later there is often a dark red or blue mottled appearance.
- Typical skin appearances are critical to making a clinical diagnosis of Scl. The skin may be initially puffy but later shiny and tight and, with progression, atrophic with contractures.

Note any muscle wasting
Wasting may be due to a degree of chronic denervation (e.g. the thenar eminence in CTS), disuse atrophy (e.g. painful polyarthropathy, joint hypomobility), or ↑ catabolism of muscle (e.g. polymyositis, RA). In the elderly there may be age-related muscle loss.

Note any deformity of digits
- Deformities tend to occur with long-standing polyarticular joint disease, e.g. OA, severe RA, and psoriatic arthritis.
- Isolated deformities may be due to previous bone or tendon trauma, severe neurological lesions and Dupuytren's contracture. A mallet finger (loss of active DIPJ extension) is due to rupture of the distal extensor tendon expansion usually 2° to direct trauma.

Inspect the palm and dorsum of the hand
- Palmar erythema is not specific but is associated with autoimmune disorders of connective tissue and joints.
- Check for Dupuytren's contracture (fascial thickening on ulnar side).
- On the dorsum of the hand, ganglia and swelling of the common extensor tendon sheath are usually easily noted. Swelling of the extensor tendon sheath is commonly associated with RA in adults.

Palpation of joints and nodules
Palpation of joints and nodules is best done using thumb pads with the patient's wrist supported.
- Swelling should be noted for site, consistency, tenderness, and mobility. Osteophytes and exostosis are periarticular or at sites of pressure, may be tender, but are always fixed (see Plate 16d).

- Ganglia are hard and usually quite mobile (can occur anywhere).
- Rheumatoid nodules (occur anywhere but typically on the dorsum of the hand and the extensor surface of the elbow) and tophi (usually distal) are rubbery, hard, relatively fixed, but may be moved (see Plate 16a).
- Synovitis is often represented by soft ('boggy'), often springy, swelling around a joint. It may be tender and warm but this is not invariable.
- Synovitis in a single joint may be due to autoimmune rheumatic disease, OA, infection, or foreign-body synovitis (e.g. rose thorn synovitis).

Palpate tendons in the palm or on the volar aspect of the phalanges

- Thickening, tenderness, and crepitus suggest tenosynovitis but tenosynovitis can be hard to spot if it is mild. Tethering and thickening of tendons in the palm associated with excessive digital flexion when the hand is at rest and a block to passive finger extension suggests chronic flexor tenosynovitis (take care to note any contributory joint damage).
- Passive tendon movement by gently flexing/extending a proximal phalanx may disclose palpable tendon nodules, crepitus and tenderness.

Discriminate Dupuytren's contracture from flexor tendonopathy

Dupuytren's contracture typically involves the fourth/fifth fingers (40% bilateral). It is common in males aged 50 to 70. The fascia extends to the second phalanx, thus, if severe, the condition causes fixed flexion of MCPJs/PIPJs. It is associated with epilepsy, diabetes, and alcoholism though is not usually painful.

Investigation of wrist and hand disorders

Radiographs

- An AP view of the hand and wrist is a useful screening investigation to characterize a polyarthropathy and diagnose traumatic and metabolic bone lesions (see Table 2.8).
- Radiographs may reveal soft tissue swelling around joints compatible with a diagnosis of synovitis.
- Radiographs are insensitive for identifying erosions in early autoimmune joint disease.
- An oblique view of the hand may add information about joint erosions if an erosive MCPJ arthritis is considered.
- Lateral and carpal tunnel views of the carpus can be obtained by varying the degree of X-ray projection angle; however, unless searching for evidence of fracture these views are rarely needed.

Further imaging: US, MR, and scintigraphy

- In experienced hands, US patterns of abnormality in association with median nerve entrapment and some soft tissue lesions can be detected.
- In experienced hands, US is a useful way of looking for small hand joint synovitis and erosions in suspected 'early' RA.

Table 2.8 Some conditions/features that may be diagnosed on simple AP hand/wrist radiographs

Bone conditions	Fractures (e.g. scaphoid, base of first metacarpal)
	Tumours
	Metabolic bone diseases (e.g. rickets, hyperparathyroidism)
	Avascular necrosis (e.g. post-traumatic—lunate, sickle cell disease)
	Sarcoidosis (may also have arthropathy)
Specific features	Cartilage damage (joint space loss and subchondral bone changes)
	Articular erosions
	Osteophytes
	Infection (cortex loss, patchy osteolysis)
	Calcium deposition in joint (e.g. triangular ligament chondrocalcinosis)
	Soft tissue swelling (e.g. over ulnar styloid in wrist synovitis)
	Periarticular osteoporosis (associated with joint inflammation)
	Carpal dislocation (e.g. lunate displacement in chronic carpal pain)
Polyarticular/ overall patterns of radiological abnormality	OA (distribution of osteophytes and subchondral bone changes)
	RA, JIA (e.g. deformities, erosion appearance/distribution)
	Psoriatic arthritis (e.g. deformities, erosion appearance—DIPJs)
	CPPD arthritis/gout (e.g. erosion appearance in gout)

- MR may demonstrate a torn or avulsed triangular cartilage in patients with a post-traumatic painful wrist or with carpal instability.
- MR images of the carpal tunnel are especially useful in confirming median nerve compression/tethering and soft tissue wrist pathology, particularly in recurrence of symptoms post-decompression surgery.
- MR can provide valuable information about the degree and distribution of inflammatory disease in joints and tendons, particularly in children and patients where history and examination are difficult.
- MR is more sensitive than radiography in identifying joint erosions in RA. Choosing MR over US depends on availability and sonographer experience.
- Bone scintigraphy is not specific for any single condition but in young adults (after closure of epiphyses and before OA is likely) it may be useful for disclosing patterns of inflammation at and around joints. ^{99m}Tc-labelled human immunoglobulin may be more specific at detecting patterns of synovitis in children and adults.

Laboratory investigations

- FBC, ESR, CRP. The characteristic, though non-specific, picture in patients with a systemic inflammatory condition such as RA or polyarticular JIA, is mild anaemia with normal red cell indices, high or high normal platelets, and ↑ acute phase response. Lymphopenia frequently accompanies autoimmune disease. Neutrophils are raised in infection, with steroids and in systemic JIA or adult Still's disease.
- Blood urea, electrolytes, creatinine, and urate will detect hyperuricaemia and renal impairment associated with gout (see Chapter 15). Blood calcium, phosphate, albumin, vit D, and ALP (± PTH) will screen for metabolic bone disease.
- Rheumatoid factor (RF) can help characterize but not diagnose an arthropathy (i.e. it is not specific for any one disease). Antinuclear antibody (ANA) and a screen of extractable nuclear antibodies (ENAs) will help characterize any autoimmune connective tissue disease.
- In children with JIA a positive ANA is associated with a risk of uveitis.
- Vasculitis screen, including ANCA in cases of purpuric rash.
- Other investigations to consider: serum angiotensin converting enzyme (sACE) for sarcoidosis, glycosylated haemoglobin in diabetics, serum and urinary protein electrophoresis for myeloma.

Other investigations

- Neurophysiology is a useful adjunct to clinical examination in diagnosis of upper limb neuropathies.
- Joint/bursa fluid aspiration is mandatory in suspected cases of sepsis and should be sent for culture and microscopy. Crystal arthropathy should also be considered.

Treatment of wrist and hand disorders

Treatment for specific diseases is considered in Part 2. Management of the soft tissue lesions in the hand and wrist, like elsewhere, combines periods of rest and splinting with active physiotherapy, avoidance of repetitive activity, and analgesia. In most cases the condition will resolve spontaneously, but severe or persistent pain and disability may warrant input from a hand Occupational Therapist, local steroid injections, or occasionally surgical soft tissue decompression.

- Conditions that respond to local steroid therapy include:
  - tenosynovitis e.g. De Quervain's
  - tendon nodules and ganglia
  - flexor tenosynovitis (and trigger finger)
  - Dupuytren's contracture
  - carpal tunnel syndrome
  - synovitis: radiocarpal and radioulnar at the wrist, MCPJs and PIPJs, first carpometacarpal.
- The accuracy of needle placement is likely to be improved by US guidance; however, greater efficacy from such an approach over blind injection has not yet been shown.
- The principles of steroid injection and rehabilitation are dealt with at the end of this chapter pp.148–53.

- Radiation synovectomy using erbium-169 colloid may be considered useful and, in some cases, may be superior to injecting steroid alone. US guidance of injection of radiocolloid is mandatory.
- Functional evaluation (from a physiotherapist and occupational therapist) is likely to be of use in cases of polyarthropathy. Early use of splints, orthotics, and exercises may lead to greater functional ability and a decrease in symptomology.
- Surgical options for the hand and wrist may include:
  - fusion or resection of the carpal bones
  - ulna styloidectomy and wrist synovectomy (RA)
  - tendon repair and transfer operations (RA)
  - synovectomy of joints and/or tendons (RA)
  - fusion of small joints
  - PIPJ/MCPJ replacements
  - Dupuytren's release/fasciectomy
  - carpal tunnel release
  - trapeziectomy for thumb CMC joint OA

Upper limb peripheral nerve lesions

Background

- Upper limb peripheral nerve lesions are common. Most are entrapment neuropathies. Occasionally, nerve trauma may present to Primary Care physicians or rheumatologists with (primarily) regional muscle weakness.
- Although not specific for its diagnosis, the triad of pain, parasthesiae, and weakness is suggestive of nerve entrapment. Features may be considered more specific for nerve entrapment if there is a history of acute or overuse trauma proximal to the distribution of the symptoms.
- Lesions may characteristically occur in association with specific activities, occupations, or sport (e.g. ulnar neuropathy in cyclists).
- Accurate diagnosis relies on demonstration of the anatomical lesion. Useful in this respect is knowledge of likely sites of entrapment or damage and, in the case of entrapment, the ability to elicit a positive Hoffman–Tinnel sign—percussion over the site of entrapment eliciting sensory symptoms in the appropriate nerve distribution.
- Always compare examination findings in both upper limbs.
- Neurophysiological examination is an adjunct to clinical diagnosis. It should not be relied on to make a diagnosis in the absence of good clinical data.
- MR techniques and their interpretation are becoming increasingly more sophisticated in identifying patterns of abnormality in these disorders.

The long thoracic nerve

- Entrapment is in the differential diagnosis of the cause of painless 'shoulder' weakness. The nerve origin is at C5–C7, and its course runs beneath subscapularis and into serratus anterior.
- Muscle paralysis is often painless and implies loss of the last 30° of overhead arm extension, disrupted scapular rhythm and scapula winging; the latter demonstrated by inspection from behind with the patient pressing against a wall with an outstretched arm.
- Damage to the nerve occurs typically from an anterior direct blow or brachial plexus injury. Damage sometimes occurs after carrying heavy backpacks (e.g. army recruits) or after surgical resection of a cervical rib.
- It can occur spontaneously after infection. There is no specific treatment.

The suprascapular nerve

- The nerve origin is at roots C4–C6, its course is lateral and deep to the trapezius, through the suprascapular notch, terminating in the supraspinatus and posteriorly in the infraspinatus. It carries pain fibres from the glenohumeral joint and ACJ.
- Impingement of the nerve at the suprascapular notch is a cause of shoulder pain where examination and imaging may not reveal an obvious musculoskeletal lesion.
- Injury to the nerve often gives diffuse shoulder pain though painless paralysis of the muscles can occur.

- Injury is often thought to occur from repeated stretching of the nerve at the notch. Weightlifters are prone to bilateral injury and volleyball players prone to dominant side injury.
- Compression by ganglia/tumours occurs and can be confirmed by MR.

Ulnar nerve

The ulnar nerve originates from C8 and T1. It lies along the medial side of the brachial artery in the upper arm, then above the medial humeral epicondyle where it passes posteriorly, piercing the medial intermuscular septum. It then runs behind the elbow in a groove between olecranon and medial epicondyle covered by a fibrous sheath and arcuate ligament (cubital tunnel). Following the line of the ulna in the flexor compartment of the forearm, branches supply flexor digitorum profundus (FDP) and flexor carpi ulnaris (FCU). The nerve enters the hand on the ulnar side dividing into superficial (palmaris brevis and skin over the medial one and a half digits) and deep (small muscles of the hand) branches.

- Lesions are usually due to entrapment.
- The ulnar nerve is occasionally damaged in the relatively exposed cubital tunnel (cubital tunnel syndrome) resulting in pain and parasthesiae along the medial forearm, wrist, and fourth/fifth digits. Damage may occur from direct trauma, compression, or recurrent subluxation. The Hoffman–Tinnel test at the elbow may be positive and there might be sensory loss over the palmar aspect of the fifth digit.
- There are a number of sites where entrapment of the ulnar nerve may occur around the wrist, either proximal to the volar carpal ligament or beneath it or the pisohamate ligament. External compression, acute or recurrent trauma, and ganglia are the usual causes. Symptoms have been noted in cyclists, users of pneumatic or vibrating tools, and in avid videogame players. Entrapment of the purely sensory cutaneous branch can occur from excessive computer mouse use.
- Motor weakness may be most evident by observing general muscle wasting in the hand (hypothenar eminence, interossei, adductor pollicis) and flexion deformity of the fourth and fifth digits—the latter caused by third and fourth lumbrical weakness (see Plate 6).
- Flexion of the wrist with ulnar deviation (FCU) and thumb adduction may be weak (adductor pollicis weakness will be evident if you ask the patient to 'run the thumb across the base of the fingers' as normally it can sweep across touching the skin).
- Froment's sign also signifies weakness of adductor pollicis and is demonstrated by a weakness in holding paper between the thumb and the index finger when both are in the sagittal plane.
- Discrimination of a wrist site from an elbow site of nerve entrapment is helped by the site of a positive Hoffman–Tinnel test, preservation of power of wrist flexion/medial deviation (FCU) in a wrist lesion and electrophysiology.
- Rest, analgesia and occasionally local steroids are helpful. A review of posture, repetitive activity, and a biomechanical assessment with changes in activities and technique are recommended. Surgical decompression may also be necessary.

Radial nerve

The nerve origin is at roots C5–C8, and its course runs anterior to subscapularis then passes behind the humerus in a groove that runs between the long and medial heads of triceps. It then winds anteriorly around the humeral shaft to lie between brachialis and brachioradialis. In the flexor compartment of the arm it divides at the level of the lateral epicondyle into superficial branch (cutaneous/sensory) and the posterior interosseous nerve (PIN), which runs through the supinator muscle into the forearm to supply the extensor compartment muscles.

• Entrapment needs to be considered in those cases of shoulder/ upper arm trauma where subsequent presentation includes arm/ wrist weakness.
• Compression of the radial nerve in the upper arm causes stiffness in the dorsal arm and forearm, weakness of the wrist, and little finger extension. The triceps is usually unaffected as nerve supply to the muscle leaves the radial nerve proximally.
• Transient compression of the nerve at the site of the medial head of triceps has been described in tennis players.
• Compression can occur as the nerve pierces the lateral intermuscular septum just distal to the radial head and also where the PIN pierces the supinator.
• At this lower site, compression is often a consequence of trauma, may be associated with a positive Hoffman–Tinnel test and local tenderness, and the pain may be reproduced by extreme passive forearm pronation combined with wrist flexion. Symptoms may mimic those of lateral epicondylitis. Surgical exploration may be necessary to confirm a diagnosis.

Median nerve

The nerve origin is from C6–T1 nerve roots. Its course from the brachial plexus runs together with the brachial artery in the upper arm (supplying nothing) then enters the forearm between the two heads of pronator teres (from medial humeral epicondyle and coronoid process of the ulna). It runs deep in the forearm dividing into median and anterior interosseous branches. The median branch enters the hand beneath the flexor retinaculum on the radial side of the wrist. All pronator and flexor muscles in the forearm (except FCU and the medial half of FDP) are supplied by the two branches. The median supplies sensory nerves to the radial side of the hand.

• Entrapment syndrome at the wrist is very common.
• In the rare pronator syndrome, trauma, swelling, or masses between the two pronator heads can cause entrapment giving lower arm pain, parasthesiae, and weakness of forearm pronation. There is local tenderness and reproduction of pain from resisted forearm pronation or wrist flexion.
• Pain in CTS is often present at night and relieved by exercising the hand. Daytime symptoms can persist. Pain can be referred up the arm even to the shoulder. Sensory symptoms are confined to the radial three and a half digits.
• Motor inco-ordination (clumsiness) is a common early feature of CTS.

- Symptoms reproduced by a positive Hoffman–Tinnel's sign (percussion over the volar aspect of the wrist) and Phalen's manoeuvre (volar aspect of the wrist rested on the back of a chair and the hand allowed to fall loosely under gravity, held for one minute) indicates nerve compression.
- A severe or chronic lesion is associated with sensory testing abnormality (see Fig. 2.9) and motor weakness of abductor pollicis brevis (APB), opponens pollicis, and first/second lumbricals.
- Nerve conduction studies are indicated if the diagnosis is uncertain, or if the condition is progressive, motor neuron disease is suspected (thenar muscle wasting marked/progressive with minimal sensory symptoms), dual pathology is suspected, surgical decompression is being considered, and in cases of surgical failure. False negative results occur in 10% of cases.
- MR appears to be more sensitive than US for detecting abnormalities involving the median nerve in/around the carpal tunnel.
- Aetiology of CTS is debated but probably multifactorial. The following are associated: Colles' fracture, trauma, carpal OA, diabetes, inflammatory joint/tendon disease (e.g. RA, scleroderma), ganglia, menopause and pregnancy. Also, hypothyroidism, acromegaly, amyloid, and benign tumours.

Treatment of carpal tunnel syndrome

- Night splinting may be curative, especially early in the condition.
- NSAIDs are helpful if there is underlying inflammatory disease.
- Local steroid injections are of value. If partial remission is achieved consider repeating the injection (see Plate 15).
- Surgical decompression is indicated when there is failure of conservative therapy, progressive/persistent neurological changes, or muscle atrophy/weakness.
- Failure of surgical release of the carpal tunnel requires further consideration of underlying causes such as a ganglion or other soft tissue lesion. Reconsider also whether there really is a mechanical/local or perhaps a more subtle cause (e.g. mononeuritis or peripheral neuropathy, entrapment at the pronator or nerve root lesion).

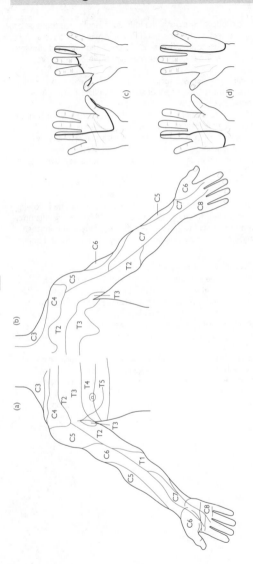

Fig. 2.9 Approximate distribution of dermatomes on the anterior (a) and posterior (b) aspects of the (right) upper limb. Approximate area of sensory change in lesions of the median (c) and ulnar (d) nerves

Thoracic back and chest pain

Background

- The typical thoracic spine (T1–T12) moves less than the lumbar and cervical vertebrae. Segmental movement in any direction is about 6°. However, given the number of segments this can add up to appreciable mobility overall. Less segmental movement results in reduced frequency of problems overall (only 6% of patients attending a spinal clinic have thoracic spine problems).
- Ribs (1–10) articulate posteriorly with vertebrae at two points: the articular facet of the rib head with the costovertebral facet on each vertebral body and the articular facet of the rib tubercle with the costotransverse facet on each vertebral lateral process. These are both synovial joints. Ribs 11 and 12 do not have costotransverse joints.
- The ribs, each continuous with its costal cartilage, articulate anteriorly by synovial joint with manubrium (1–2), sternum (2–7), each costal cartilage above (8–10), or do not articulate (11/12—'floating ribs').
- A massive block of spinal extensor muscles is responsible for maintaining the body against gravity. Some extend over some distance (e.g. the spinalis thoracis from the upper thoracic to the mid-lumbar spinous processes).
- Dermatomes are circumferential and extend from T2 at the clavicles to T10 at the umbilicus. However, up to five nerve roots may contribute innervation of any one point in a truncal dermatome.

Taking a history

The interpretation of cardiac, oesophageal, or pleural chest pain as musculoskeletal in origin is a common occurrence. It may result in missing a serious condition. Take a good history (see Tables 2.9 and 2.10).

- A review of the patterns of quality and radiation of cardiac and oesophageal pain in the clinical context should always be considered.
- Pleuritic pain is common. Recurrent pulmonary emboli are probably underdiagnosed, are difficult to diagnose, and have serious consequences. Any inflammatory, infective, or infiltrative pleural lesion will be painful.
- Lesions confined to pulmonary parenchyma do not produce pain.
- Pericardial pain can be misinterpreted as musculoskeletal or pleuritic.
- Mediastinal abnormalities can produce pain that is often referred.

The interpretation of neurogenic or musculoskeletal chest pains as cardiogenic, oesophageal, or pleural is a common occurrence and may lead to unnecessary investigations. Take a good history (see Table 2.10).

- Thoracic spine lesions can result in referred anterolateral chest pain.
- Costovertebral and costotransverse joint dysfunction is relatively common and is generally age-related but can occur in anyone with spinal deformity. It may produce thoracic spine pain alone or result in an extensive pattern of radiation of pain over the back, lateral, and anterior chest wall.

Table 2.9 Characteristics of chest pain from non-neurological and non-musculoskeletal pathology.

Process	Characteristics of pain
Angina	Gradual onset often related to exercise, a heavy meal, or emotion. Squeezing, strangling, or constriction in chest, can be aching or burning in nature. Commonly substernal but radiates to any of anterior chest, interscapular area, arms (mainly left), shoulders, teeth, and abdomen. Reduces with rest and sublingual nitrates
Myocardial infarction	Similar to above regarding quality and distribution. Longer duration. Less easily relieved
Pericardial inflammation	Sharp or steady substernal pain. Can be referred to shoulder tip, anterior chest, upper abdomen, or back. Often has a pleural component and is altered by change in position—sharper more left-sided when supine but eased by leaning forward
Aortic dissection	Acute onset with extremely severe peak. Felt in centre of chest or back. Lasts for hours
Pleuritic inflammation	Common. Sharp, knife-like, superficial. Aggravated by deep inspiration, sneezing, or coughing. If accompanied by haemoptysis consider pulmonary embolism
Mediastinal conditions	Empyema or surgical emphysema may be intense and sharp and radiate from substernal to shoulder area. Associated with crepitus. Mediastinitis and tumour pain resembles pleural pain. May have constant feeling of constriction/oppression
Peptic disease	Penetrating duodenal ulcers can cause intense, persistent mid-thoracic back pain
Oesophageal reflux	Persistent retrosternal burning is typical. Often post-prandial, when lying or at night/early morning. Oesophageal spasm can be similar to angina and can cause mid-thoracic back pain but reflux symptoms often coexist

Table 2.10 Painful neurological and musculoskeletal conditions of the thoracic spine and chest wall

Thoracic vertebral disease	Osteoporotic or pathological fracture
	Tumours, e.g. osteoid osteoma, metastasis
	Osteomyelitis
	Paget's disease
	Osteomalacia, rickets
	Costovertebral joint dysfunction
Nerve irritation	Root irritation/compression from disc prolapse or osteophyte at exit foramen, from structure distal to exit foramen, or from neuroma
Biomechanical/ degenerative	Scoliosis (non-structural compensatory, structural)
	Diffuse idiopathic skeletal hyperostosis (DISH)
	Calcium pyrophosphate dihydrate disease (of ligamentum flavum)
Herpes-Zoster of intercostal nerve	
Chest wall/superficial lesions	Rib fracture
	Other rib lesions, e.g. tumours, fibrous dysplasia, osteomalacia
	Costochondritis/enthesitis
	Intercostal muscle tear/strain
	Mastitis or fibrocystic disease of the breast
	Myofascial pain and fibromyalgia
	Parietal pleural inflammation/infection/infiltration
Spondylarthropathy (e.g. ankylosing spondylitis)	Spinal inflammation
	Acute discitis
	Chronic indolent discitis
Scheuermann's osteochondritis	In adolescents only

- Lower cervical spine lesions can refer pain to the anterior chest wall.
- Many painful chest conditions are associated with radiation of the pain down the left arm. This pattern is not specific for myocardial ischaemia.
- Lower cervical pain may be referred to the interscapula region.
- Interscapular pain may also be associated with mechanical lumbar disorders. Unlike infection, tumours, and fracture, referred pain is eased or abolished by changes in position or posture.

If there is thoracic back pain alone and it is acute and/or severe consider osteoporosis, tumours, and infection.

- Osteoporotic vertebral collapse is common in post-menopausal women. An acute, non/minimal-trauma-associated severe pain is typical. Fractures occur in many other situations, e.g. AS or a neoplastic bone lesion.
- Spinal infections should not be missed. All are usually associated symptoms. The commonest are *Staphylococcus aureus*, *Brucella*, and *Mycobacterium tuberculosis* (see Chapter 17).

Ask about the quality of pain

- Musculoskeletal pain (local or referred) generally associates with specific movements, positions, or postures and is reproducible.
- Pain which increases with coughing, sneezing, or deep inspiration, is suggestive of, but not specific for, pleural lesions. Rib and intercostal lesions or costovertebral joint dysfunction are possibilities.
- Early morning stiffness is not specific for spondylitis and is common. It may be due to muscle spasm associated with a painful lesion.

Ask about other symptoms and risk factors

- The pain from a fracture/lesion (osteoporotic, malignancy, infection) is often localized and extreme, waking the patient at night.
- Acute or chronic thoracic spine lesions may be associated with cord compression. Ask about recent change in sphincter function and progressive lower limb stiffness or heaviness.
- Risks for osteoporosis (see Chapter 16).
- Systemic symptoms of fever (osteomyelitis).
- Bone pain elsewhere (metastases, osteomalacia, Paget's disease).
- Spinal pain in adolescence (for an adult with kyphosis/spinal pain).
- A positive family history is recognized in idiopathic juvenile scoliosis, osteoporosis, and generalized osteoarthritis (see Chapter 6).
- Depression and anxiety are important modulators of pain. However, though thoracic back and chest pains may be psychogenic, it is imprudent to settle on this diagnosis without excluding musculoskeletal conditions and diseases of viscera that can cause referred pain.

Examination

Visual inspection

Observe the patient (who has undressed down to their underwear) from back and front. Look for deformity, asymmetry, swellings, and note the respiratory pattern.

- Any scoliosis should be noted. Non-structural scoliosis is frequently due to posture, severe back or abdominal pain, leg length discrepancy, and, rarely, can be psychogenic. Structural scoliosis may be 2° to various lesions at any age.
- There is a normal mild thoracic kyphos; however, marked kyphos in adults (particularly post-menopausal women) might suggest multiple osteoporotic vertebral fractures, though degenerative disc disease often results in kyphosis development in old age. A loss of normal kyphosis (flat spine) may be seen in spondylitis or possibly severe muscle spasm.
- Loose folds of skin on the back might denote multiple vertebral fractures.
- Costochondral swelling occurs in some cases of costochondritis or rickets ('rickety rosary') in children. Look for synovitis of costosternal or sternoclavicular joints (pattern associated with spondylarthropathy).

Palpation

Palpate over the vertebrae, paravertebral joints, and back musculature with the patient prone. Palpate the anterior chest wall.

- Spinal osteomyelitis may be associated with obvious skin swelling and erythema, exquisite focal tenderness, and extensor spasm. Tumours may give similar signs, though skin erythema is not likely.
- Costotransverse joints may be tender (4–5 cm from midline). Discomfort at any costovertebral joint and its referred pain can be elicited by individual rib manipulation (downward pressure on the rib lateral to its vertebral joints when the patient is prone).
- Identify any trigger points that reproduce myofascial pain in back muscles.
- Tender swelling of the sternoclavicular, costomanubrial or sternocostal joints may suggest spondylarthropathy or SAPHO (synovitis, acne, pustulosis (palmoplantar), hyperostosis and (aseptic) osteomyelitis).
- Inflammation of costal cartilages is often associated with painful swelling and tenderness. Rib/intercostal lesions should be easily discriminated from referred pain by eliciting local tenderness.

Check thoracic spinal movement

Movements of the thoracic spine should be checked. Ask the patient to sit on the couch with their arms folded in front of them. Guided by movements of the spinous processes gauge the range of thoracic spine movement.

- Approximate normal ranges of movement in the above position are extension 30°, lateral flexion 30°, flexion 90°, and rotation 60°.
- Scoliosis is often associated with rotation that is accentuated on flexion.

- Abnormal mobility will not be specific for any underlying condition but may draw attention to the major affected spinal segment (painful segments are 'guarded' and may appear hypomobile).
- Spondylitis may become obvious if there is extensive spinal hypomobility.
- Chest expansion should be measured from forced expiration to complete inspiration measuring at expansion, with a tape, at the level of the xiphisternum. Normal young adult chest expansion should measure at least 3 cm.

Other examination

- Given the range of serious conditions causing chest pains, a full medical examination is important and should always be considered.
- Neurological examination of the legs should be considered in anyone who is at risk of spinal cord compression. Look for ↑ tone, pyramidal weakness, ↑ reflexes, and extensor plantars.
- Breast and axillary lymph node examination should be done.

Investigations

Radiographs

- Lateral view radiographs generally provide more information about thoracic spine lesions than anteroposterior views; however, together, both views should confirm osteoporosis, degenerative disease (e.g. previous Scheuermann's osteochondritis, ochronosis, DISH), and Paget's disease (see Chapter 16).
- Look for vertebral squaring (in AS) and either marginal or non-marginal syndesmophytes as in psoriatic spondylitis (See Plate 7) or other SpA (see Chapter 8).
- Discriminate enthesitis from DISH at the corners of vertebrae by the presence of erosions with bone reaction (enthesitis) compared with bone proliferation alone (DISH). Enthesitis, associated with chronic spondylodiscitis is part of the SpA spectrum of diseases.
- Normal radiographs do not exclude malignancy.
- Bone lesions can be well characterized by CT (e.g. osteoid osteoma).

MR

- MR is important in discriminating tumour from infection.
- Disc lesions, spinal canal, and cord are well visualized with MR.
- Fat suppressed or gadolinium-enhanced MR sequences may be necessary to discriminate enthesitis or spondylodiscitis associated with SpA.

Bone scintigraphy

- A bone scan is a sensitive test for infection and malignancy.
- In suspected cases of (previously undiagnosed) malignancy, it is more sensitive than radiographs, can often confirm the lytic or sclerotic nature of a lesion, and will identify any other skeletal sites of disease.
- It is a useful investigation in patients with malignancy who present with back pain. A lack of additional lesions strongly suggests against a single spinal abnormality being malignancy-related.
- Tomography can discriminate abnormality in the pars interarticularis, facet joint, and disc/vertebral body.

- Bone scintigraphy sensitively identifies rib and, in most cases, inflammatory intercostal lesions. If solitary the differential diagnosis is of a metastasis, 1° malignant or benign bone tumour, healed rib fracture, fibrous dysplasia, Paget's bone disease, hyperparathyroidism, or infection.

Other investigations to consider in patients with chest pain

- CXR, then consider pulmonary ventilation/perfusion scintigraphy and spiral CT (?PEs).
- CT of the chest in patients with unexplained pleural pain.
- ECG (EKG) and an exercise ECG or coronary perfusion scintigraphy for patients with possible cardiac ischaemia.
- Transthoracic echocardiography to show thickened pericardium or an effusion associated with pericarditis.
- Upper gastrointestinal endoscopy in suspected cases of peptic ulceration.
- Diagnostic trial of a proton pump inhibitor in cases of reflux oesophagitis.

Treatment

For treatment of thoracic and chest wall lesions see the next section on Low back pain and also Chapter 20.

Low back pain and disorders in adults

Epidemiology

- The lifetime prevalence of back pain is 58% and the greatest prevalence is between 45 and 64 years of age.
- There are 12 million primary care consultations and over 2.4 million adult outpatient visits to hospitals annually for low back pain in the United Kingdom (population 65 million).
- Estimated annual financial costs of back pain to the United Kingdom National Health Service are more than £500 million. Indirect costs are estimated to be more than £5 billion for lost work.
- The financial health care and indirect employment costs of low back pain in the United States are estimated to be more than $24 billion.

Lumbar and sacral spine anatomy

- There are normally five lumbar vertebrae. Anomalies are not uncommon at the lumbosacral junction.
- The transition between the mobile lumbar spine (flexion, extension, and lateral flexion) and fixed sacrum together with high weight-loading combine to make the region highly prone to damage.
- The facet joints are sharply angled, effectively reducing rotation in lumbar segments.
- The sacroiliac joints (synovial) are held firmly by a strong fibrous capsule and tough ligaments. The amount of normal movement (essentially rotation) is normally inversely proportional to age.
- The spinal cord ends at L1/L2. Nerves then run individually, are normally mobile in the spinal canal, and together are termed the cauda equina.
- Each nerve exits its appropriate lateral intervertebral exit foramen passing initially superior and then laterally to the disc, e.g. L4 from L4/L5 exit foramen. However, in the spinal canal each nerve descends immediately posterior to the more proximal intervertebral disc before it exits. Thus, for example, L4 root symptoms can occur from either lateral herniation of the L4/5 disc or posterior herniation of the L3/L4 disc (or from both).
- Facet joint innervation is from posterior 1° rami, each of which supplies the corresponding joint at its level, one higher and one lower.

Basic principles of assessment

- Low back pain can arise from damage or inflammation of the thoracic or lumbar spines or from the posterior pelvis. Pathology in retroperitoneal abdominal and pelvic viscera can result in referred pain to the low back.
- A simple way of categorizing back pain is to consider its cause to be primarily mechanical or inflammatory, due to bone pathology, as referred pain, or from intrinsic neurological disease (see Table 2.11).
- Over 90% of episodes of low back pain in adults are mechanical, self-limiting, and do not require investigation.

Table 2.11 Common and/or serious causes of low back pain in adults

Mechanical/degenerative (very common)	Hypermobility (see Chapter 16)
	Facet joint arthritis
	Disc disease (annular tear, internal disruption, prolapse)
	Scoliosis/kyphosis
	Spinal stenosis
	Sacroiliitis
Inflammatory (uncommon)	AS (Chapter 8)
	Sacroiliitis (e.g. AS, brucellosis)
Infection (rare)	Osteomyelitis (e.g. Staphylococcus aureus, TB, brucellosis) (see Chapter 17)
Bone disease (common)	Osteoporotic fracture (see Chapter 16)
	Paget's disease
	Osteomalacia
Neoplasia (rare)	Secondary metastases
	Multiple myeloma
Other	Sickle cell crisis
	Renal disease (e.g. tumours, infection)
	Gynaecological disease
	Fibromyalgia (see Chapter 18)

- Indicators for further investigation include age > 55 years of age, stiffness, focal pain, pain that disturbs sleep, nerve root symptoms, and chronic persistent (> 6 weeks) pain.
- The low back is often a focus for those who may use pain (consciously or unconsciously) as a protective device in the face of domestic, emotional, or occupational stress. These stresses commonly influence the description and impact of pain but rarely act alone in causing pain—there is usually some underlying organic pathology.

Taking a history
Differentiate whether the pain is likely to be primarily mechanical or inflammatory, due to bone pathology or referred
- The site and extent of the pain does not easily discriminate the cause. All disorders may be associated with mechanical deformity and/or muscle spasm that may cause pain in a more diffuse distribution.
- Generally, pain due to mechanical lesions is often acute in onset whereas patients with pain from inflammatory lesions often present after symptoms have been present for some time.

- Inflammatory pain is often worse at night, is associated with stiffness at night/rest or on waking, and is eased by movement. Mechanical lesions often settle at night and worsen with (at least some or certain) movements. Many 'mechanical' or 'degenerative' lesions may have an inflammatory component, e.g. internal disc disruption causing discogenic pain.
- Intrinsic bone pathology often causes severe, unremitting, focal pain. Sleep is disturbed. Pain does not ease substantially with movement.
- About 3% of patients presenting with back pain have non-muscu-loskeletal causes. In the low back (in women) a significant proportion have pelvic conditions such as ovarian cysts or endometriosis. Pain may be cyclical.
- For those aged over 55 with no previous similar episodes of pain—increase suspicion of an underlying neoplastic lesion. Investigation is required.
- Associated systemic symptoms are common in osteomyelitis and may be present if a malignancy has disseminated.

Ask about pain radiation and symptoms in the legs

- Progressive neurological leg symptoms suggest a worsening/expanding lesion such as a tumour, infection/vertebral collapse, Paget's disease, or lumbosacral spinal stenosis.
- Pressure on neural elements of the cauda equina sufficient to cause a disturbance in perineal sensation and/or bowel/bladder paralysis is a neurosurgical emergency (cauda equina syndrome).
- Leg pain caused by nerve root irritation/compression is often clearly defined and sharp, often accompanied by numbness or parasthesiae. The commonest involved nerve roots are L4, L5, or S1. Pain generally radiates to below the knee and often, but not always, to the heel and big toe.
- Sciatic nerve entrapment at the level of the piriformis muscle can produce identical radicular symptoms to L5 or S1 nerve root entrapment.
- Neurological symptoms in the distribution of the femoral nerve (primarily anterior thigh musculature) might suggest a high lumbar nerve root lesion (L1–L3 for example).
- Disc prolapse is the commonest cause of nerve root pain but bony encroachment at the nerve root exit foramen by vertebral end-plate or facet joint osteophytes and/or soft tissue thickening or fibrosis can cause similar pain too (foramenal stenosis).
- Discs do not need to prolapse to cause pain. Annular tears and internal disruption (?microfractures in vertebral end-plates) can cause a pattern of pain, termed discogenic pain, characterized by low back and referred buttock/posterior thigh pain aggravated by movement.
- Generally, all mechanical lesions of the lumbar spine can result in referred pain around the pelvis and anterior thighs. However, pain from lumbar facet joints and probably other segmental structures can be referred to the lower leg.

- Aching in the back and posterior thighs after standing is typical of, but not specific for, spondylolisthesis. There are often added spasms of acute pain, especially if there is segmental instability.
- The symptoms of spinal stenosis are often relieved by sitting bent slightly forward (spinal canal dimensions increase in this position).
- Sacroiliitis often causes referred pain to the buttocks and back of thighs. It occurs commonly in spondylarthropathy (see Chapter 8).
- Sacroiliac pain can occur in multiparous women—the condition may be associated with hypermobility.

Note the description of the pain

- Pain may be 'severe' whatever the cause; however, note whether the patient's descriptors of it suggest non-organic influences.
- Sharp, lancinating leg pains suggest nerve root irritation/compression (radicular pain) whereas leg pain referred from other structures within a lumbar segment is generally deep and aching. Distribution may be similar (see above). More persistent, rather than episodic, radicular pain may denote stenosis of the nerve root exit foramen.
- A description of bilateral buttock/leg pain that worsens on walking is consistent with spinal stenosis, especially in those with normal peripheral pulses and no bruits.
- A change in the description of pain in someone who has an estab-lished diagnosis may be important, e.g. subacute, severe, unremitting localized pain in a patient with AS who normally has mild inflammatory pain might reflect a superadded discitis; or, acute severe unremitting sleep-disturbing pain in an elderly woman with known chronic mechanical pain associated with OA might suggest osteoporotic fracture.
- Florid descriptions of the pain and its severity are associated with psychological modulators of pain.

Previous back pain and trauma, occupation, and family history

- Scheuermann's disease causes spinal pain in adolescence. It is a risk for spinal degeneration and kyphosis in adults.
- Previous trauma may have caused pars interarticularis fractures (an ante-cedent of spondylolisthesis), vertebral fracture (risk of further mechanical damage), or ligament rupture (subsequent segmental instability).
- It is generally accepted that the high prevalence of disc disease amongst manual workers at a relatively young age provides some evidence for a causal relationship.
- It is often the case that patients with chronic pain following (sometimes trivial) trauma may be dissatisfied with the quality of care received at the time of the injury. Be aware that many believe, and there is some evidence to support this, that the way in which spinal pain is handled at its onset significantly influences its subsequent course.
- Sacroiliitis is an early part of brucellar arthritis (20–51% of patients). Poor animal- or carcass-handling hygiene or ingestion of infected foodstuffs/milk can lead to infection. Spondylitis is a late feature and is characterized by erosions, disc infection, and abcesses.
- A positive family history of low back pain might, in context, suggest SpA (sacroiliitis), hypermobility (see Chapter 16), or generalized osteoarthritis (see Chapter 6).

Examination

Inspect the undressed patient from the side and behind

- Note the fluidity of movement when the patient is undressing.
- Check the skin for redness, local swelling, and skin markings. Redness and swelling occasionally accompany osteomyelitis.
- Lipomata, hairy patches, café-au-lait patches, or skin tags often reflect underlying structural nerve or bone abnormality, e.g. spina bifida, diastematomyelia, neurofibromatosis.
- Skin folds often suggest an underlying significant structural change such as osteoporotic fracture or spondylolisthesis.
- Note any deformity: hyperlordosis (associated with L5/S1 damage and weak abdominal musculature), prominent thoracolumbar kyphosis (multiple disc degeneration or vertebral fractures), scoliosis (degenerative, compensatory muscle spasm for unilateral pain).
- Look from the side. A gentle lordotic curve is normal. Flattening suggests muscle spasm or fusion in SpA. With major spondylolisthesis, a step between spinous processes can sometimes be seen.

Observe active movements whilst the patient is standing

Lumbar forward flexion ('…with your legs straight, slowly reach down to try and touch your knees/ankles…'), lateral flexion ('…with your legs and back straight, tip sideways and run your hand down your leg towards your knee…') and extension ('…with your legs straight, slowly bend backwards…'). Note: flexion can be mediated by the hip joints; extension can be effected by slight pelvic tilt and body sway. Ask what can be achieved normally and what is painful.

- Abnormal movements are not specific for any condition though they may help to localize a problem.
- Pain in extension is characteristic of retrospondylolisthesis, facet joint arthritis, or impinging spinous processes. All may be relieved by flexion.
- Failure of the spinous processes to separate in a patient who manages good forward flexion would be consistent with permanent spinal stiffness, e.g. AS, with flexion mediated by the hip joints.
- Forward flexion can be measured using the modified Schöber's test. When erect, mark the skin at the point midway between the posterior superior iliac spines (Venus' dimples) and again 10 cm above and 5 cm below. Measure the increase in distance between the outer marks at full forward flexion—in a young adult this is normally more than 6 cm.
- Ask the patient to stand on one foot then lift onto their toes a few times. Weakness might imply an L5 nerve root entrapment (gastrocnemius/soleus).

Observe the gait pattern

Abnormality of gait may reflect any spinal or lower limb problem:
- An antalgic gait.
- A wide-based gait suggests unsteadiness (due to dizziness, muscular weakness, proprioceptive, or cerebellar deficit etc.).

- Leaning forwards/stiff legged—though not specific, in older people this may denote spinal stenosis.
- Shuffling, which could suggest Parkinsonism (back pain/stiffness is a recognized early sign).
- Foot drop, which could suggest L5 or S1 nerve root compression.
- Flat feet, hind feet valgus, and genu recurvatum on stance phase, might suggest general hypermobility—associated with various low back lesions.

Check extension and lumbar rotation (patient seated)

With the patient seated on the couch, check lumbar extension and rotation (the pelvis is now fixed).

- Typically, combined rotation and extension can elicit pain from arthritic facet joints. It is a sensitive though not specific test.
- Slumping forwards (see Fig. 2.10) stretches the dura. Increased lumbar pain may be elicited in cases of disc prolapse but, more importantly, leg pain can be elicited in cases of nerve root entrapment. A more provocative test can be done by gently extending each knee in turn in the slump position. Look for asymmetry.

Examine the sacroiliac joints and hips (patient supine)

With the patient supine, examination of the sacroiliac joints and an examination of the hips should be done to exclude pain arising from these structures.

- Test flexion and the rotational range of each hip by lifting the leg, flexed at the knee, so that the upper leg is vertical. Passive movement should normally be pain-free.
- No SIJ stress test is specific. Tests are designed to reproduce pain in cases of SIJ dysfunction or sacroiliitis. Here are two:
  - press down/out reasonably firmly over both anterior superior iliac spines at the same time.
  - lift one leg, flex, and abduct the hip slightly. Exert an axial force into the acetabulum at two or three different angles. This test is considered by many to be more useful and probably stresses both the joint and many of the sacral ligaments though is less specific if the hip joint is abnormal.

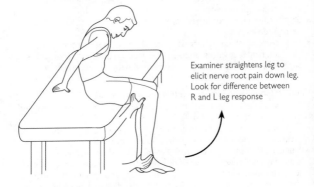

Examiner straightens leg to
elicit nerve root pain down leg.
Look for difference between
R and L leg response

Fig. 2.10 The slump test identifies pain from lumbar disc and nerve root irritation
or compression (see text).

Straight leg raise (Laseague's test)

The normal variation in straight leg raise ranges from 60° to more than
90° in adults. Compare sides.

- Discomfort from normal tightening of the posterior thigh or calf
  muscles must be discriminated from a positive test. A positive test
  (leg raising restricted to 40° or less by the radicular pain) is most
  specific in patients aged <30 years and for L5 or S1 nerve root lesions.
- A crossed straight leg raise (pain elicited by raising the unaffected leg)
  is even more specific for nerve root entrapment.
- To identify more subtle cases of nerve root entrapment, apply
  additional foot dorsiflexion at the maximum possible angle of
  (pain-free) leg raise.
- Laseague's test does not always reproduce pain in every patient who
  has sciatica. It is also often negative in older patients with the condition
  when it is chiefly due to foramenal stenosis and when central posterior
  disc prolapse occurs (giving bilateral sciatica but no root compression).

Neurological examination

- Neurological examination of the legs is essential in suspected cases of
  nerve root entrapment, cord compression, spinal stenosis and cauda
  equina syndrome.

Table 2.12 lists tests for muscle strength in the lower limbs—weakness
may denote nerve root entrapment—and Table 2.13 lists the principal
signs of lumbar nerve root lesions.

Table 2.12 Testing muscle strength in the lower limbs (patient supine unless otherwise stated). Weakness may denote nerve root entrapment

Muscle or muscle group	Nerve roots	Test*
Hamstrings (knee flexion)	L5, S1, S2	Ask patient to flex the knee to 45°, hold patient's ankle and ask them to bend the knee further against your hold
Iliopsoas (hip flexion/internal rotation)	L1, L2, L3	Ask patient to lift the leg with a bent knee, hold up the upper leg and resist your push. Try to push the leg down and slightly outwards
Quadriceps femoris (hip flexion, knee extension)	L2, L3, L4	1. Hold the patient's relaxed upper leg above the couch (grasped underneath above the knee). The lower leg should drop loosely. Ask them to straighten the lower leg against your resistance
		2. From patient standing test repetitive squatting for more subtle weakness
Tibialis anterior (ankle dorsiflexion).Tibialis posterior (ankle inversion and dorsiflexion)	L4, L5	1. With the knee straight ask the patient to pull back their foot (show them first) against your pull. Resist dorsiflexion
		2. Standing or walking on heels tests for more subtle weakness. Note: if the hind foot rests in valgus or the patient significantly everts the foot during dorsiflexion, the test may also recruit peroneal muscles (L5, S1)
Extensor hallucis longus	L5, S1	Ask the patient to pull their big toe back against your finger (at the base)
Gastrocnemius and soleus (ankle plantar flexion)	S1, S2	1. Ask the patient to point their toes. Resist the movement by pressing against the ball of the foot
		2. Standing or walking on the toes tests for more subtle weakness

* Compare sides. Score according to scale, for example: 0 = no muscle contraction; 1 = contraction visible; 2 = active movement, gravity eliminated; 3 = active movement against gravity; 4-/4/4+ = active movement against slight/moderate/strong resistance; 5 = normal power.

Table 2.13 An *aide-mémoire*: principal combinations of signs used for identifying lumbar nerve root lesions

Nerve root	Parasthesiae and sensory change	Muscle weakness	Tendon reflex changes
L2	Upper thigh: anterior, medial + lateral surfaces	Hip flexion and adduction	None
L3	Anterior surface of lower thigh	Hip adduction + knee extension	Knee jerk possibly reduced
L4	Anteromedial surface of lower leg	Knee extension, foot dorsiflexion + inversion	Knee jerk decreased
L5	Anterolateral surface of lower leg + dorsum/medial side of foot/toe 1	Hip extension and abduction. Knee flexion. Foot/toe 1 dorsiflexion	None
S1	Lateral border + sole of foot. Back of heel + calf	Knee flexion. Plantar flexion and eversion of foot	Ankle jerk decreased

Examination of the prone patient

Ask the patient to turn to lie prone. Palpate low back and over sacrum.

- Diffuse tenderness may be due to muscle spasm.
- Superficial tenderness over the spinous processes or interspinous interval might suggest interspinous ligament disruption or impinging processes.
- Paravertebral bony tenderness may suggest facet joint arthritis.
- Loin tenderness could indicate renal pathology.
- Tenderness over the SIJs is not specific for sacroiliitis.
- A positive femoral stretch test reproduces L1–L4 (especially L3) radicular pain in the anterior or medial part of the thigh. Flex the patient's knee to 90° and passively extend the hip.

Other examination

- In suspected cases of spinal stenosis or cauda equina syndrome it is essential to check for sensory loss in the sacral nerve dermatomes. Also check anal sphincter tone by rectal examination (S5).
- In suspected cases of spinal stenosis, the patient can be asked to walk until limited by pain then re-examined. If there is any ischaemia of the cauda equina or of a nerve root (from foraminal stenosis) nerve root signs may become more obvious.

Investigations

- There are two important initial steps in investigating low back pain. First deciding whether radiographs will help. Second, though relatively rare in practice, the possibility of infection, malignancy, and cauda equina compression always needs to be borne in mind. Simple radiographic views are insensitive indicators of these conditions and, in most cases, are not specific although most radiologists would agree they are desirable in addition to CT or MR. Laboratory tests are mandatory in all suspected cases of inflammation, infection, and malignancy.

Radiographs—decision-making in requesting them
(Table 2.14)

- Lumbar spine radiographs are not always helpful. Remember that nine out of ten cases of back pain in the primary care setting are mechanical and self-limiting. Features on a plain radiograph of the lumbar spine correlate poorly with the presence or pattern of pain.
- Spondylosis is common, age-related, and often isn't symptomatic.
- Children, athletes, and young adults with back pain need prompt radiographic investigation. Failure to detect and treat a pars interarticularis fracture may lead on to a spondylolysis. Abnormalities are more readily appreciated in these age groups as the frequency of age-related degenerative changes in the spine is low.
- Obtaining radiographs to help in the management of patients is a different issue to obtaining them to aid diagnosis and one that requires careful thought, e.g. is the patient likely to perceive that they have received suboptimal care if a radiograph is not requested?

- Spondylolysis may be seen on a lateral view but is more easily seen on oblique views. Oblique views will also show pedicle stress fractures in athletes.
- Spondylolisthesis may be identified and graded by a lateral film. Flexion and extension views may be helpful in delineating subtle cases and instability (spondylolytic).
- General osteopenia is a risk factor for low bone mass; however, it is not a sensitive indicator of low bone mass.
- Look for vertebral squaring (in AS), non-marginal syndesmophytes (other SpA e.g. psoriatic) or the flowing or exuberant syndesmophytes of DISH.
- Consider obtaining an AP view of the pelvis. Established, but often not early, sacroiliitis can be ruled-out. A further 'coned' view is often helpful.
- Sacroiliitis (periarticular osteoporosis, erosion, sclerosis of bone, widening joint space) occurs in all types of SpA. It can be unilateral.
- Sclerosis of the SIJ on the lower iliac side alone suggests osteitis condensans ilii. Joint space is normal and joint margin well defined.
- Patterns of metabolic bone disease, Paget's disease and hip pathology are usually readily identifiable on a pelvic film.

Bone scintigraphy
- A bone scan is an extremely sensitive test for infection or malignancy. It is a useful investigation in patients with previously diagnosed malignancy who present with back pain, especially in those who have had no previous skeletal metastases. A lack of additional lesions strongly suggests against a single spinal abnormality being malignancy-related.
- It is not specific for the various degenerative lesions but can help localize the site of a lesion.
- Bone scan SIJ appearances in sacroiliitis can be unreliable.

CT or MR?
The choice of imaging depends largely on likely clinical and radiographic differential diagnosis:
- For spondylolytic spondylolisthesis, CT shows the exact site of pars' defects. The usual appearance is of sclerotic irregular edges.
- Nerve impingement can be shown by CT or MR.
- Intervertebral disc prolapse, both posterior and posterolateral, can be shown by either technique. Prolapse material is of similar CT density and MR signal to the disc and well-defined against epidural fat.
- Changes in the normal disc signal pattern are associated with age-related disc degeneration. Discogenic pain has been associated with MRI abnormalities classified according to Modic.
- On T_2-weighted MR, disc material is usually of higher signal than 'scar' (e.g. fibrosis from a previous lesion), in which signal decreases with aging. Recent scarring enhances immediately but old scarring does so only slowly. This discrimination requires gadolinium-enhanced MR.
- CT or MR shows early sacroiliitis in AS when X-rays are normal.

Table 2.14 Commonly reported patterns of radiographic abnormality in adults, the interpretation, and suggested reaction.

Radiographic abnormalities	Lesion suggested	Sensible further action
Lumbosacral anomalies	Risk for future back pain	May not be clinically significant. Risk for low back pain (esp. if hypermobile)
Generalized osteopenia	Osteoporosis	Measurement of bone density. Rule out secondary causes, e.g. myeloma
Narrowed disc space, marginal vertebral end-plate osteophytes or both	Intervertebral disc disruption	MR if persistent symptoms or signs of same level nerve root entrapment, spinal or nerve root exit foramen stenosis
Localized lucent or sclerotic lesion, loss of cortex	Tumour, infection, or fracture	Discuss case with radiologist. MR or CT may be advised. A bone scan may be helpful. Initiate appropriate laboratory tests immediately
Facet joint OA	Facet joint syndrome	Consider whether there is associated spinal/nerve root exit foramen stenosis (?radicular symptoms) or symptoms suggestive of spondylolisthesis. CT or MR is then likely to be appropriate
Pars interarticularis defect	Spondylolysis/ ?spondylolytic	Probable prior fracture. Further oblique film centered on suspected level or CT should confirm. Association with symptoms or signs of disc disease or spondylolisthesis suggests an unstable segment. Flexion and extension lateral view radiographs may show instability. MR helpful for imaging soft-tissues including nerves
Short lumbar pedicles	Spinal stenosis	Consider MR if symptoms suggest spinal stenosis
Mixed patchy sclerosis and lucency in entire (enlarged) vertebra(e)	Paget's disease	Neurological leg symptoms suggest spinal/exit foramen stenosis or vascular 'steal'

- Shape and outline of the spinal canal are ideally shown on CT but are also seen simply with MR. It is difficult for MR to distinguish fibrous structures from sclerotic or cortical bone, though it discerns intrathecal contents more readily which is an advantage in identifying intradural tumours. CT is perhaps the preferred choice for investigating canal stenosis.
- Spondylodiscitis (part of SpA), if chronic, may be difficult to discriminate from degenerative disc/vertebral end-plate disease. Fat-suppressed or gadolinium-enhanced sequences may show high signal at the anterior disc vertebral end-plate junctions.

Myelography and CT myelography (using non-ionic contrast)
- Myelographic patterns of abnormality of nerve root entrapment from posterolateral and posterior disc prolapse and spinal stenosis are well-recognized. However, both CT and MR have superceded myelography in most cases.
- Myelography or a combination of CT with radiculopathy is occasionally requested and is useful in patients in whom technical or personal considerations preclude MR examination (about 15% of people).

Screening for infection, malignancy, or metabolic bone disease
- In cases where the history and examination suggest a mechanical condition, but where the clinician wishes to be more confident of excluding an inflammatory condition, an ESR (or plasma viscosity) is suggested.
- A raised ESR would point towards further laboratory investigation.
- An infection screen should include an FBC for anaemia and leucocytosis, CRP, blood and urine cultures. If spinal tuberculosis is suspected a plain CXR should be taken and serial (over 3 days) early morning urine samples taken.
- Urine Bence-Jones proteins and serum immunoglobulin electrophoresis are essential tests in the 'work-up' for myeloma. Serum bone biochemistry and plasma U&E are also important as hypercalcaemia and acute renal impairment have prognostic significance in this condition.
- Serum bone biochemistry may point to an underlying metabolic bone disorder such as Paget's disease or osteomalacia. Bone biochemistry is normal in post-menopausal osteoporosis.
- If osteoporosis is diagnosed (see Chapter 16) a screen for 2° causes should include ESR (and if raised, serum and urinary protein electrophoresis), bone biochemistry, and sex hormones, but also serum 25-hydroxyvitamin D and PTH, TFTs, LFTs, and Cr.

Treatment (also see Chapter 20 for greater detail)
- An important therapeutic intervention in the case of acute pain is to take the patient seriously, take a positive view, and in the absence of sinister signs e.g. nerve root pain, urge early mobility.
- Analgesics and antispasmodics can be used in the short term, initially regularly, then as required.
- Physical therapy with graded-activity programmes may be of value, certainly early in disc disease or spondylosis.

- Cord compression 2° to bone collapse from a tumour is an acute emergency and should be discussed immediately with an oncologist or radiotherapist, and a spinal orthopaedic or neurosurgeon.
- Cases with disc prolapse failing to respond to conservative therapy, or cases where there is ongoing or rapidly progressive neurological deficit, should be referred for surgery.
- Available surgical techniques for acute or persistent disc disease include decompression procedures (e.g. nerve root decompression and partial facetectomy), prosthetic intervertebral disc replacement, intradiscal thermocoagulation, and intradiscal steroid injections though evidence for long-term efficacy is lacking for all these procedures.
- Surgery for spinal stenosis is useful for relieving leg neurogenic features but not indicated, even when stenosis proved with MR, if there is no significant leg/sphincter neurocompromise. Surgery is not usually done if the only effect of spinal stenosis is back pain.
- In chronic back pain, aerobic exercises combined with behavioural methods may be more effective than exercise alone and can help reduce 'sickness behaviour'. Methods may also incorporate psychological and social assessment and management.
- The common treatments available for chronic back pain include:
  - analgesics and muscle relaxants
  - antiepileptics/antidepressants for neuropathic pain
  - local anaesthetic/steroid injections
  - acupuncture
  - transcutaneous electrical nerve stimulation (TENS)
  - physiotherapy
  - ergonomic advice
  - multidisciplinary programmes:
    — counselling
    — cognitive therapy
    — education
    — relaxation
    — corsets and belts.
- Timely surgery for structural scoliosis (more common in JIA than the general population) can lessen spinal curvature.

Spinal disorders in children and adolescents

(See also Chapter 20.)

Background

- Common conditions in adults such as degenerative back pain and intervertebral disc disease are rare in childhood or adolescence.
- In hospital series upto 85% of referred children have identifiable causes (see Table 2.15) though spinal hypermobility in the context of generalized hypermobility and fibromyalgia has not been adequately addressed.
- Not all presentations are with pain. Some children present with either deformity or neurological symptoms.
- A diagnosis must be firmly established or at least rigorously sought because serious disease can present with few symptoms.

Taking a history

Keep an open mind as to whether a history from the child, parent/s, or 1° care-giver provides the most useful information. There are merits in consulting all of them. The process may be time-consuming.

Table 2.15 Cause of childhood back pain. Experience of an orthopaedic clinic (a review of 233 referrals)

Cause of back pain	Frequency (%)
Non-specific (i.e. no cause found)	32
Scoliosis	21
Spondylolysis/'listhesis (non-trauma)	11
Scheuermann's disease	7
Infection	6
Tumours, e.g. osteoid osteoma	4
Psychogenic	4
Disc prolapse	3
Inflammatory, e.g. spondylarthropathy	3
Trauma (excluding strains)	2
Limb length inequality/biomechanical	2
Renal pain	<1
Rickets	<1
Congenital anomalies	<1

Severity, distribution, and quality of pain
- Pain may be mild even though there is a serious underlying disorder.
- If the pain occurs, or initially occurred, during sport, consider pars interarticularis fractures, spondylolytic spondylolisthesis or Scheuermann's disease (vertebral epiphyseal osteochondritis).
- Persistent pain, unrelieved by rest and disturbing sleep, requires consideration of a bone tumour, bone and/or disc infection, or osteoporotic fracture (steroid-related or juvenile idiopathic osteoporosis (JIO)).
- JIO is rare, occurs between 6 and 13 years of age and is more common in boys. The main differential diagnosis is osteogenesis imperfecta (see Chapter 16).
- Although uncommon, neurological symptoms such as burning pain, parasthesiae, and weakness in the legs, suggests nerve root irritation.
- Spinal stiffness in a child (typically between 2 and 6 years of age) associated with irritability and a diffusely tender back may be due to infective discitis (though organisms are only found in 50%). In an older child or adolescent (typically 10–15 years of age) and with a less striking history, immobility-related stiffness could represent juvenile enthesitis related arthritis (ERA).

If pain is absent ...
Spinal conditions are not always associated with pain. Occasionally a child may present with back deformity or neurological symptoms in the legs alone.
- The history may be non-specific and, for example in a very young child, nothing more than a refusal to walk.
- Scheuermann's disease commonly presents in teenagers with a painless thoracic kyphosis. Pain is more likely to be present if the chondritis is thoracolumbar rather than thoracic. The condition is often asymptomatic.
- Spinal dysraphism (bony abnormality—usually spina bifida, associated with neural anomaly—invariably cord tethering) and spinal cord tumours can often present with neurological leg symptoms/signs alone without back pain. Symptoms may be mild initially.
- Scoliosis is usually pain-free. Pain with scoliosis usually indicates significant underlying pathology. The differential is wide (see Table 2.16).
- The most frequent single cause of a scoliosis in schoolchildren (40%), found from radiographic screening, is pelvic tilt due to leg length inequality.

Table 2.16 Causes of scoliosis in children and adolescents

Structural scolioses (vetebral rotation, vertebral structural change, and loss of normal spinal flexibility)	Idiopathic: infantile (0–3 years); juvenile (3–10 years); adolescent (> 10 years)
	Neuromuscular
	Congenital: failure of vertebral formation, segmentation, or both
	Neurofibromatosis
	Heritable disorders of connective tissue, e.g. osteogenesis imperfecta
	Trauma: fracture; surgical (e.g. post-laminectomy); irradiation
	Spondyloepiphyseal dysplasia
	Metabolic bone disease
	Lumbosacral anomalies (e.g. spondylolytic spondylolisthesis)
	Cervicothoracic anomalies (e.g. cervical fusion (Klippel–Feil))
	Rheumatoid arthritis
	Extraspinal contractures (e.g. post-empyema, post-burns)
Non-structural scolioses (lateral spinal curvature but no vetebral rotation)*	Postural
	Nerve root irritation associated
	Abdominal pain associated (e.g. appendicitis, renal pain)
	Associated with local inflammation
	Spinal infection
	Spinal tumours
	Secondary to leg length discrepancy
	Related to soft-tissue contractures around the hip
	Psychogenic

* It is characteristic of non-structural scolioses that if the underlying cause is successfully dealt with, the scoliosis resolves.

Past developmental, medical, family, and social history
- Ask about milestones in musculoskeletal development. Abnormality or delay might suggest spinal dysraphism or neuromuscular conditions.
- Osteoporosis may be evident from previous fragility fracture— axial or appendicular—or may be intimated from risk factors, e.g. steroid use.
- Previous low back trauma may have been pars interarticularis fractures preceding (the current) vertebral slip or disc prolapse.
- Irradiation (e.g. of previous Wilms' tumour) is a cause of scoliosis.

- Ask about previous TB or immunization against it in patients you think are at risk of TB osteomyelitis.
- Torticollis may be associated with chronic squint, previous trauma (?psychogenic component) and neuroleptic drugs. It can be a sign of an underlying neurological or inflammatory lesion or occurs because of an underlying structural anomaly.
- A history of a heritable disease of connective tissue can often be elicited from the family of a child with structural scoliosis.
- A history of back pain is sometimes elicited from families of children with non-specific back pain. Joint dislocation and multiple soft-tissue musculoskeletal injury (especially overuse) in family members raises the possibility of general hypermobility (either joint hypermobility syndrome or a heritable connective tissue disease, e.g. Marfan syndrome (see Chapter 16).
- There is often a family history of back pain associated with investigation-negative, non-specific spinal pain (more frequently diagnosed in girls than in boys) that is considered to have a psychogenic component.
- The existence, or child's perception, of social disharmony at home or school is likely to be more important in influencing the impact of back pain rather than a cause of it. Nevertheless in children with non-specific spinal pain or fibromyalgia especially, social conflict resulting in stress and anxiety may be very important in generating symptoms.

Examination

It is best, and certainly ultimately more informative, to undertake the examination only when the child is comfortable with the situation, with their modesty and dignity preserved, and with consent to go ahead after a reassurance that the examination will be stopped if it is painful. With younger children there may be 'an examinable moment', usually after the child has gained confidence in the surroundings and with the situation. Observing the young child whilst playing is a considerate way of starting the examination.

Age-related variations in biomechanical development and gait patterns

- Walking whilst holding a hand or furniture develops by 12 months and normally independent walking by 18 months.
- Until 3 years the stance is broad-based in relation to pelvic width, the knee may not fully extend and the ankle may be plantar flexed at foot-strike.
- Climbing stairs is usually done using alternate feet by age of 3 years.
- Tiptoe walking is not abnormal at first but should disappear by 2 years. If this pattern remains consider spasticity, tethered cord, or muscle weakness.
- Flat feet up to age 5 are normal (a consequence of the distribution of fat and paucity of muscle development). Only investigate if symptomatic.
- Leg alignment often concerns parents. Up until 2 years of age it is normal to have genu varum. From 2–5 years mild genu valgum may occur. Angles of >10° or asymmetry may be associated with underlying disease.
- Regression of motor development is a clue to the presence of disease.

Observation

Observe children unclothed to underwear if possible; initially at play then look from behind. Look for weakness, scoliosis, kyphosis, and swellings.

- The main cause of spinal asymmetry will be scoliosis (see Table 2.16).
- Localized soft tissue swelling may denote soft tissue extension of a spinal tumour though an 'apparent' kyphosis associated with scoliosis is usually a result of spinal rotation.
- In children with neck pain look for a short neck (?Klippel–Fiel) or asymmetric scapulae (Sprengel's deformity: a higher, hypoplastic scapula).
- Adolescent kyphosis may be due to Scheuermann's disease or fractures. Unless there has been steroid use, the former is more likely.
- Note any skin markings such as café-au-lait spots, skin indents (lumbar area) and lumbosacral hair. They may be markers of bony abnormality.
- Note any muscular weakness. With truncal weakness (e.g. DM, (see Chapter 13)) the child may have to roll over before getting up from a supine position. Hip girdle weakness may be present in a child unwilling to squat and unable to stand from squatting without exhibiting Gower's sign (unable to stand up from the floor without using hands to push off).

Examine the gait pattern

- Look for asymmetry and a limp.
- Back or leg pain from any cause can give rise to a limp. Also, limp may be the only feature of a serious underlying neurological or bony deformity.
- Asymmetry of shoulder height, transverse posterior skin folds, pelvic tilt, and arm swing may be a clue to spinal pathology.

Spinal examination with the child standing

Examine the whole spine whilst the child is standing. The immature spine is usually far more flexible than an adult's.

- Ask about the presence and site of neck or low back pain during forward flexion, extension, and lateral flexion (and rotation for neck). Experienced examiners should be able to detect significantly limited movements.
- Palpate along the line of (lumbar) spinous processes. An inward step may be caused by spondylolisthesis.
- Palpate any swellings. Lipomata are painless. Soft tissue tumours may be, but are not necessarily, tender and fixed.

Examine the sitting patient

Examine the child who is sitting on the couch, legs hanging over the side.

- This is the best way to elicit pain from posterior vertebral structure pathology in thoracic or lumbar segments (e.g. pars osteoid osteoma, pars fracture). Combine extension and rotation movements. Ask if the pain is worse on one side than the other.

Examine the supine patient

Examine the child or adolescent when supine. Look for leg length discrepancy, lower leg asymmetry, and do a neurological examination.

- Measure and determine actual or apparent leg length discrepancy. True leg length discrepancy is a cause of non-structural scoliosis. Apparent leg length discrepancy/pelvic tilts can occur to compensate for scoliosis caused by spinal lesions.
- Different foot or leg sizes/appearances are a non-specific sign of spinal dysraphism.
- Hip and sacroiliac examination should be done routinely in children with low back pain. Tests for dural irritation and neurological examination are essential (see section on Low back pain and disorders in adults, pp.74–87).
- Though limb pain, weakness and other neurological symptoms occur, the majority of children with intradural tumours have none of these features. A normal examination does not rule out serious pathology.

Examine the prone patient

- Palpate over the spinous processes, interspinous spaces, paracentrally between spinous processes (over facet joints) and in the sacroiliac area.
- Diffuse tenderness may only be a reflection of muscle spasm and its extensive mechanical effect. Where there are isolated areas of tenderness feel for skin warmth, as this may be a site of infection.

Investigations

Radiographs

- Radiographs have a characteristic appearance in certain cases of bone tumour but may also, in some cases, be normal (see Table 2.17).
- A normal bone scan rules out most serious pathology.
- A widened interpedicular distance on an AP film is a sign of meningo-myelocele or spinal dysraphism, also of an intraspinal mass.
- Posterior vertebral scalloping on a lateral radiograph is most obviously seen in lumbar or cervical spines, most prominent in association with lesions occurring in childhood and most commonly due to spinal tumours, neurofibromatosis, osteogenesis imperfecta, Ehlers–Danlos, and Marfan syndrome.
- Spondylolysis/pars fractures may be visible on lateral X-rays but are best characterized by oblique films (see Plate 8). Associated internal disc derangement or radiculopathy is best characterized using MR.
- Appearances of Scheuermann's disease (multiple irregular vertebral endplates, with anterior ring epiphyseal fragmentation and vertebral wedging) are an occasional incidental X-ray finding.
- Radiographs of the neck may show a degree of cervical fusion (Klippel–Feil). Suspect hypermobility in non-affected segments and investigate C1/C2 with MR if there are high cervical pain or myelopathic symptoms.

Table 2.17 Radiographic features of spinal tumours in children (see also Table 20.7)

Tumour type	Notable clinical features and radiological appearances
Osteochondroma	Has the appearance of an exostosis
Osteoid osteoma	Radiographs often normal. Bone scintigraphy will localize lesion and CT sharply define it
Osteoblastoma	Lytic with central ossification on radiograph. Can metastasize
Aneurysmal bone cyst	Lucent lesion with central trabeculae on radiographs. MR important to document soft-tissue expansion
Langerhan's cell histiocytosis (eosinophilic granuloma)	Either solitary, polyostotic, or associated with systemic illness. Lytic lesion can cause solitary vertebral collapse, even collapse of adjacent bones. Used to be called histiocytosis X
Myeloma	Rare in children. Lytic lesions on radiographs. Distribution of lesions can be shown with bone scintigraphy but use as adjunct to radiographs
Ewing's sarcoma	Age 5–20 usually. 'Moth-eaten' destruction of bone on radiograph
Lymphoma	Sclerotic ('ivory') vertebra on film
Osteosarcoma	Mixed lytic/sclerotic appearance on radiographs
Metastases	Most likely are from leukaemia or neuroblastoma
Intra- and extramedullary tumours	Delay in diagnosis common. Up to 50% have abnormal films: widened spinal canal, pedicle erosions, scalloping of vertebral bodies. MR usually characterizes the lesion

- Bone scintigraphy is sensitive to detect spinal bony abnormality and a –ve test rules out most subtle lesions e.g. osteoid osteomas.
- Consider SIJ radiographs and MR in patients with prominent immobility-related low back pain and stiffness (commonly due spondylarthropathy-related conditions).

Investigating scoliosis
- The cause of painful scoliosis must be determined. Consider MR or CT of any localized area of pain. Idiopathic scoliosis is asymptomatic and is a diagnosis of exclusion.
- Mild idiopathic scoliosis (5–10°) can be determined on a posteroanterior thoracolumbar radiograph and is relatively common in the school population (7%). A scoliosis of > 20° occurs in 1 in 500 people and is three to four times more common in girls than boys.
- In 10–20% of those with a trunk inclination of > 5°, the scoliosis progresses at least a further 5°. Most have a non-progressive scoliosis.

Laboratory investigations

Laboratory investigations should be sought if infection, inflammation or malignancy is considered (see section on low back pain and disorders in adults).

The management of various spinal disorders in adults and children is included in Chapter 20.

Pelvic, groin, and thigh pain

Anatomy

Anatomy of the pelvis and hip region

- The bony pelvis consists of two inominate bones (ilium above the acetabulum and ischium below it) that articulate with each other at the anterior symphysis pubis and posteriorly with the sacrum at the SIJs.
- SIJs are initially synovial but become fibrous with age. A few degrees of rotation can be demonstrated in children and young adults.
- Strong ligaments stabilize the posterior pelvis through sacroinominate, lumbo(L5)–sacral, and lumbo(L5)–iliac attachments.
- The symphysis pubis is a cartilagenous joint and normally does not move.
- When standing, weight is transferred through the head of the femur that is stablized in the acetabulum and its surrounding fibrous labrum by strong pericapsular ligaments.
- The ligamentum teres crosses the hip joint and carries blood vessels to the head of the femur in children and young adults. In old age, blood supply is largely via vessels that enter the femoral neck.
- Bursae are associated with gluteus maximus at its insertion: one behind, and separating it from, the greater trochanter; the other in front of the bone separating gluteus maximus from part of the origin of vastus lateralis.
- The ischial bursa separates gluteus maximus from the ischial tuberosity and can become inflamed from frictional injury.

Anatomy of pelvic musculature

- Three groups of muscles move the hip joint: gluteals, flexor muscles, and the adductor group.
- The major gluteal group muscles are:
  - gluteus maximus (L5, S1/2): arises mainly from ilium and sacrum, swathes down posteriolaterally and inserts into the posterior femur (20% of it) but mainly into the lateral tensor fasciae latae. It extends and externally rotates the hip (hamstrings also extend the hip).
  - gluteus medius (L4/5, S1): lies deeper and more lateral. It inserts into the lateral greater trochanter and abducts and internally rotates the hip.
  - piriformis, obdurator internus, and quadratus femoris arise deep in the pelvis and insert into the posterior greater trochanter. All externally rotate the hip.
- The major hip flexor, psoas major (L2/3), is a massive muscle that arises from the lateral part of the vertebrae and intervertebral discs (T12–L5) and lateral processes of the lumbar vertebrae. It runs anteriorly over the iliac rim, across the pelvis, under the inguinal ligament, and inserts into the lesser trochanter. Iliacus (L2–L4) arises from the 'inside' of the iliac blade, passes under the inguinal ligament medially to the lesser trochanter. Both flex but psoas also internally rotates the hip.

- Psoas is enveloped in a fascial sheath. Retroperitoneal or spinal infection which tracks along soft tissue planes sometimes involves the psoas sheath and can cause inflammation in the psoas bursa, which separates the muscle from the hip joint which it overlies.
- All adductor muscles arise from the pubis or ischiopubic rami. Adductor longus and gracilis are the most superficial, arise most medially—from the pubis—and insert into the femoral shaft and pes anserinus ('goose's foot') below the knee, respectively. Adductor magnus (L4/5) is the largest of the deeper adductors and inserts into the length of the medial femoral shaft.
- Adductors stabilize movement about the hip towards the end of the stance phase of the gait. Body weight is transferred onto one leg during this action, thus adductors need to be strong, especially for running.

Functional anatomy of the hip
- With a flexed knee the limit of hip flexion is about 135°.
- Hip extension (at 30°), and internal (at 30–35°) and external (at 45–55°) rotation is limited by strong, pericapsular ligaments.
- Abduction is limited to 45–50° by contact between the greater trochanter and acetabular labrum rim and adduction to 20–30° (leg swung across other) with a fixed pelvis (see Plate 9). These are adult ranges.
- Greater femoral neck anteversion (angulation of neck compared to a line drawn through the femoral condyles in the coronal plane) allows greater internal rotation of the hip (and reduced external rotation). Tibial torsion can compensate but often this and hip anteversion results in a toe-in gait. Femoral neck retroversion (if the angle is posterior to the femoral intercondylar plane) allows greater external rotation of the hip, usually resulting in a toe-out gait (see Fig. 2.21).
- Normally infants have more anteversion than older children or adults (30–40° at age 2 compared with 8–15° at age > 18).

Neuroanatomy
- The femoral nerve is formed from L2–L4 nerve roots and supplies mainly muscles of the quadriceps group and some deeper hip adductors.
- With contributions from L4–S3 roots, nerves from the plexus converge at the inferior border of the piriformis to form the sciatic nerve. This is at a foramen formed by the ilium (above and lateral), sacrum (medial), sacrospinous ligament (below), and sacrotuberous ligament (posteromedial).
- In about 10% of people the sciatic nerve divides before exiting the pelvis. In some a branch exits above the piriformis muscle. Nerve entrapment and trauma from intramuscular injections at this site is recognized (Piriformis syndrome).

Taking a history

Age

Age is a risk factor for some conditions:

- Congenital hip dislocation is common (prevalence 1:500) and more so in girls vs. boys (8:1). It should be considered in toddlers if there is delay in motor milestones or pain on 'weight-bearing'.
- The commonest cause of hip pain in children aged 2–12 years is transient synovitis (unilateral, self-limiting). The differential diagnosis includes Legg–Calvé–Perthes' disease (osteonecrosis of femoral head) and Lyme or post-streptococcal arthritis.
- Legg–Calvé–Perthes' disease (age 3–12 years) is four to five times more common in boys and bilateral in 10–20% of cases.
- Slipped capital epiphysis is rare in children aged <8 and > 16 years. It is associated with obesity and endocrine disorders (4% are hypothyroid).
- Unless there has been previous hip disease (e.g. osteonecrosis, synovitis), trauma, or a long-standing biomechanical abnormality
- (e.g. epiphyseal dysplasia, heritable disease of connective tissue), hip osteoarthritis (OA) is uncommon in adults <55.
- Paget's disease of bone is rare in adults <50.

Distribution and type of bone and soft tissue pain

- All mechanical lesions of the lumbar spine can result in referred pain around the pelvis/thighs. It is often bilateral, localizes poorly, and is aching in nature.
- Lateral pelvic pain is often referred from the lumbosacral spine. If pain localizes well (i.e. patient points) to the greater trochanter, it may be due to trochanteric bursitis, enthesitis, or meralgia parasthetica (see Table 2.18).
- Hip joint pain is felt in the groin, though it can be located deep in the buttock when ischial bursitis and sacroiliac pain should also be considered. It may be referred distally to the anteromedial thigh and knee.
- Groin pain on weight-bearing suggests hip pathology such as synovitis; osteonecrosis or OA but is not specific. Tendonitis of adductor longus, osteitis pubis, a femoral neck stress fracture (4% of all stress fractures), osteoid osteoma, or psoas bursitis can give similar symptoms.
- Bone pathology typically gives unremitting pain. Sleep is often disturbed.
- Pain from deep musculoskeletal pelvic structures is typically poorly localized though can be extremely severe. If the pain appears to be 'catastrophic' consider pelvic bone disease (tumours, infection, Paget's disease, osteomalacia, osteoporotic fracture)(see Chapters 16 and 17), or an unstable pelvis (chronic osteitis pubis with diastasis/laxity of the symphysis pubis and SIJs).
- Enthesitis and osteitis pubis associated with spondylarthropathy (SpA) (see Chapter 8) are probably under-recognized.

Table 2.18 Patterns of pain around the proximal leg and their major causes

Pattern of pain	Causes
Pain in buttock and posterior thighs	Referred pain from: lumbar spine e.g. facet, OA, spondylolisthesis; SIJ inflammation; lower lumbar nerve root irritation; sciatic nerve entrapment (piriformis syndrome)
	Localized pain: ischial bursitis/enthesitis or fracture; coccidynia
	Diffuse muscular pain/stiffness: myositis or PMR
	Paget's or other bone lesion of sacrum
Lateral pelvic pain	Referred from lumbosacral spine
	Trochanteric bursitis/enthesitis
	Gluteus medius tear
	Lateral hip joint pain, e.g. osteophyte
Groin pain	Hip disease, e.g. OA, osteonecrosis, synovitis
	Psoas bursitis
	Adductor tendonitis, osteitis pubis
	Pelvic enthesitis
	Paget's disease (pelvis or femur)
	Femoral neck or pubic ramus fracture
	Hernia
Anterior or medial pain	Referred from: lumbar spine, e.g. facet OA, thigh spondylolisthesis; upper lumbar nerve root; hip joint, femoral neck, psoas bursa
	Myositis, PMR, diabetic amyotrophy
	Meralgia parasthetica (anterolateral)
	Adductor tendonitis, osteitis pubis
	Ischaemia (claudication)
	Lymph nodes

- Aching in the back of the legs after standing is typical of, but not specific for, spondylolisthesis.
- Sacroiliac pain and stiffness radiates to the buttocks and posterior thighs.

Pain in a muscular distribution

- Diffuse pain in the buttocks and thighs occurs in polymyalgia rheumatica (PMR). It is often sudden or subacute in onset, associated with stiffness, and may give similar symptoms to those caused by sacroiliitis but invariably occurs for the first time in a much older age group.
- Pain from autoimmune myositis (see Chapter 13) is unlikely to be confined to pelvic musculature or be unilateral, but should be considered where acute or subacute onset diffuse pelvic girdle/thigh pain accompanies weakness.

Quality and distribution of nerve pain
- Nerve root pain is often clearly defined and sharp. It may be burning in quality and is often accompanied by numbness or parasthesiae. L5 or S1 lesions generally cause pain below the knee though can cause posterior thigh pain. L1–L3 root lesions can cause pain in the anteromedial thigh.
- Pain with parasthesiae on the anterolateral part of the thigh may be due to entrapment of the lateral cutaneous nerve of the thigh under the lateral part of the inguinal ligament (meralgia paraesthetica). Symptoms may be referred to this area with L2 or L3 nerve root lesions as these roots are from where the nerve originates (see Fig. 2.11).
- Diabetics with uncontrolled hyperglycaemia are at risk of amyotrophy. Acute unilateral or bilateral thigh pain with muscle wasting occurs. It should not be misdiagnosed as PMR, in which weakness/wasting does not occur, or autoimmune myositis.
- Soccer players are at risk of adductor tendonitis (often an adductor apophysitis) and osteitis pubis owing to substantial mechanical forces placed on pelvic structures during running and kicking.
- Though hip fractures usually present obviously and acutely, be aware that they can present subacutely with patients still able to walk (particularly stress fractures and in the elderly).

Previous trauma, low back, and musculoskeletal problems
- Previous trauma/disease causing permanent deformity of any lumbosacral or hip joint structure can be considered a risk for further trouble (see Table 2.19).
- Multiparity is a risk for osteitis pubis, sacroiliac, and pelvic pain.
- Trochanteric bursitis may coexist with referred back pain.
- Tears of the gluteus medius can occur at its greater trochanter insertion and give similar symptoms to those caused by bursitis.
- Historically, tailors were at risk of ischial bursitis because of sitting on the floor continually crossing and uncrossing their legs, which causes friction irritation of soft tissues overlying the ischial tuberosity.

Examination

The reader is referred to the sequence of examination for the low back including sacroiliac and lower limb neurological examination (see pp. 80–83). Always consider lower spinal, muscle, or neurological pathology when assessing weakness and pain around the pelvis.

Observation and palpation
For observation and palpation the patient should be supine on a couch:
- Look for leg length discrepancy (hip disease, scoliosis) and a leg resting in external rotation (hip fracture).
- Psoriasis over the knees might be associated with sacroiliitis.

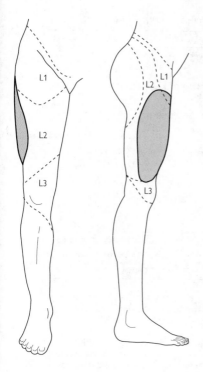

Fig. 2.11 The approximate areas within which sensory changes may be found in lesions of the lateral cutaneous nerve of the thigh (hatched area) and high lumbar radiculopathy (broken line). Shaded area-sensory symptoms distribution from Meralgia Parasthetica.

Table 2.19 Risk factors for painful pelvic or hip lesions

Risk factor	Pelvic/hip pathology
Mechanical abnormality of the low back	Referred pain
	Trochanteric bursitis
Mechanical abnormality of the hip (e.g. Perthes', slipped epiphysis, epiphyseal dysplasia, Paget's)	Hip OA
Corticosteroid use	Osteoporotic fracture
	Osteonecrosis of the femoral head
Autoimmune rheumatic disease (e.g.RA, JIA, AS)	Synovitis hip
	Secondary OA of the hip
	Pyogenic arthritis of the hip
	Osteoporotic fracture
Maternal history of hip fracture; low body mass index; low bone mass; falls	Osteoporotic hip fracture
Multiple pregnancies	Osteitis pubis (± pelvic instability)
Soccer players	Adductor tendonitis/apophysitis
	Osteitis pubis

- Swelling in the groin may be a hernia (?reducible or cough impulse), lipomata (soft/non-tender/diffuse), a saphenous varix, or lymphadenopathy (hard/rubbery and invariably mobile). A hip joint effusion cannot be felt.
- Tenderness over the hip joint in the groin is not specific for joint pathology (the joint is deep, muscles and psoas bursa overlie it).
- If the groin is very tender with slight touch, consider hip fracture or infection. Hyperpathia (and allodynia) is consistent with algodystrophy (see Chapter 18).
- Numbness over the anterolateral thigh suggests meralgia paraesthetica (see Fig. 2.11).
- The adductor longus tendon can be palpated at its insertion at the pubic tubercle and distally along the upper medial thigh. The pubic tubercle is found by palpating slowly and lightly downwards from umbilicus over the bladder until bone is reached.
- Pain from osteitis pubis or adductor apophysitis is often ↑ with abdominal rectus contraction (ask the patient to slowly lift their head and shoulders off the couch keeping your finger on the pubic tubercle).

Hip examination

The patient is supine. Tests generally help to discriminate intra-from extra-articular disease but not causes of intra-articular disease:

- Measure and determine actual or apparent leg length discrepancy: measure from the anterior superior iliac spine to the medial tibial malleolus then, by flexing hips and knees, the site of shortening should become apparent.

- A fixed loss of extension is a sign of intra-articular hip disease. The patient flexes the hip and knee on one side until normal lumbar lordosis flattens out (confirmed by feeling pressure on your hand placed under their lumbar spine during the manoeuvre). If the other hip flexes simultaneously, it suggests hip extension loss on that side (Thomas' test).
- Using the patella or tibial tubercle as pointers, test the rotational hip range in extension by rotating the straightened legs holding the heels.
- Rotational movements are also tested by lifting the leg, flexed 90° at the knee, and swinging the foot out (internal rotation) or in (external rotation). Hip flexion can be tested in this position too (see Plate 9). Patients without intra-articular pathology should have a pain-free range of movement.
- Rotational ranges in hip flexion and extension may differ between left and right in an individual. Also, variations in femoral neck anteversion contribute to variations in rotation range.
- To test hip abduction/adduction, fix the pelvis to avoid pelvic tilt by placing one hand firmly over the iliac crest (see Plate 9). Occasionally, pain at the end of abduction or internal rotation occurs with a bony block (solid 'end-feel'). In an older patient this might suggest impingement of a marginal joint osteophyte.
- Barlow's manoeuvre checks for congenital dislocation of the hips in babies. Flex and adduct the hips exerting an axial force into the posterior 'acetabulum' to demonstrate posterior dislocation.
- Greater retroversion (allowing excessive hip external rotation) usually occurs in cases of slipped femoral epiphysis. External rotation is accentuated when the hip is flexed. The slip (usually inferoposterior) is thought to occur in association with a period of rapid growth.

Muscle activation tests

Specific muscle activation against resistance can be used to elicit pain, but results need to be interpreted cautiously in the context of known hip disease:

- Hip adduction against resistance (sliding their leg inwards towards the other against your hand) reproducing pain is a sensitive test for adductor longus tendonitis but may be positive in osteitis pubis, hip joint lesions, and other soft tissue lesions in the adductor muscles.
- Test psoas by resisted hip flexion in slight internal rotation. Psoas bursitis or infection tracking along the psoas sheath is likely to give intense pain with minimal resistance.
- Hip abduction (sliding the leg outwards against your hand) may be particularly painful in cases of gluteus medius tears but also in trochanteric bursitis or intra-articular pathology.

Palpate posterolateral structures

Ask the patient to lie on their side and palpate the posterolateral structures (see Fig. 2.12):

- Tenderness over the greater trochanter is usually well-localized although it may be anterior or posterolateral to the trochanter and refers a small way down the leg.

- The ischial tuberosity and its overlying bursa lie at the apex of the buttock.
- The soft tissues overlying the point where the sciatic nerve exits the pelvis is found midway between the ischial spine and the greater trochanter. There may be tenderness as a result of soft tissue lesions or trauma causing sciatic nerve entrapment (painful foot drop—piriformis syndrome).
- A tender coccyx (coccidynia) can be palpated in this position. It can also be palpated and the sacrococcygeal joint moved from a bidigital examination, though this requires the index finger to be placed inside the rectum, the thumb outside, the two digits then holding the joint.

Investigations

Radiographs

An AP radiograph of the pelvis is a good initial screening test in patients with pelvic, hip, or thigh pain. AP and lateral lumbar spine films may be warranted.

- The pelvis is a common site of involvement in myeloma, metastatic malignancy, and Paget's disease of bone (see Chapter 16).
- Established, but often not early, sacroiliitis can be ruled out. The main differential diagnoses of the causes of sacroiliitis are: AS, psoriatic or reactive arthritis, enteric arthropathy including Whipple's disease, brucellosis and other infections, hyperparathyroidism and osteitis condensans ilii (sclerosis of the SIJ on the lower iliac side).
- Widening of the symphysis in children may be a sign of congenital disorders of development (e.g. epispadias, achondrogenesis, chondrodysplasias, hypophosphatasia), trauma and hyperparathyroidism (see Chapter 16).
- Widening of the symphysis pubis, osteitis pubis (bone resorption and sclerosis) and osteitis condensans ilii are signs associated with chronic pelvic pain in multiparous women.
- General osteopenia may be reported and is a risk factor for general low bone mass measured by densitometry; however, it is not a sensitive or specific indicator of osteoporosis (e.g. may be osteomalacia or rickets).
- Regional osteoporosis confined to the femur is non-specific but may reflect hip synovitis, infection, or transient osteoporosis of the hip (rare).
- Early synovitis and infection may be demonstrated through subtle radiological signs such as joint space widening and change in soft tissue fat planes.
- A 'frogs' legs' (lateral) view of the hip shows the anterior and posterior femoral head more clearly than an AP view (useful in early osteonecrosis/Perthes', slipped epiphysis).

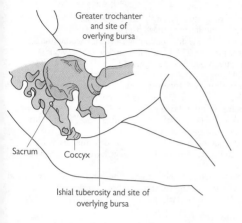

Greater trochanter
and site of
overlying bursa

Sacrum   Coccyx

Ishial tuberosity and site of
overlying bursa

Fig. 2.12 Bony anatomy of the posterior hip and pelvis, showing the position in which lesions around the greater trochanter and ischial bursa can be palpated

- The acetebulae are best visualized on 45° oblique views (acetebular fractures can be missed on a conventional AP view).
- 'Stork' views of the symphysis pubis (standing on one leg) are useful for confirming diastasis of the joint.

Diagnostic ultrasound

- US is a sensitive and simple way of confirming a hip joint effusion. Fluid can be aspirated for culture relatively easily and an assessment of the extent of synovial thickening can be made.
- Tendon damage in the groin area should be identifiable with US alone (guided steroid injection can then be done if necessary) but MR may be needed either to characterize pathology further or rule out joint pathology.

Bone scintigraphy

Bone scintigraphy is a useful screening test though is often nonspecific:

- Characteristic, though non-specific, patterns of bone scan abnormality are recognized in the hip/pelvic area. The following conditions can be recognized: sacroiliitis, bone malignancy, myeloma, Paget's disease, hip fracture, femoral head osteonecrosis (see Plate 10), osteoid osteoma, OA and synovitis of the hip, osteitis pubis/adductor apophysitis (requires special seated 'ring' view), and bursitis/enthesitis at the greater trochanter.
- Bone scintigraphy is a useful investigation in children and adolescents as a screening investigation if radiology is normal and symptoms remain.

CT and MR

- CT/MR of the high lumbar region should be considered to confirm a nerve root lesion causing groin/thigh pain.
- Specific patterns of X-ray attenuation/signal change around the SIJs occur in sacroiliitis with CT/MR, though current and previous inflammation cannot easily be distinguished.
- A suspicion of bony malignancy from radiographs of the pelvis requires further characterization. CT is the technique of choice for characterizing bone lesions around the hip such as femoral neck stress fracture, osteoid osteoma, or other bone tumours. CT may give more information about the lesion (and is valuable in 'guided biopsy') but MR is useful in checking for pelvic visceral lesions.
- MR is the technique of choice if hip infection or osteonecrosis is suspected. In adults, patterns of signal change have been correlated with prognosis.
- During a single examination the pattern of hip synovitis (vascularity and thickness), cartilage loss, and subchondral bone erosion can be documented. This is particularly useful in children with JIA.

Laboratory investigations

- ESR and CRP may be normal in inflammatory SIJ, lumbar vertebral disc, and pelvic enthesis disorders.
- PMR is invariably associated with an acute phase response.
- Myeloma is unlikely if the ESR is normal.
- A high ALP is typically associated with an acute phase response, although association with pelvic pain in the elderly might suggest Paget's disease.
- ANA and RF are unlikely to help diagnostically.
- Major metabolic bone disease such as osteomalacia and hyperparathyroidism is usually excluded by a normal serum calcium and phosphate.

Treatment

Treatment of spinal and neuropathic pain is covered in the section on Low back pain and disorders in adults (pp.74–87).

- Simple and NSAID analgesia may be required for a number of the conditions described above, particularly OA, hip synovitis, and tendon inflammation.
- Physiotherapy and rehabilitation play a vital and early part in management, maintaining mobility, preventing tissue contracture, and restrengthening/stabilizing the lower back, pelvis, and hip.
- Either physiotherapists or podiatrists may help in accurately evaluating back and lower limb biomechanics. Asymmetry and muscular imbalance may be modifiable relatively simply with foot orthotics, for example.
- Steroid injections may be important in the following conditions:
  - meralgia parasthetica
  - osteitis pubis
  - trochanteric bursitis/enthesitis
  - ischial bursitis/enthesitis
  - adductor tendonitis
  - coccydinia

- hip synovitis (under imaging guidance)
- sacroiliitis—in intractable pain and under X-ray or US guidance.
- Injection techniques are covered at the end of this chapter, p.148.

Surgery

- When the hip has been damaged by an inflammatory arthritis or OA the principal surgical intervention is joint replacement. Osteotomy has been mainly superceded by more reliable replacement.
- Surgical synovectomy of the hip is a difficult procedure and opening the hip carries a risk of avascular necrosis. This procedure is very rarely done.
- Excision arthroplasty is only really necessary where infection or poor bone stock make reconstruction unwise. Power is often greatly reduced and even the previously fit young patient will often require two sticks as walking aids.
- In children in particular, it is important to assess spinal and knee disease, especially contractures, before embarking on hip surgery as the 1° cause for flexion deformities or hip damage may be at these levels.

Knee pain

Anatomy of the knee

- The knee extends, flexes and also rotates.
- The main extensor quadriceps consists of four muscle segments—rectus femoris, vastus lateralis, medialis, and intermedius—which converge to form a tendon containing the patella which then inserts into the tibia. Rectus femoris arises from the pelvis and vastus muscles from the upper femur.
- The hamstring muscles (biceps femoris, semitendinosus, semi-membranosus) all arise from the ischial tuberosity and flex the knee. Biceps femoris inserts around the fibular head. The other two muscles insert into the tibia on the medial side and can externally rotate the femur.
- In the knee the femoral condyles articulate within semicircular fibrocartilage menisci on the tibial condyles (see Fig 2.13). Only the peripheral 10–30% of the menisci is vascular and innervated and can potentially repair.
- As the knee approaches full extension the femur internally rotates on the tibia (biceps femoris action) tightening each pair of ligaments relative to each other (see Fig. 2.13). This configuration confers maximum stability.
- As flexion is initiated a small amount of femoral external rotation on the tibia occurs. This 'unlocking' is done by popliteus—a muscle which arises from the posterior surface of the tibia below. It passes up obliquely across the back of the knee and inserts, via a cord-like tendon, into the lateral femoral condyle. The tendon partly lies within the knee joint capsule.
- Grooves on the femoral condyle articular surfaces allow tight congruity with the anterior horns of the menisci when the knee is extended. If full extension—and this optimal articulation configuration—is lost then articular cartilage degeneration invariably follows (important in inflammatory arthritis).
- The cruciate ligaments are the principal joint stabilizers. The anterior cruciate attaches above to the inside of the lateral femoral condyle and below to the tibia in front of the tibial spines though a slip attaches to the anterior horn of the lateral meniscus. Its main role is to control and contain the amount of knee rotation when the joint is flexed.
- The posterior cruciate attaches above to the inside of the medial femoral condyle. Below it attaches in a (posterior) groove between tibial condyles. Its main role is to stabilize the joint by preventing forward displacement of the femur relative to the tibia when the knee is flexed.
- The cruciates are extra-articular and are covered by a layer of vascular synovium. Bleeding usually accompanies disruption.
- The tibial or medial collateral ligament (MCL) has superficial and deep layers (see Fig. 2.14). It stabilizes the knee against valgus stresses mostly during flexion. The superficial MCL overlies, and moves relative to, the deep part and is separated from it by a bursa. The lower part of the superficial MCL is covered by the long adductors, gracilis,

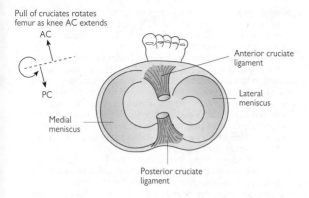

Pull of cruciates rotates
femur as knee AC extends

AC

PC

Anterior cruciate
ligament

Lateral
meniscus

Medial
meniscus

Posterior cruciate
ligament

Fig. 2.13 Axial section of the right knee joint (looking down on the tibial plateau, where the foot is fixed on the floor). The femoral condyles articulate within the menisci. As the knee extends the cruciate ligaments tighten and pull the femoral condyles acting to internally rotate the femur through the last few degrees of extension. The knee therefore 'locks' and is stable when the leg is straight

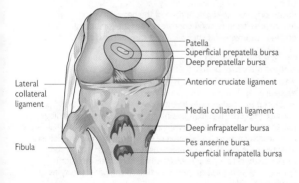

Patella
Superficial prepatella bursa
Deep prepatellar bursa

Lateral
collateral
ligament

Anterior cruciate ligament

Medial collateral ligament

Deep infrapatellar bursa

Pes anserine bursa

Superficial infrapatella bursa

Fibula

Fig. 2.14 Anterior knee structures

semitendinosus, and sartorius, as they merge (as the pes anserinus) before inserting into the tibia. The MCL and pes anserinus are separated by the anserine bursa. Deeper MCL fibres attach to, and stabilize the medial meniscus.

- The fibular or lateral collateral ligament (LCL) joins the lateral femoral condyle to the fibular head and is separated from it by a bursa. It stabilizes the knee on its lateral side. It has no meniscal attachment. A small bursa separates it from the overlapping tendon insertion of biceps femoris.
- The patella is a sesamoid bone that articulates in the femoral condylar groove and makes quadriceps action more efficient. Patella articular facet configuration can vary, though not convincingly consistently with any specific condition; however, congenital bi/tripartite patellae are associated with anterior knee pain.
- The strongest force on the patella is from vastus lateralis (see Fig. 2.15). Mechanical factors which increase the ratio of lateral to medial forces during patella tracking such as a wide pelvis, a more lateral origin of vastus lateralis, femoral neck anteversion, external tibial torsion and a weak vastus medialis are risk factors for patella maltracking and anterior knee pain.
- There are bursae (see Fig. 2.14) between the quadriceps tendon and the femur (suprapatellar), the patellar tendon and tibial tubercle (deep infrapatellar), and overlying the patella (prepatellar) and patellar tendon insertion (superficial infrapatellar). The suprapatellar bursa communicates with the knee joint and large joint effusions invariably fill it.
- Posteriorly, bursae separate each of the heads of gastrocnemius (which arise from femoral condyles) from the joint capsule. The bursae communicate with the knee joint and can fill from joint effusions.

Taking a history
Ask about the site of pain
Try to establish whether pain is from articular, soft tissue, or anterior knee structures. Is it referred pain?

- Bursa, tendon, and most ligament lesions cause well-localized pain.
- Localized tibiofemoral joint line pain suggests meniscal pathology.
- Localized medial knee pain has a number of possible causes: MCL tear or chronic inflammation (calcification of MCL origin termed the Pellegrini–Stieda phenomenon), medial meniscus tear, meniscal cyst, anserine tendonitis, bursitis, or enthesitis (?semimembranosus insertion).
- Enthesitis of structures at their insertion to the patella margins can result in considerable pain.
- Overuse in runners and cyclists can cause localized inflammation and pain of the iliotibial band (ITB) or its underlying bursa over the lateral femoral condyle (as the band moves across the bone as the knee flexes).
- Anterior pain in children, adolescents, and young adults invariably suggests an underlying mechanical abnormality. In older adults the commonest cause is patellofemoral OA (see Table 2.20).
- Anterior knee pain may be referred from the hip or L3 nerve root. Hip pain is an aching pain, root pain is sharp often with parasthesiae.

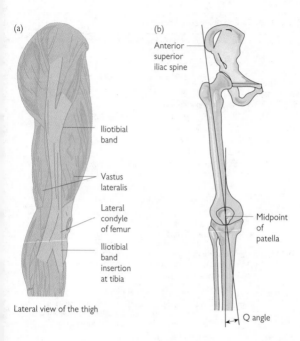

(a)

Iliotibial
band

Vastus
lateralis

Lateral
condyle
of femur

Iliotibial
band
insertion
at tibia

Lateral view of the thigh

(b)

Anterior
superior
iliac spine

Midpoint
of
patella

Q angle

Fig. 2.15 (a) The iliotibial band. (b) The patella Q angle (normal values—men 10°, women 15°)

- Posterior knee pain associated with 'a lump' is often due to synovitis in the posterior knee compartment with popliteal cyst formation (Baker's cyst).

Ask about injury

Knee injuries are common, the most significant is anterior cruciate injury. Ask about injury and whether the knee feels unstable or 'gives way'.

- Anterior cruciate injuries are invariably associated with a haemarthrosis, thus a painful effusion will have occurred immediately. Meniscus tears can cause immediate pain but synovitis and swelling are delayed for about 6 h.
- Patients may volunteer that the knee 'keeps going out'. This feeling may be the pivot shift phenomenon caused by reduced anterior cruciate stability against a valgus stress as the knee is flexing.
- Anterior cruciate and MCL injuries often coexist (they are attached). Ask about medial knee pain originally and subsequently.

Table 2.20 Causes of anterior knee pain

Commonly in adults	Patellofemoral OA (look for mechanical factors and generalized OA)
	Referred hip pain, e.g. hip OA
	Referred pain from L3 nerve root irritation
Specific to children and adolescents	Referred pain from the hip, e.g. slipped femoral epiphysis
	Bi-/tripartite patella
	Synovial plicae (synovial shelf clicking over femoral condyle on knee flexion)
	Recurrent patellar dislocation (tissue laxity, patella alta, trauma)
	Osteochondritis at patellar lower pole—overuse injury in jumping sports*
	Osteochondritis of tibial tubercle (Osgood–Schlatter's)
	Non-specific ('chondromalacia patellae')
Causes at any age	Mechanical factors (?patellar maltracking): wide pelvis, femoral anteversion, external tibial torsion; specific strengthening of lateral structures, e.g. iliotibial band syndrome; weakness or injury of vastus medialis or medial knee structures; tissue laxity, e.g. benign joint hypermobility syndrome
	Osteochondritis dissecans of patella (average age 18)
	Enthesitis at patellar margins (may be part of SpA)
	Bursitis (prepatellar, superficial/deep infrapatellar): gout (very rare in children unless inherited metabolic deficiency); autoimmune rheumatic disease; infection
	Tear/cyst of anterior meniscal horn
	Patellar fracture
	Fat pad syndrome (recurrent retropatella tendon pain with swelling)

*Sinding–Larsen–Johansson disease.

Ask about knee locking

Knee locking is a mechanical effect of disruption of normal articulation by 'loose bodies'.

- Suspect meniscus damage in the middle aged or if the patient plays a lot of sport. A meniscus tear is the commonest cause of the knee locking.
- In adolescents, locking may be due to a tear in a discoid meniscus (>98% lateral). The morphologically abnormal discs are prone to degeneration.
- Chondral fragments (from osteochondritis dissecans lesions) can cause locking; the condition is commonest in the 5–20 year age group (boys > girls).
- Synovial chondromatosis is a rare cause.
- Some patients with anterior knee pain describe the knee locking or giving way. This is due to reflex quadriceps inhibition rather than true instability.

Ask about the initial onset of pain
- Acute pain is usual with injuries of cruciates and vertical meniscal tears.
- Acute onset pain without trauma (but always with swelling) suggests infection, crystal arthritis, or spontaneous haemarthrosis.
- In the very elderly, traumatic lesions may be missed, as presentation is not always so striking, e.g. intra-articular fracture with haemarthrosis.
- An insidious onset of pain is usual in cleavage tears of menisci (horizontal tears), which occur typically in adults where the disc is degenerate, in adolescents with discoid menisci and in early ostochondritis dissecans.

Ask about the pattern and type of pain
- Pain from synovitis is often associated with stiffness and is often worse after a period of immobility. Almost without exception knee synovitis can occur in all forms of arthritis.
- Pain from subchondral damage is almost always worse on weight-bearing, e.g. OA, but this association is not specific.
- Pain on kneeling/squatting is characteristic of anterior knee pain.
- Burning pain may be neurogenic, e.g. L3 nerve root or algodystrophy pain.
- Florid descriptors of pain are often used in algodystrophy.

Past medical, family, occupational, and leisure history
- Knee synovitis and patellar enthesitis occur in adult and juvenile enthesitis-related arthritis. Ask about previous uveitis, low back pain, urethral discharge, sexually transmitted disease, dysentery, and psoriasis.
- Gout (see Chapter 15) is not uncommon around the knee. Ask about gout risk factors and whether the patient has ever had first MTPJ pain (70% of gout sufferers).
- There may be a family history of generalized OA (see Chapter 6), a hereditary disease of connective tissue or hypermobility in young adults with OA.
- Prepatellar bursitis classically occurred in housemaids! Friction caused by repeated kneeling (occupational) can cause it.
- Sports injuries are common. Anterior cruciate injury occurs character-istically in rugby. Meniscal injuries are common in soccer. Jumping events (e.g. high jump, basketball) can lead to patellar tendon apophysitis. Cycling is associated with anterior knee pain. MCL and meniscal injuries are common in skiing and weight-bearing activities where rotation and change of direction are frequent. Cycling and running are associated with ITB/bursa pain and inflammation.

Examination
From front and behind, observe the patient standing
- Look for mechanical abnormalities that might be associated with knee lesions: patella asymmetry, prominent tibial tubercles from previous Osgood–Schlatter's (anterior knee pain), flat feet, and hypermobility (patella dislocation, hyperextension of >10°).

- Check for mechanical abnormalities which might suggest specific pathology: genu varum (bowed leg, typical appearance with primarily medial compartment OA), obvious suprapatellar knee swelling (synovitis), psoriasis (associated synovitis or enthesitis).
- Marked genu varum occurs in the rare Blount's disease (developmental abnormality of the medial tibial physis typically in Afro-Caribbean boys).

Examination of the sitting patient

Ask the patient to sit on the couch with legs hanging, knees bent. Patellar tracking and pain from medial meniscus damage can be assessed. An alternative approach is with the patient supine. Observe any muscle wasting. Palpate anterior, medial, and lateral structures.

- In patients with anterior knee pain look for symmetrical patellar alignment.
- Observe active knee extension. Patellar movement should be smooth, pain-free, and symmetrical.
- Passively externally rotate each lower leg to its extreme. This is a reasonably sensitive test for conditions of the medial knee compartment (e.g. meniscus tear) and medial knee structures. Discomfort will be felt. If the MCL is totally deficient an abnormally increased range of external rotation may occur.
- Quadriceps wasting (accentuated depression in muscle just above the patella) occurs with disuse after injuries and in chronic arthropathies.
- Sites of bursae, patellar tendon, and ligament insertions should be palpated in patients with localized pain (see Fig. 2.16).
- Tibiofemoral joint line tenderness is likely to be due to either meniscus pathology or marginal osteophytes. Osteophytes give bony swelling.
- Anterior pain from patellofemoral joint disorders may be elicited by gentle pressure down on the patella. Mobilizing the patella sideways will give an impression of tissue laxity (possible underlying hypermobility).
- Factors that predispose to patellofemoral pain syndrome include: high or lateral patella, weak vastus medialis, excessive pronation, weak ankle dorsiflexors, tight hamstrings, reduced movement at the ankle, and a wide Q-angle. The Q-angle is formed between a line from the anterior superior iliac spine to the centre of the patella, and a line extended upwards from the tibial tubercle through the centre of the patella. The larger the angle the greater the lateral tensile pull on the patella (see Fig. 2.15).
- Localized tenderness of the femoral condyle is often the only sign of osteochondritis dissecans in adolescents. The commonest site is on the inside of the medial femoral condyle (75%).

Examine for joint synovitis (synovial inflammation giving synovial thickening and/or tenderness) and an effusion

- The joint may be warm. Chronic synovitis does not always result in a warm joint but infection, crystal arthritis, and haemarthrosis usually do.
- Gross synovitis can produce obvious effusions and/or synovial thickening most easily felt around the patellar edges.
- Effusions may be confirmed by the patellar tap test (see Plate 11).

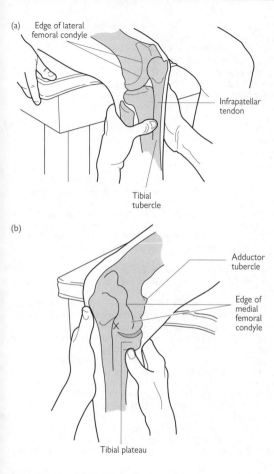

Fig. 2.16 Position of the knee for palpation of most of its structures. Palpating for enthesitis at the patellar tendon insertion (a) Palpation over the insertion of semimembranosus and pes anserinus under the tibial plateau (b) The site of the majority of osteochondritis lesions in the knee is shown by the 'X'

- Small effusions can be detected by eliciting the 'bulge sign'. Fluid in the medial compartment is swept firmly upward and laterally into the suprapatellar pouch. Firm pressure on the lateral side of the joint may then push fluid back into the medial compartment producing a bulge.
- Thickened synovium can be detected by experienced examiners in the absence of a detectable effusion. It is not always tender.
- Posterior compartment synovial thickening and popliteal cysts can be felt by wrapping the fingers around under the knee when it is slightly flexed.
- In contrast to adults, popliteal cysts in children are not usually associated with intra-articular pathology. Investigation is not always necessary.

Test the knee for stability

- There are many tests for instability: instability may be straight or rotatory and can be graded according to consensus criteria (consult orthopaedics texts).
- The Lachmann test (see Fig. 2.17) is arguably the most sensitive test for eliciting anterior cruciate disruption: hold the knee flexed between 20–30°, grasped above and below the joint. Attempt to move the tibia forwards and backwards on the femur. Ask about pain and feel for laxity or a 'clunk'.
- The anterior draw test is not as sensitive as the Lachmann test for detecting partial anterior cruciate tears but is easier to do. The patient lies flat, hip flexed, the knee flexed at 90°, with the foot flat on the couch. Fix the foot by gently sitting on it and pull the top of the lower leg forwards in the line of the thigh. Ask about pain and feel for laxity.
- The posterior draw test identifies posterior cruciate disruption: with the knee flexed to 90°, press the top of the lower leg backwards in the line of the thigh, ask about pain and feel for laxity.
- Test medial stability at 0° and 30° of flexion (MCL stabilizes maximally at 30°) by holding the upper leg still and applying a valgus force to the tibia. Laxity associated with widening of the tibiofemoral joint (with or without pain) is a positive test and suggests MCL deficiency.
- Lateral (LCL and ITB) stability is similarly tested, though using a varus force on the lower leg.
- MCL tears can accompany anterior cruciate injuries and deep lesions are associated with simultaneous tears of the medial meniscus. Such complex pathology can make specific examination manoeuvres difficult to interpret.

Test for meniscus damage

- McMurray's test (see Fig. 2.18). Flex the knee, internally rotate the lower leg, then extend the joint. Repeat with the lower leg externally rotated. The fingers (over the joint line) may feel a 'clunk' as a femoral condyle passes over a torn meniscus. It is often +ve (21–65% of cases) when surgery subsequently reveals no tear.
- Ask the patient to turn over. Lying initially on their side allows you to do Ober's test to detect lateral soft tissue injury. When prone, look and palpate for swelling in the popliteal fossa and proximal calf (low lying popliteal cyst).

Anterior draw test

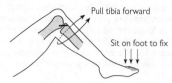

Pull tibia forward

Sit on foot to fix

Lachmann test

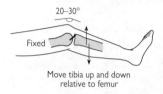

20–30°

Fixed

Move tibia up and down
relative to femur

Fig. 2.17 Dynamic tests of anterior cruciate function. Patients should be relaxed lying supine on a couch. Excessive laxity is the most important sign

McMurray's test

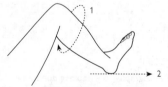

1

2

Action:	Hold the knee and the heel.
	Internally rotate the lower leg (1) then extend it (2)
Positive test:	(Palpable) clunk at joint line

Fig. 2.18 Dynamic test designed to elicit signs of meniscus damage. 'Clunks', intra-articular pain, and coarse crepitus may indicate damage. The test is not specific and is open to misinterpretation

- Inflammation of the bursa underlying the ITB may result in tenderness over the lateral femoral condyle. The ITB may be tight. This is demonstrated using Ober's test. The patient lies on their side with the lower (non-affected) leg flexed at the hip. The upper (painful) knee is flexed to 90° and the thigh is extended and adducted. The test is +ve if, when the examiner's hand is removed, the hip does not drop down (further stretching the ITB). Leg length inequality and foot over-pronation may be causative factors.
- Detecting specific structures in the posterior fossa is often difficult because of the lack of bony landmarks and overlapping soft tissue structures. Synovial cysts may form under pressure and are often hard and tender. Diffuse thickening suggests joint synovitis.

Investigations

Radiographs

AP and lateral weight-bearing radiographs are suitable screening views if the diagnosis is unclear after clinical assessment.

- Early synovitis may only be evident from the presence of an effusion, periarticular osteopenia, or soft tissue swelling. Patterns of bone damage in chronic arthropathies may be recognized.
- Signs of joint infection, which may not necessarily present acutely, are patchy bone osteolysis and irregular loss of bone cortex. Osteonecrosis is uncommon in the knee although it occurs in sickle cell anaemia.
- Loss of joint space, angulation deformity, osteophytes, subchondral bone sclerosis, and bone cysts are hallmark features of OA.
- In adults, linear or vague intra-articular calcification suggests chondrocalcinosis (associated with calcium pyrophosphate dihydrate (CPPD) arthritis). Gross 'thumbprint' calcification is typical of synovial chondromatosis (mainly in children).
- In children check for an osteochondral fragment (e.g. osteochondritis dissecans), normal epiphyses, epiphyseal plates and metaphyses, normal patella shape, and osteochondritis at the tibial tubercle (see Table 2.21).

Specialized radiographic views: tomographic views; 'skyline' (axial with knee bent) view; or lateral view taken with at least 30° of flexion

- Tomography is useful for clarifying non-peripheral osteochondral defects.
- Skyline views demonstrate anomalous patellar facet configuration and can reveal patellofemoral incongruity though multiple views may be needed. Subchondral patellar pathology is seen more clearly than on lateral views.
- Patella alta is most reliably seen on a lateral view with 30° flexion.

Further imaging

Further imaging depends on differential diagnosis and a discussion with your radiologist:

- Periarticular soft tissue lesions can be characterized with MR, though with superficial lesions adequate information needed for further management may be obtainable with ultrasound alone.

Table 2.21 Interpretation of radiographic knee abnormalities in children

Radiographic abnormality	Possible conditions (most commonly)
Intra-articular calcific fragment	Osteochondritis dissecans, traumatic avulsion, synovial tumours, or chondro-matosis (rare)
Epiphyseal defect/abnormality	JIA, sepsis, avulsion injury, bone dysplasias, rickets, haemophilia, hypothyroidism
Transverse radiolucent metaphyseal band or lysis	Leukaemia, lymphoma, neuroblastoma metastases, infections (neonates), osteogenesis imperfecta, idiopathic juvenile osteoporosis, Cushing's disease
Joint space narrowing	JIA, sepsis, PVNS, haemophilia
Diffuse low bone density	Rickets, OI, osteoporosis, mucopolysaccharidosis
Periosteal reaction	Fracture, sepsis, infarction, tumours matosis (rare)

- Patterns of meniscus damage are recognized on MR, give an indication of prognosis, and aid the surgeon's decision to proceed to arthroscopy.
- MR is essential if there is likely to be a combination of lesions, e.g. anterior cruciate, MCL, and medial meniscus lesions.
- In children, both US and MR will confirm synovitis.
- MR is more sensitive in identifying joint erosions in RA compared than are radiographs or US.
- The place of CT or MR in investigating radiographically detected bone tumours depends on the likely nature of the lesion.

Aspiration of joint and periarticular fluid collections

⚠ Early aspiration is essential if infection is suspected.

- The knee is a common site of monoarthritis. The principles behind management apply to all cases of single joint pathology.
- Send joint fluid for microscopy and culture of gonococcus in adolescents and young adults, and TB as well as routine bacterial pathogens (see Chapters 17 and 21).
- In adults, the usual differential diagnosis of sepsis of knee structures is gout, so fluid should be examined by polarized light microscopy for urate crystals.
- Blood-stained fluid either suggests a traumatic tap or chondrocalcino-sis. Frank blood suggests haemarthrosis, the major causes of which are cruciate tear, bleeding diathesis, intra-articular fracture, and pigmented villonodular synovitis (PVNS).
- Bursa fluid may be more successfully detected and aspirated using US guidance.

Laboratory investigations

These should be directed towards suspected underlying disease:

- FBC/CBC, acute phase response (ESR, CRP).
- Blood urea, electrolytes, creatinine, and urate.
- Blood calcium, phosphate, albumin, ALP, 25-OH vit D (± PTH) to screen for metabolic bone disease.
- Autoantibodies: rheumatoid factor (RF), antinuclear (ANA), and extractable nuclear antibodies (ENAs) to characterize an autoimmune process where synovitis is chronic.
- Serum angiotensin converting enzyme (sACE) for sarcoid.
- IgM *Borrelia burgdorferi* serology for acute arthropathy in Lyme disease, streptococcal antibodies for reactive strep. arthritis.

Treatment

- In general most soft tissue lesions will settle with rest and NSAIDs.
- Anterior knee pain may respond well to isometric exercises, adjustments to foot alignment, e.g. sensible shoes and foot orthoses (support insoles) and hamstring stretching exercises.
- The acute swollen knee requires aspiration, rest for 24 h and gentle mobilization. If infection is considered, broad-spectrum antibiotics against staphylococcal and streptococcal agents should be started immediately pending results of cultures. In infection, intra-articular antibiotics and steroids should be avoided. The patient should not bear weight on an acutely infected joint (see Chapter 21).
- Acute and chronic inflammation can lead to joint destruction and instability. If RA, treat early (see Chapter 5).
- Physiotherapy and splinting play an important role in maintaining function and preventing contractures etc.

Address biomechanical factors

Physiotherapy input may be helpful in cases of anterior knee pain. Success from McConnell (patellar) taping is more likely in nonpatellofemoral OA-related anterior knee pain.

- Quadriceps strengthening exercises can be reviewed and reinforced by physiotherapists in cases of knee OA.
- Knee pain, particularly anterior pain, may be linked to foot abnormalities, e.g. overpronation, and hip alignment (see Q-angle, above). Specific muscle strengthening exercises, foot orthotics, and knee braces should be considered.

Local steroid injection

Local steroid injections can be helpful in the following situations:

- Acute flare of non-infective inflammatory disease:
  - OA (especially where CPPD is present—mild OA may also respond to hyaluronate injections
  - autoimmune arthritis, e.g. RA, SpA
  - intra-articular gout
  - SpA, etc.
- Bursitis (may be gout):
  - pre- and infrapatella (superficial and deep) bursa (the latter may require US guidance)
  - anserine.

- Baker's cyst (note: the knee joint is injected at the site of the 1° pathology assuming there is intra-articular communication between joint and cyst. Direct popliteal cyst injection should be under US guidance only).
- Enthesopathy, e.g. semimembranosus insertion.
- Trauma, e.g. pain over medial collateral ligament insertion.
- Other soft-tissue: ITB syndrome.

The reader is referred to p.148 for steroid injection techniques and to part 2 chapters for specific diseases.

Joint injection therapies

- Needle arthrocentesis with saline irrigation may be helpful in treating knee OA.
- Radiation synovectomy using yttrium-90 (Y-90) colloid or dysprosium-165 ferric hydroxymacroaggregates given before there is evidence of advanced chondral loss are useful adjuncts in managing inflammatory arthritis. Long-acting steroid should be co-injected.
- Y-90 has been shown to be effective in CPPD and, in uncontrolled series, in haemophilic arthritis.
- There is anecdotal evidence for the efficacy of intra-articular osmic acid injection (chemical synonectomy) in inflammatory arthritis. It may be preferred to Y-90 in juvenile idiopathic arthritis given the risks of using radiation in children.

Note: all intra-articular injection therapies are more effective when patients' knees are immobilized (bed rest or strong splint) for 48 h following the procedure.

Drugs

- NSAIDs will invariably be helpful in cases of inflammatory and infective arthritis.
- Colchicine 0.5 mg up to 2–3-hourly is often useful in relieving pain from crystal arthritis in patients intolerant of NSAIDs.
- In randomized trials, paracetamol is as effective as NSAIDs.
- Glucosamine has been shown to have an analgesic effect and improves function in OA. It may slow the rate of cartilage loss.

See part 2 chapters for specific treatment of chronic autoimmune arthritides.

Surgery

- Arthroscopy is often used as a diagnostic tool in cases of undiagnosed monoarthritis and to confirm and trim cartilage tears. Synovium and synovial lesions (e.g. PVNS, synovial chondromatosis) can be biopsied or excised (synovectomy) and the joint can be irrigated.
- In appropriate cases joint replacement can be remarkably successful and is an important option to consider in OA and inflammatory arthritis where pain is severe and present at rest, and when mobility is substantially restricted.
- Arthrodesis is rarely indicated.
- Unicondylar osteotomy can aid realignment of the tibiofemoral joint, e.g. in metabolic bone disease such as Paget's disease.

Other

- In OA, capsaicin cream applied three or four times daily to painful superficial structures, e.g. patellar margins or marginal tibiofemoral joint pain, can ease symptoms. Response may not occur for 6–8 weeks.
- There is anecdotal evidence for external beam radiotherapy in treating inflammatory lesions, e.g. enthesitis. In appropriate patients the relative risks are negligible (e.g. the elderly and those at high risk from systemic medications).

Lower leg and foot disorders (adults)

Anatomy

Anatomy of bones and joints

- The leg absorbs six times the body weight during weight-bearing. Strong ligaments secure the ankle (formed by tibia above/medially and fibular malleolus laterally) and talocalcaneal (subtalar) joints and bones of the midfoot (see Fig. 2.19).
- Anomalous ossicles in the foot are common. Some are associated with specific pathology. There are many potential sites, though the sesamoids in flexor hallucis brevis (FHB) are invariable.
- The foot is an optimal mechanical device to support body weight when walking or running over flat, inclined, and uneven types of terrain. The configuration of, and synchronous movements between, bones at synovial articulations allows dorsal flexion (foot pulled up), plantar flexion (to walk on toes), inversion (foot tips in), eversion (foot tips out), and small degrees of adduction and abduction. Midfoot movements allow pronation and supination.
- The normal ankle joint range is about 25° of dorsal flexion and 50° of plantar flexion from neutral (foot 90° to leg). The range of subtalar inversion–eversion is normally 10–15°.

Anatomy of the long muscles and tendons

- In the lower leg a strong fascia connects the tibia and fibula. Lower leg muscles primarily move the foot. They are separated into compartments by fasciae and are prone to pressure effects.
- The foot dorsal flexors—tibialis anterior, extensor digitorum longus (EDL), extensor hallucis longus (EHL) and peroneus tertius—lie adjacent to the anteromedial side of the tibia. Their tendons pass in front of the ankle in synovial sheaths held down by strong retinaculae (see Fig. 2.20). Tibialis anterior, the bulkiest, inserts into the medial midfoot (medial cuneiform).
- In the posterior lower leg gastrocnemius (and plantaris), which arises from the femur, plantar flexes the foot by levering up the back of the calcaneum. Soleus, which arises in the lower leg, merges with them in the Achilles' tendon. The tendon has a deep and superficial bursa at its insertion site.
- Plantar flexion is assisted weakly by long muscles, which arise in the lower leg, pass behind the medial malleolus in synovial sheaths (see Fig. 2.20), and insert into the sole. They mostly invert the foot. Tibialis posterior, the most bulky, inserts into the plantar surface of the navicular.
- Peroneus longus and brevis arise from the fibular side of the leg and pass around the lateral malleolus in a common synovial sheath held by a retinaculum. Longus passes into the sole and inserts into the medial cuneiform. Brevis inserts into the fifth metatarsal base. Both evert the foot.
- The tibial nerve and artery follow the course of the medial tendons under the flexor retinaculum (see Fig. 2.20).

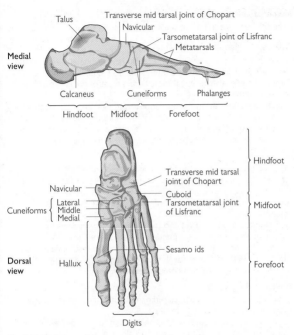

Fig. 2.19 The bones of the foot

Anatomy of intrinsic foot structure

- Intrinsic foot structures have been greatly modified during evolution to combine provision of a sprung platform for support and a rigid lever for thrusting body weight forward when walking.
- In the sole of the foot, muscles are aligned longitudinally in four layers. The deepest layers include phalangeal interossei in the forefeet, tibialis posterior, peroneus longus, adductor hallucis, and FHB—which has two insertions into the proximal great toe phalanx, each containing a sesamoid.
- The superficial layers include flexor digitorum longus (FDL), which inserts into the lateral four distal phalanges, the phalangeal lumbricals, flexor digitorum brevis, and abductor hallucis. The latter two muscles arise from the plantar surface of the calcaneum deep to the plantar fascia.
- Flexor tendons merge with the deeper part of the plantar fascia, a swath of tissue that extends from os calcis to the metatarsal area.
- Longitudinal muscles, ligaments, and fascia contribute to stabilize the foot with a longitudinal arch—its apex at the talus but also with some effect laterally. The foot arches transversely—its apex at medial cuneiform level.

Neuroanatomy

- The sciatic nerve splits into tibial and common peroneal nerves above the knee. The common peroneal is prone to pressure neuropathy as it runs superficially around the fibular head. The nerve then divides. A deep branch runs distally with EDL under the extensor retinaculum to the foot. It supplies tibialis anterior, EHL, and EDL. A superficial branch supplies the peroneal muscles and most of the skin over the dorsum of the foot.
- The tibial nerve runs in the posterior lower leg compartment supplying gastrocnemius and soleus. It then passes under the medial flexor retinaculum dividing into medial and lateral plantar nerves, which supply the intrinsic plantar muscles of the foot and skin of the sole.

Functional anatomy

- In a normal gait pattern the foot is dorsiflexed and invertors/evertors stabilize the hindfoot for heel strike. As weight is transferred forwards the foot plantar flexes and pronates, the great toe extends (optimally between 65 and 75°), and push off occurs through the medial side of the forefoot.
- All metatarsals bear weight and can suffer weight-bearing injury.
- Ligamentous attachments around the hindfoot are strong. A fall on a pronated inverted foot without direct trauma can result in a fracture of the distal fibula. This is probably a consequence of the relative strength of the talofibular ligaments compared with bone.

Developmental factors

- Developmental characteristics often imply that different age groups are prone to a different spectrum of conditions.
- Due to ligamentous laxity, when babies begin to walk the midfoot is flat to the floor. A longitudinal arch usually develops by 5 years.
- During growth, tendon insertions (apophyses) are often weaker than the tendons themselves. Traction strain on tendons can lead to apophysitis (osteochondritis). This is a common pattern of injury in the foot in active older children.

Conditions of the lower leg

- Patients with lower leg conditions may present with pain or deformity alone. In children, deformity may typically be due to spinal dysraphism (from birth), rickets (acquired age 1 year plus), or osteogenesis imperfecta (see Chapter 16).
- Pains in the calf may be due to local soft tissue or muscle conditions but in adults are commonly due to referred lumbosacral pain. These pains are often described by patients as 'cramps'—suggesting a muscle problem at first. A detailed history may suggest nerve root pathology.

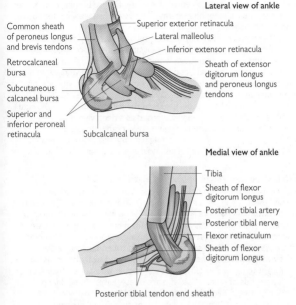

Lateral view of ankle

Common sheath of peroneus longus and brevis tendons

Retrocalcaneal bursa

Subcutaneous calcaneal bursa

Superior and inferior peroneal retinacula

Subcalcaneal bursa

Superior exterior retinacula

Lateral malleolus

Inferior extensor retinacula

Sheath of extensor digitorum longus and peroneus longus tendons

Medial view of ankle

Tibia

Sheath of flexor digitorum longus

Posterior tibial artery

Posterior tibial nerve

Flexor retinaculum

Sheath of flexor digitorum longus

Posterior tibial tendon end sheath

Fig. 2.20 Tendons, retinaculae, and bursae of the hindfoot

- Imbalance of muscles in the foot can lead to ↑ tension at tendon and fascial insertions in the calf and shin, resulting in 'shin splints'. Shin splints usually present after activity and are relieved by rest. Conditions to consider include:
  - stress fractures of the tibia of fibula
  - tibialis posterior fasciitis—often associated with a flat, pronated foot
  - compartment syndrome (soft tissue and vascular swelling)
  - popliteal artery stenosis
  - referred nerve pain (spinal claudication)
  - peripheral vascular disease (intermittent claudication).

Taking a history
Ask about site and quality of pain in the lower leg
- Localized anterior pain occurs in bony lesions of the anterior tibia, e.g. stress fractures, periositis etc. (see 'shin splints' above).

- Burning pain suggests a neurogenic cause. Diffuse burning pain may be caused by peripheral neuropathy, algodystrophy (see Chapter 18), or erythromelalgia.
- Most commonly occurring in the elderly, bilateral leg pain with 'heaviness' or 'stiffness' limiting walking distance is typical of lumbosacral canal stenosis. An alternative would be vascular claudication where often pain is more overt, and critical ischaemia can give night pain eased by hanging the legs over the side of the bed (gravity effects).
- Simultaneous knee problems may be relevant. Escape of synovial fluid from the knee into the soft tissues of the calf can present with acute pain and swelling and be misdiagnosed as a deep vein thrombosis. Often a history of preceding joint effusion can be elicited.
- Low-lying synovial cysts connecting with the knee can cause calf pain (with or without swelling). This invariably occurs only with chronic synovitis.

Establish possible causes of hindfoot pain (Table 2.22)

- Establishing the cause of hindfoot pain from the history alone is difficult. There are important clues, mainly from patterns of injury/overuse.
- Posterior heel pain has a few causes. Often clinically indistinguishable from Achilles tendonitis or retrocalcaneal bursitis, enthesitis is usually associated with SpA (see Chapter 8). An os trigonum may become damaged especially in soccer players and ballerinas (see below).
- The origin of plantar heel pain is varied. Mechanical plantar fasciitis is thought to occur more frequently in people who are on their feet for long periods of time, those who are obese, have thin heel fat pads, or poor footwear. Symptoms of arthritis and enthesopathy elsewhere, low back pain (sacroiliitis), eye inflammation (iritis), psoriasis, or previous gut or 'urethral' infection, might suggest a link of 1° inflammatory plantar fasciitis with SpA.
- Less common causes of plantar heel pain include fracture through a calcaneal spur and lateral plantar nerve entrapment between the fascia of abductor hallucis and quadratus plantae muscles (causing pain/parasthesiae on the lateral side of the sole).
- In the elderly and postmenopausal women calcaneal stress fractures are a recognized feature of osteoporosis (see Chapter 16) and can present with heel pain.
- Ankle and talocalcaneal synovitis, OA, ankle osteochondritis dissecans, and tendonitis around the hindfoot may be difficult to distinguish from the history alone. Synovitis or an effusion often accompanies OA of these joints.

Establish possible causes of midfoot and first MTP pain

- Gout (see Chapter 15), OA (see Chapter 6), enthesitis, and referred L5 nerve root pain are the likeliest diagnoses of midfoot and first MTP pain.
- Any joint may potentially become involved in the major chronic arthropathies.

Table 2.22 Common conditions causing localized foot pain in children, adolescents, and adults

Site of pain	Common lesions
Ankle region	Ankle or talocalcaneal joint: synovitis (e.g. gout), OA. L4/L5 root pain
Posterior heel	Achilles tendonitis. Retrocalcaneal bursitis. Achilles enthesitis. Osteonecrosis of os trigonum
Medial side of heel	As for ankle region. Calcaneal fracture. Tibialis posterior tendonitis. Plantar fasciitis.
Lateral side of heel	As for ankle region. Calcaneal fracture. Peroneal tendonitis. Fifth metatarsal base fracture*
Underneath heel	Plantar fasciitis. Calcaneal fracture. Infracalcaneal bursitis. Lateral plantar nerve entrapment
Top of foot	Midfoot joint synovitis (e.g. gout), OA. Navicular osteochondritis. Enthesitis. L5 root pain
Sole of foot	S1 root pain. Plantar fasciitis. Metatarsal stress fracture. Tibial/plantar nerve entrapment
Toes	MTPJ synovitis (e.g. RA, gout). MTPJ OA. Morton's metatarsalgia. Bursitis. Enthesitis/dactylitis

*Robert–Jones fracture from an inversion–pronation injury.

- Gout should always be considered a possible cause of painful lesions in the foot in people at risk. Gout is not always intra-articular, intrabursal, or intratendonal. Local or diffuse soft tissue inflammation is common and often misdiagnosed as cellulitis. Swelling is usually marked.
- L5 pain is referred to the top (dorsum) and S1 pain to the sole of the foot.
- In older adults OA of midfoot joints is common. Mild synovitis can occur with it and may be caused by CPPD crystals (see Chapter 15).

Establish possible causes of forefoot pain
- In those with forefoot pain, typically referred to as metatarsalgia, establish whether the condition is focal or due to arthropathy.
- Pain under the ball of the foot whilst walking is non-specific but might suggest any MTPJ abnormality, distal metatarsal stress fracture, Freiberg's disease, planter nerve neuroma, or bursitis.
- Patients with RA often describe pain under the MTPJs and a feeling of 'walking on pebbles' (due to joint swelling and/or subluxation). Synovitis of the MTPJs is a very common feature of early RA.
- Acute pain under the forefoot spreading into one or more (adjacent) toes and worse on walking suggests a plantar nerve neuroma (Morton's metatarsalgia) or intermetatarsal bursitis.
- Pain associated with parasthesiae or numbness under the forefoot might be due to S1 root irritation (common) or entrapment of the tibial nerve in the hindfoot (rare). Ask about back pain and other hindfoot problems.

- Non-traumatic toe pain associated with entire toe swelling suggests a dactylitis (associated with SpA). Although many toes may be affected, the dactylitis may be unilateral and affect just one toe.
- The development of hallux valgus is associated with tight footwear. The established deformity is associated with altered weight-bearing and a second toe (hammer) deformity. Big toe pain might be due to hallux rigidus. It is usually 2° to OA and important to recognize as it may prevent toe dorsiflexion sufficiently to lead to a compromised gait pattern.
- Pain specifically under the hallux may be due to damage of the sesamoids in the flexor hallucis brevis tendon and be misdiagnosed as a joint problem.

Ask for a description of the pain

- As in the hand, neurogenic pain is common and typical.
- Severe or unremitting pain when at rest suggests intrinsic bone pathology. Consider osteonecrosis, infection, fracture, and tumours, e.g. osteoid osteoma.
- Neurogenic pain may be sharp and well-defined (e.g. in acute L5 or S1 root pain, (see p.82)), deep, achy, and less well-defined (e.g. chronic nerve root symptoms as in spinal or foraminal stenosis) or burning in quality. Parasthesiae and numbness may accompany both.
- If swelling accompanies neurogenic pain, consider algodystrophy. There are numerous triggers, e.g. trauma, surgery. Patients may be unwilling to walk and apparent disability may appear profound.

Weakness (?)

If true weakness is the major problem rather than pain, the diagnosis is usually between a spinal and peripheral nerve lesion (see Examination, below).

Examination

Observation

Observe the lower legs and feet from front and back whilst the patient is standing. Note any swelling, deformities, or rashes:

- Lower leg deformities to note: tibia varum (or bow legs) in an older adult may be due to Paget's disease of the tibia. Muscle wasting might suggest disuse atrophy, old polio, or lumbosacral spinal canal stenosis (bilateral and subtle usually in older adults).
- Oedema or soft tissue swelling may be relevant to an underlying condition, e.g. RA. Although it may cause discomfort, oedema from cardiac failure, venous congestion, and hypoproteinaemia and lymphoedema is not painful unless there are ulcers or thrombophlebitis.
- Gout can cause swelling anywhere.
- Calf swelling may be due to vein thrombosis or ruptured popliteal cyst.
- Common patterns of foot deformity are:
  - flat feet (pes planus)
  - high-arched feet (pes cavus) with high medial arch
  - hallux valgus and rigidus
  - overriding, hammer, and claw toes.
- Skin conditions from venous abnormalities are common in the elderly. Other skin lesions which may be relevant include purpura, panniculitis—which is often subtle and over the shins—and pyoderma gangrenosum.

Ask the patient to walk in bare feet

Gait patterns should be noted:

- An antalgic ('limp and wince') gait is a non-specific indicator of pain.
- A wide-based gait (>10 cm wider than normal) suggests instability: joint instability, muscle weakness, or neurological lesions may be the cause.
- A foot that slaps down or a high stepping gait suggests tibialis anterior weakness (L4 nerve root or common peroneal nerve lesion).
- Significant weakness of gluteus medius and gluteus maximus in L5 and S1 root lesions respectively can result in lurching during gait. In the former, as weight is taken on the affected side, gluteus medius may be weak in controlling the small 2–3 cm lateral displacement in the weight-bearing hip that normally occurs. This can be compensated for if the body centre of gravity is brought over the hip by lurching the upper body over the affected side. With gluteus maximus lesions (S1) extension of the hip, which helps mediate motion through the stance phase prior to toeing-off, may be weak. Thrusting the thorax forward with an arched back (forward lurch) compensates for the weakness and helps to maintain hip extension.
- A flat-footed gait with little or weak toe-off may suggest an S1 root lesion; however, 'flat-foot' (loss of the medial arch) with associated hind foot eversion and heel pain (plantar fasciitis) is extremely common. Often the arch weakness corrects when the patient is asked to walk.

Examine the lower leg

With the patient supine on the couch, examine the lower leg:

- After a ruptured popliteal cyst, calf tissues are often diffusely tender and swollen. Calf circumferences can be compared (e.g. 10 cm below tibial tubercle). There may also be mild skin erythema. Findings are not specific. Gout and infection (see Chapter 17) are the main alternatives if there is marked tenderness. A DVT causes relatively painless swelling.
- Check for bruising, swelling, and tenderness around the fibula head in patients with foot drop (possible peroneal nerve palsy). Neurological examination may be done at this point.
- Localized anterior tibial tenderness is often found in patients with stress fractures or with pseudofractures (osteomalacia—see Chapter 16).
- Tibial deformity in adults may be associated with diffuse bony tenderness and heat (arteriovenous shunting) in Paget's disease (see Chapter 16).

Examine the ankle and hindfoot

At the ankle and hindfoot, examine for joint and tendon synovitis, palpate specific structures and test passive hindfoot joint mobility:

- Synovitis of hindfoot joints is not always easily detected. With ankle joint synovitis, thickened tissue may be felt anteriorly in the ankle crease (where there may be a 'springy fullness') or laterally around the malleoli.

- Posterior tibial and peroneal tendonitis are associated with soft tissue swelling of the medial and lateral hindfoot respectively. Synovial thickening from ankle and talocalcaneal joints may also be felt here and synovitis of structures may coexist in RA or SpA. Pain from resisted movement of tendons may not be specific.
- Pathology of medial hindfoot structures may be associated with tibial nerve entrapment resulting in sensory symptoms on the sole of the foot. There may be a positive Tinnel's sign.
- Posterior heel pain may be due to Achilles' tendonitis, enthesitis and mechanical damage to the tendon, and retrocalcaneal bursitis. Deep tenderness may suggest an os trigonum lesion.
- The loss of passive hindfoot movements is not specific and can be associated with any cause of ankle or subtalar arthritis (20–30° of dorsiflexion and 45–55° of plantar flexion is average for the ankle and a 10–20° inversion–eversion range is average for the subtalar joint). Subtalar joint movement can be difficult to test accurately.
- The pain of plantar fasciitis may be elicited by firm palpation of the medial underside of the calcaneum. A negative test does not rule out pathology, as often the history is more sensitive. Full musculoskeletal examination is required to check for features of SpA such as arthritis/enthesitis elsewhere and sacroiliitis.

Examine for midfoot lesions

Identifying specific midfoot lesions is difficult, though bony landmarks and discrete tender areas can be noted:

- Twisting the midfoot may elicit pain non-specifically. Common lesions include gout, OA, and synovitis associated with RA and SpA.
- Bony tenderness alone without soft tissue swelling does not rule out synovitis of an adjacent joint.
- The midfoot is a typical site for neuroarthropathy in diabetes.
- Bony lumps (exostoses) that may have formed at sites of pressure are common in the foot (e.g. medial or dorsal aspect of the first MTPJ, base or head of the fifth metatarsal, distal talus, or over the midfoot). In the elderly bony pain and skin sores may form at these sites.
- Both gout and infection result in swelling, skin erythema and localized tenderness. Gout of the first MTPJ occurs at any one time in 70% of patients with the condition. It can occur anywhere in the foot.

Examine the forefoot

Check for bony or other swelling, digit separation, and examine the sole of the foot. Squeezing the whole forefoot at the line of the MTPJs is a non-specific but useful screening test for painful forefoot lesions:

- Tender swelling of the whole toe (dactylitis) occurs in SpA (see Chapter 8), sarcoid (see Chapter 18), and HIV infection (see Chapter 17). Swelling is soft not bony. Tender bony swelling suggests a bunion and is common on the dorsal aspect of the toes and the first and fifth MTPJs.
- Forefoot splaying and interdigital separation suggests MTPJ synovitis or interdigital bursitis. MTPJs may be individually tender (simultaneously palpated with thumb below and finger above).

- Tenderness between metatarsal heads is typical in Morton's metatarsalgia. There may be a sensory deficit in the interdigital cleft. The differential diagnosis (in adolescents) may be osteochondritis of the second and third metatarsal head.
- Check for hallux rigidus—passive dorsiflexion should be at least 50°. Extending the big toe passively can reveal an ability to form a medial longitudinal arch in patients with flat feet (Jack's test).
- Discrete bony tenderness without swelling occurs with stress fractures.
- Uneven callus distribution under the forefoot may suggest an abnormally focused area of weight-bearing and an underlying mechanical abnormality.
- Rashes on the sole of the foot are uncommon but important to consider are: pompholyx, pustular psoriasis, and keratoderma blenhorragica (see Reactive arthritis p.306).
- Loss of sensation under the forefoot may be due to an S1 root lesion, peripheral neuropathy (e.g. diabetes), mononeuritis (e.g. vasculitis—see Chapter 14), Sjögren's syndrome (see Chapter 11), mixed connective tissue disease), or, rarely, tibial nerve entrapment (examine hindfoot).

Neurological examination

Neurological examination is essential in cases where pain is neurogenic or there is weakness, numbness, or parasthesiae (see Table 2.23).

Investigations

Imaging of the lower leg

- Suspected tibial abnormalities such as stress fractures and pseudofractures in osteomalacia and Paget's disease have characteristic radiological appearances.
- Periosteal changes occur in trauma, psoriatic arthritis (above ankle), HPOA and pachydermal periostitis
- In athletes with exercise-related pain a three-phase bone scan is part of the work-up for anterior shin pain.
- In suspected (though radiograph-negative) cases of bony disease such as cortical stress fracture, periostitis, or cortical hyperostosis a bone scan is a useful investigation as it is sensitive for these conditions.

Imaging of the foot

Information available on radiographs of the hindfoot includes:

- Increased soft-tissue attenuation around the tendon insertion in cases of Achilles tendonitis or retrocalcaneal bursitis.
- Erosions or periostitis at the Achilles tendon insertion in enthesitis associated with SpA.
- Erosions in gout and RA-associated retrocalcaneal bursitis.
- Axial radiographs of the hindfoot are useful in showing talocalcaneal joint abnormalities, e.g. in RA.
- If radiographs are normal in patients with posterior heel pain, US can show patterns of tendon and bursal inflammation. MR characterizes any discrete pattern of tendon injury further.

Table 2.23 Patterns of common abnormal examination findings in lower lumbar nerve root lesions

Nerve root	Abnormal finding
L4	Weakness of ankle dorsiflexion (tibialis anterior)
	Patient finds walking on their heel difficult (strong ankle dorsiflexion needed)*
	Reduced knee reflex (L3 and L4)
L5	Weakness of big toe dorsiflexion (extensor hallucis longus)
	Weakness of foot eversion (peroneal muscles, also S1)
	Sensory deficit over dorsum of foot
	Reduced ankle reflex (L5 and S1)
S1	Weakness of ankle plantar flexion (gastrocnemius and soleus)
	Patient finds walking on, or repeatedly rising onto, tiptoe difficult*
	Sensory deficit over sole of foot
	Reduced ankle reflex

*Manoeuvres may be affected by pain, making interpretation difficult.

- Osteonecrosis of an os trigonum or posterior talar process or tarsal navicular may be identified by radiographs. It is invariably located by bone scintigraphy and can be characterized further, usually with soft tissue swelling, by MR.
- A plantar spur does not denote current plantar fasciitis.
- Plantar heel pain may be due to a fracture in a spur. Erosions just above the spur may be seen. The thickness of heel fat pad can be gauged from its X-ray attenuation (thin = risk for plantar fasciitis). A fat pad >23 mm thick in men and >21.5 mm thick in women is associated with acromegaly.
- Calcaneal fractures or an osteoid osteoma can be seen in some cases with radiographs alone. Bone scans/CT are more sensitive.
- Patterns of joint, enthesis, and tendon inflammation can be documented using MR but also with a well-executed bone scan. This is useful information when characterizing an arthropathy.
- Bony abnormalities in the mid and forefoot are generally revealed by radiographs alone, though metatarsal stress fractures may be missed. MR can discriminate a plantar neuroma from interdigital bursitis and MTPJ synovitis. The former are probably best initially demonstrated by US.

Other investigations
- Neurophysiology is a useful adjunct to clinical examination in diagnosis of lower limb neuropathies and can help discriminate between peripheral (common peroneal or sciatic) or nerve root causes of foot drop, and also S1 root or tibial nerve entrapment causes of paraesthesiae of the sole of the foot.

- Joint/bursa fluid aspiration is mandatory in suspected cases of sepsis and should be sent for culture (remember to consider gonococcus in young adults and TB in patients from endemic or inner-city areas). Fluid should be sent for polarized microscopy if a crystal-induced disease is suspected.
- Laboratory tests requested should reflect suspicion of specific infective, inflammatory, metabolic, or malignant pathology.

Treatment

Lower leg disorders

- Anterior shin pain should be treated according to cause. If there is also a problem of foot alignment then orthoses that support both the hind foot and mid arch may be very useful. Patients may volunteer that good 'training' shoes help (as is the case with plantar fasciitis).
- Exercise-induced lower leg pain has a number of causes and includes shin splints and compartment syndrome. The latter may require further investigation with pressure readings or exercise scintigraphy (^{99m}Tc-MIBI). In cases resistant to rest, analgesia, and modification of triggering factors, decompressive surgery may be required.
- Patients with Paget's disease of the tibia may require treatment with high-dose bisphosphonates and will need a biomechanical assessment.

Ankle and hindfoot disorders

- Tendonitis around the ankle should respond to treatment of its underlying cause. Chronic posterior tibial tendonitis left untreated will eventually accelerate the development of hindfoot valgus. Consider heel and arch support orthotics early.
- Plantar fasciitis may respond to a number of conservative measures:
  - heel pads and/or supportive shoes ('trainers')
  - modification of weight-bearing activity
  - Achilles tendon stretching
  - hindfoot strapping
  - resting night splint (preventing ankle plantar flexion)
  - steroid injection around medial calcaneal tubercle
  - external beam radiotherapy
  - surgery.

Forefoot disorders

- Localized forefoot pain, e.g. metatarsalgia, may respond to support pads and a change to a wider, more supportive, low-heel shoe. A podiatry/chiropody opinion should be sought as required.
- Forefoot stress fractures and metatarsal head osteochondritis require rest, supportive footwear and time to heal.
- Patients with chronic forefoot pain may benefit from a podiatric assessment. 'Stress offloading' foot orthoses for metatarsalgia and other biomechanical abnormalities (e.g. hallux rigidus) can be individually moulded using thermoplastic materials.

Steroid injections (see also p.148)

Steroid injections may be of value in the following:
- Ankle joint inflammation (e.g. RA, OA, gout)
- Subtalar joint inflammation

- Tarsal tunnel syndrome
- Achilles peritendonitis (local steroid injections for Achilles' nodules should be avoided if possible as the risk of rupture is high. The same concern, though probably lesser risk, applies to Achilles' peritendonitis)
- Calcaneal apophysitis (Sever's disease—Achilles' tendon insertion)
- Retrocalcaneal bursitis
- Plantar fasciitis
- Gout/OA/enthesitis at first MTPJ.

Surgery
- Minor surgical techniques can be curative in tarsal tunnel syndrome and in excising an interdigital (Morton's) neuroma. Consider excision of painful exostoses and troublesome rheumatoid nodules and amputation of deformed or over-riding toes.
- Major surgical procedures with good outcomes in appropriate patients include fusion of hindfoot joints and forefoot arthroplasty in chronic inflammatory arthritides. Osteotomy realignment of a hallux valgus deformity can be successful in the long term.

Child and adolescent foot disorders

For a review of classification criteria of autoimmune juvenile arthritides see Chapter 7 p.193.

Background

Lower limb and foot deformities of babies may be noticed first by parents. Diagnostic evaluation needs to focus on ruling out major congenital disease and exploring biomechanical factors.

- Neonatal deformities of the leg are uncommon.
- Talipes equinovarus (club foot) is an important deformity, which presents at birth. It is most commonly idiopathic and it is associated with wasting of the lower leg muscles. Causes to consider and rule out are spina bifida, spinal dysraphism, cerebral palsy, and arthrogryposis.
- With babies, persistence of certain sleeping postures is associated with patterns of angular and torsion deformity involving the whole leg. Postures include prone sleeping with knees tucked up under the chest, hips extended, or in a 'frog's-legs' position.
- In children able to walk, the commonest conditions that present to paediatric orthopaedic clinics are in-toeing and flat feet, though serious causes of flat feet usually affect only older children. Important points in evaluating an in-toeing deformity and flat feet are shown in Table 2.24. Some deformities in this group have been associated with persistence of sitting postures, e.g. cross-legged or 'reverse tailor' (floor sitting, knees bent and legs splayed out/back) positions.
- Achiness in the feet is the typical symptom in young children with torsional leg deformities of significance. If the biomechanical problem is sufficiently severe, shoes can rapidly deform.
- Regional musculoskeletal lesions in children <3 years of age are rare but most inflammatory arthritides can affect foot joints. Pain from an inflamed joint results in a miserable child and a refusal to walk.
- Periosteal pain (hyperostosis) in the tibiae and other long bones occurs in Caffey's disease. There is usually symmetrical limb enlargement in this rare condition, which usually occurs before the baby is 6 months old.

Table 2.24 Common patterns of foot deformity in babies and infants

Deformity	Commonest causes	Features
In-toeing	Metatarsus varus	Presents age 0–3 months or when starts to walk. Examination: forefoot varus only (heel is in neutral or valgus). Over 80% correct without surgery though predicting which will is difficult: 'wait and see until age 3' is appropriate
	Torsional lower limb deformity—medial tibial torsion and/or excessive femoral anteversion	Often related to regular prone knee–chest (fetal) sleeping position in babies and toddlers, and persistently sitting on the floor with legs forward internally rotated and knees bent out/backwards in children (see Fig. 2.21)
	Cerebral palsy	Most often caused by excessive femoral anteversion
	Spinal dysraphism	Rare
Flat feet (pes planus)	Idiopathic or familial, hereditary connective tissue diseases, hindfoot disease: tarsal coalitions, arthritis, tumour, osteochondritis, infection etc.	Very common—often asymptomatic. Children often develop medial arch with time (passive big toe extension or standing on toes often reveals it). It is associated with conditions of general tissue laxity. If it occurs with pain and/or stiff flat feet look for peroneal muscle spasm and hindfoot pathology as the cause
Talipes equinovarus (club-foot)	Idiopathic, spina bifida, spinal dysraphism, tibial dysplasia, cerebral palsy, arthrogryposis	Incidence 1–2:1000 overall. Presents at birth. Idiopathic (aetiology unknown) is commonest. Often a family history. Examination: calf wasting, hindfoot and forefoot in equinus (plantaris) and varus
Pes cavus	Idiopathic, peroneal muscular atrophy	High arch (medial and lateral sides), toe clawing. Associated with neurological disease rarely e.g. Friedrich's ataxia

Taking a history

Ask about the site and quality of the pain

- Lower leg pain may be due to one of the causes of 'shin splints', a bone lesion, or algodystrophy.
- Localized anterior lower leg pain occurs in lesions of the anterior tibia e.g. stress fractures, periositis, tibial tubercle osteochondritis, but deeper more diffuse anterior pain (often also medial) occurs in 'shin splints' (see below).
- Minimal or non-traumatic tibial fracture associated with fracture or bony deformity elsewhere raises the possibility of osteogenesis imperfecta.
- Localized or diffuse burning pain suggests a neurogenic cause. In children, disc prolapse is rare. Superficial burning pain may be due to peripheral neuropathy or algodystrophy.
- Algodystrophy (see Chapter 18) typically gives burning pain although it can occur with dull, aching pain or paroxysms. Pain often disturbs sleep. In children it is more common in the lower leg and foot than in the upper limb. Diffuse swelling and skin changes may be present. In many cases trauma is a triggering event but anything from simple sprains to arthroscopic knee surgery can trigger it and 25% are idiopathic cases.
- In children, algodystrophy may occur in the limb distal to an arthritic joint.
- Unremitting, sleep-disturbing pain that is worse on weight-bearing suggests bone or bone marrow pathology e.g. bone tumours, osteomyelitis, or periositis (hypertrophic osteoarthropathy, Gaucher's disease).

Ask about pain onset during sport

There are typical sports injuries of the lower leg that occur relatively often in active children and adolescents. Ask about pain onset during sport or recurrence during or after specific activities:

- Adolescents may refer to 'shin splints'. Possible conditions include: tibial stress fracture, Osgood–Schlatter's disease, tibialis posterior fasciitis, compartment syndrome, popliteal artery stenosis, and malalignment of the hind- and midfoot.
- Tibial fascial inflammation and pain typically occurs as running begins, though patients can run through it, but it often returns severely after exercise and takes days to wear off. It is associated with hyperprona-tion of the foot (which increases stretch forces on the tendon).
- Compartment syndrome may be acute (due to muscle necrosis) or chronic. The chronic form occurs almost exclusively in endurance sports. Pain is absent at rest but builds as exercise progresses. It diminishes gradually—usually within a few hours. The pattern of pain and findings from perfusion scintigraphy suggest the cause of pain is ischaemic. Increased compartment pressures can be demonstrated by invasive monitoring.

- Pain from major vessel ischaemia occurs typically with walking. Muscle or a fibrous band in the popliteal fossa can compress the popliteal artery.
- Stress fractures occur in young athletes. In girls there may be an association with amenorrhea and generalized osteopenia.

Are there regional traumatic lesions?

In the foot, regional traumatic lesions are quite common, particularly in active children and athletes. Chronic arthritides should be considered:

- Apophysitides (osteochondritides) are quite common (see Table 2.25). Most present with localized pain during exercise. There is tenderness and often swelling and pain on resisted movement of the appropriate tendon.
- Proximal midfoot pain may be caused by an accessory navicular, navicular osteochondritis (Köhler's disease), and tarsal coalitions (abnormal joins between bones leading to joint hypomobility, bilateral in 50% of cases). All lesions may be associated with a rigid flat foot (peroneal spastic flat foot) and will be more painful on weight-bearing.

Table 2.25 Localized painful foot disorders specific to school-age children and adolescents. Tumours are rare but osteoid osteoma should be considered

Site of pain	Disorder	Characteristics of disorder
Posterior heel	Calcaneal apophysitis (Sever's disease)	Traction osteochondritis. Both sexes age 8–10 years
Dorsal midfoot	Accessory navicular	Common finding in all children (50%). In 75% it fuses with main navicular. Majority not painful. Rarely it is associated with exercise-related pain
	Navicular osteochondritis (Köhler's disease).	Boys > girls. Presents with pain, limp and weight bearing on the outside of the foot
	Tarsal coalitions	Asymptomatic or with 'peroneal spastic' (rigid) flat foot (8–16 years)
Medial side of foot (may be diffuse)	Hypermobile flat foot	Children 1–5 years. May have generalized tissue laxity
Lateral side of foot	5th metatarsal base osteochondritis (Iselin's disease)	Children 10–12 years. Possibly due to 2° tendon ossification centre and related to tight shoes
Dorsal and plantar distal midfoot	Stress fracture (rare)	Adolescents—2nd/3rd metatarsal
	Metatarsal head osteochondritis (Freiberg's disease)	Commonly 2nd metatarsal head. Affects active adolescent girls most frequently

- Joint synovitis (pain with immobility-related stiffness) is often difficult to detect clinically. Ankle synovitis is the easiest to be confident about. Soft or springy swelling with tenderness over the dorsal skin crease often suggests an effusion. Synovial thickening can be felt in florid cases circumferentially or just around the lower margins of the malleoli. In oligoarticular JIA the ankle joint is sometimes painlessly swollen.
- Juvenile SpA/ERA is rare in children aged <8, and up until that age oligo/polyarticular JIA is a more likely cause of joint synovitis in the foot. Juvenile SpA/ERA may present with synovitis in a single lower limb joint, enthesitis at the Achilles tendon insertion or plantar fasciitis.
- Dactylitis ('sausage toe') raises the possibility of psoriatic arthritis or sarcoid. History usually discriminates the pattern of arthritis that helps in the differential diagnosis.
- The most common other arthritides to involve foot joints are viral and post-streptococcal arthritis and Lyme disease.
- Diffuse foot swelling occasionally occurs with synovitis in oligo/polyarticular JIA. The major differential is algodystrophy. Both pains are worse at night. Sensory symptoms are prominent and skin changes common in established algodystrophy.
- Forefoot pain in adolescents may be due to an interdigital neuroma (Morton's metatarsalgia) or osteochondritis of a metatarsal head (Freiberg's osteochondritis). Neuroma pain is often associated with dysaesthesia and numbness between the toes.
- Big toe pain from hallux rigidus (<50° passive dorsiflexion) is rare but can occur after injury and prevent running.
- Unlike in adults, gout occurs rarely in children and usually only in the context of renal failure, glucose 6-phosphatase deficiency (von Gierke's), malignancy, or X chromosome-linked disorders of uric acid metabolism.

Examination

Observe the lower legs from front and back whilst the patient is standing:
- Lower leg muscle wasting occurs in hereditary sensorimotor neuropathy (bilateral) and typically accompanies spinal dysraphism. Diffuse muscle hypertrophy might suggest muscular dystrophy.
- Extremity swelling occurs in some forms of JIA (see Chapter 7), vasculitis (e.g. Henoch–Schönlein purpura (HSP)—see Chapter 14) and sepsis (see Chapter 17).
- Note the appearance and distribution of any rashes. Skin conditions from venous abnormalities are common. Other skin lesions which may be relevant include purpura (?HSP) and panniculitis over the shins (?erythema nodosum/sarcoid—see Chapter 18).

Observe the feet from front and back whilst the patient is standing
- Look for swelling and patterns of deformity. Patterns of deformity may require detailed orthopaedic assessment. Check the gait.
- Look for localized oedema—an occasional sign of underlying JIA but also present in nephrotic syndrome and in systemic vasculitides.
- Some torsional leg deformities are clinically significant. The commonest pattern is with the hip internally rotated (usually excessive femoral

anteversion), the tibia compensating in external rotation, and associated hindfoot valgus and forefoot varus.

- Torsional deformities will not spontaneously correct if they've not done so by the age of 7. There is speculation (based on the rationale of joint incongruity), but no proof, that torsional deformities in children are a risk for early OA.
- Flat feet are often asymptomatic and familial, and regress as the child grows (the medial arch becomes evident standing on tiptoe and with passive big toe dorsiflexion). Hindfoot pathology may be a cause.

Examine the sitting patient

With the patient sitting on the edge of the couch, check for tibial torsion:

- Tibial torsion is measured as the angle between an imaginary line through the tibial tubercle in the sagittal plane and the perpendicular of an imaginary line through the malleoli (see Fig. 2.21).

Examine the supine patient

With the patient supine on the couch, examine the lower leg:

- Check for bruising, swelling, and tenderness around the fibular head in patients with foot drop (?peroneal nerve palsy).
- Localized anterior tibial tenderness is often found in patients with stress fractures.
- The purpuric rash of HSP invariably occurs over the back of the calves.

Examine for swellings in the foot

- Bony lumps (exostoses) that may have formed at sites of pressure (e.g. posterior heel—'pump bump').
- Swelling, skin erythema and localized tenderness suggests infection, although synovitis, skin vasculitis and panniculitis (e.g. erythema nodosum) should also be considered.

Examine the hindfoot

In the hindfoot, examine for joint and tendon synovitis, palpate specific structures, and test passive hindfoot joint mobility:

- Synovitis of hindfoot joints is not always easily detected. With ankle joint synovitis thickened tissue may be felt anteriorly in the ankle crease (where there may be a 'springy fullness') or laterally around the malleoli.
- The pain of plantar fasciitis may be elicited by firm palpation of the medial underside of the calcaneum. ERA should be ruled out.
- Posterior tibial and peroneal tendonitis are associated with soft tissue swelling of the medial and lateral hindfoot respectively. Synovial thickening from ankle and talocalcaneal joints may also be felt there and synovitis of structures may coexist in JIA or ERA. Resisting a tendon's movement aiming to elicit specific tendon pain may not be a specific test.
- Painful posterior heel structures are usually easily palpated, though pain may be due to a number of causes including Achilles' enthesitis, mechanical damage to the tendon, retrocalcaneal bursitis, and apophysitis.

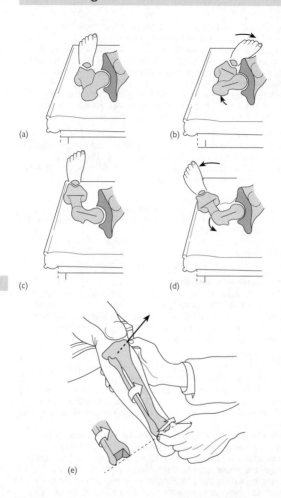

(a)

(b)

(c)

(d)

(e)

Fig. 2.21 Femoral anteversion, retroversion, and tibial torsion. (a) Where the femoral neck angulates excessively forward relative to an imaginary axis through the femoral condyles, the hip is anteverted. (b) Femoral neck anteversion can lead to a greater than usual range of hip internal rotation and a toe-in gait. (c) and (d) Retroversion, where the femoral neck angulates posteriorly relative to a femoral condyle axis, can cause a toe-out gait. (e) Toeing can also be caused by excessive medial tibial torsion. Normally the ankle mortise faces 15° externally relative to a sagittal plane axis through the tibial tubercle (arrow) but in medial torsion it faces forward or internally.

- The loss of passive hindfoot movements is not specific. Often due to ankle synovitis, stiffness may also occur in other causes of joint pain (e.g. osteochondritis dissecans) and cases of peroneal spastic flat foot. The hindfeet of children are more mobile than those of adults.
- Peroneal 'spastic' (rigid) flat foot syndrome should be distinguished from flexible flat foot (when the medial longitudinal arch reappears when standing on the toes or with passive big toe dorsiflexion). Pain is centred on the dorsomedial side of the foot. The medial longitudinal arch is deficient. Associated peroneal muscle spasm may be painful. The age of presentation depends on the aetiology, the commonest cause being tarsal coalition. It is always important to consider cerebral palsy and spinal dysraphism as well as local lesions: tumours (e.g. osteoid osteoma of calcaneum); navicular osteochondritis (Köhler's); local osteomyelitis or pyogenic arthritis; ankle or talocalcaneal joint synovitis (e.g. JIA). The diagnosis is of underlying cause but AP, lateral, oblique, and axial talocalcaneal radiographs, a three-phase bone scan and hindfoot CT may all be useful in defining associated hindfoot lesions.

Examine the midfoot

In the midfoot determine any sites of tenderness and stiffness:

- Twisting the midfoot may elicit pain from lesions, though non-specifically.
- The major condition to rule out in teenagers is tarsal coalitions. These are fibrous, cartilagenous, or osseous joins between bones resulting in no or little mobility. The commonest involved joints are calcaneonavicular and talocalcaneal. They may be tender. Passive movement with inversion is usually painful and increases spasm in peroneal muscles.
- A tender navicular may also be due to osteochondritis.
- Synovitis associated with some forms of JIA can occur at any joint. Precise location is often difficult to identify clinically.

Examine the forefoot

Check for bony or other swelling, look for digit separation, examine the digits and the sole of the forefoot. Squeezing the whole forefoot at the line of MTPJs is a useful but non-specific screening test for painful forefoot lesions:

- Dactylitis (psoriatic arthritis or sarcoid) swelling is soft, not bony.
- Forefoot splaying and interdigital separation suggests MTPJ synovitis. MTPJs may be tender when palpated (simultaneously with thumb below and finger above).
- Tenderness between two metatarsal heads is typical in Morton's neuroma. The differential (in adolescents) may be osteochondritis of the second or third metatarsal head.
- Extending the big toe passively can reveal an ability to form a medial longitudinal arch in patients with flat feet (Jack's test).
- Discrete bony tenderness without swelling may occur with stress fractures.
- Loss of sensation under the forefoot is rare. Full back and neurological leg examination may be necessary.

Investigations
Imaging of the lower leg
- Radiographs of the lower leg have characteristic patterns of abnormality in osteogenesis imperfecta, rickets, and some periosteal conditions, e.g. from stress fracture or periostitis, etc.
- Bone scintigraphy is a sensitive investigation for radiograph-negative cases of suspected bone disease. It is also a useful initial investigation in adolescents with shin splints as it will rule out stress fractures and can show tibialis fasciitis.
- Treadmill or cycle ergometer exercise scintigraphy using ^{99m}Tc-MIBI can be useful in revealing compartmental perfusion defects in athletes with ischaemic-type pain during exercise (another cause of shin splints).

Imaging of the foot
Local lesions require investigation with radiographs, though in patients with inflammatory or bony lesions further imaging may be necessary:
- Routine AP and lateral hindfoot radiographs will reveal most cases of Sever's disease and osteochondritis dissecans of the ankle. Some cases of talocalcaneal coalition will require extra views and CT for diagnosis.
- In patients with a rigid flat foot additional oblique and axial view radiographs of the hindfoot help to show osteoarticular abnormalities if routine AP and lateral views do not. The gold-standard investigation is CT which is used prior to, and to plan, surgery.
- Forefoot radiographs are a good screening test in those with forefoot pain. Though insensitive for detecting early synovitis, osteochondritides, hallux abnormalities, and the pattern of established arthritis can be identified.
- It is important to check a radiograph for first MTPJ osteochondritis dissecans in those with hallux rigidus.
- Isolated soft tissue swelling may be due to algodystrophy, underlying synovitis, or infection. Radiographs are mandatory. Bone scintigraphy may be non-specific in this setting though the three-phase pattern of abnormality is characteristic in algodystrophy if synovitis can be ruled out.
- MR of the whole foot or swollen area is the quickest way to an advanced differential diagnosis.
- Where swelling, pain, and tenderness coexist infection must be ruled out using imaging. If it cannot and suspicion remains, tissue or fluid sampling should be undertaken. In most cases it is appropriate to do this under general anaesthesia. Algodystrophy should be excluded before any intervention.

Laboratory tests
Any possibility of joint synovitis (most likely to be ankle), enthesitis, tendonitis, or infection requires investigation with laboratory tests:
- ESR and CRP are likely to be raised in cases of autoimmune arthritis and infection and are more likely to be normal or only slightly ↑ in oligoarticular JIA and juvenile ERA compared with polyarticular and systemic JIA or infection.

- Normochromic anaemia (± mild microcytosis) is a non-specific sign of a systemic condition. FBC/CBC may be normal in oligoarticular JIA. Leucoctosis is typical with infection, with steroids and in systemic JIA.
- Moderately ↑ titres of ANA may be present in 40–75% of patients with oligoarticular JIA and is a risk factor for associated uveitis that is not necessarily acute and painful but left unchecked can still threaten sight.
- Check for circulating rheumatoid factor (RF) in cases of synovitis. High titres are a necessary part of, though not specific for, (RF+) polyarticular JIA.

Treatment

Lower leg disorders

- Anterior shin pain should be treated according to cause.
- Treat foot alignment problems with appropriate orthotics.
- Avoid NSAIDs if possible.
- Review diagnosis if conservative treatment fails, e.g. is there an underlying stress fracture or periostitis? (get a bone scan if not already done).

Ankle and foot disorders

- The management of bony anomalies/deformities should be discussed with an orthopedic surgeon and physiotherapist early, to avoid missing an opportunity to prevent growth abnormalities.
- Be aware that soft-tissue steroid injection of a presumed local lesion may impair healing/growth at apophyses and may aggravate the symptoms of (missed) algodystrophy.
- Consider intra-articular steroid injection of specific joints in oligoarticular JIA if joints can be clearly identified by scintigraphy or MR. Injection under sedation (adolescents) or light general anaesthesia (toddlers/children) is appropriate.

Corticosteroid injection therapy

Background

- Local anaesthetic and steroid injection into joints or soft tissues is a very effective treatment for localized pain.
- Injection offers a local maximal anti-inflammatory effect with minimal systemic absorption.
- The indications for local steroid injection include: to reduce inflammation in joints, entheses, tendon sheaths and bursae; to relieve pain from inflammatory ligament lesions; to relieve any inflammation at sites of nerve compression; to attempt to reduce the size of nodules and ganglia; to relieve pain at trigger points; and as part of epidurals.
- The contraindications are:
  - Absolute:
    —septic arthritis/septicaemia
    —febrile patient, cause unknown
    —serious allergy to previous injection
    —sickle cell disease
  - Relative
    —unknown cause of monoarthritis
    —neutropenia, thrombocytopenia
    —anticoagulation or bleeding disorder.
- Hydrocortisone acetate is a short-acting, weak anti-inflammatory, useful for superficial lesions such as tendons and bursae. A dose of 25mg is typical.
- Methylprednisolone acetate (40mg/ml), prednisolone acetate (25mg/ml), and triamcinolone acetonide (10 and 40mg/ml) are long-acting synthetic agents suitable for joint injections.
- Small joints accept only a small volume thus for IPJs, MCPJs, MTPJs, ACJs, and TMJs, 0.5 ml of triamcinolone acetonide (10mg) is appropriate. All other joints should accept at least 1ml. Choice of strength of steroid remains empirical. There may be merit in diluting the steroid in sterile saline, to increase volume for better distribution in larger joints.
- The patient should be warned of potential, though uncommon, side-effects:
  - exacerbation of pain for 24–48 h
  - septic arthritis and reactivation of TB
  - tissue atrophy (less likely with hydrocortisone than others)
  - depigmentation
  - anaphylaxis
  - nerve damage
  - tendon rupture
  - avascular necrosis
  - cartilage damage
  - soft-tissue calcification
  - temporary exacerbation of glycaemia in diabetes.
- As a general rule it is recommended that any one joint should not be injected > four times in 12 months and there are at least 6 weeks between injections.

- Children and some adolescents usually require a light general anaesthetic for most joint injections given the procedure can be quite traumatic. An alternative for older or more robust children or those who have had many injections done before, is to use local anaesthetic gel pads to numb skin adequately before the injection.

Principles of injection techniques

The procedure need not necessarily be done in a sterile environment. Some steps below illustrate the need to maintain relatively aseptic conditions:

- Mark the exact spot of needle insertion.
- Wash hands. Use gloves for procedure (preferably sterile).
- Clean the skin with alcohol.
- Anaesthetize the skin (either with local anaesthetic or refrigerant alcohol spray).
- Insert clean needle with empty syringe and aspirate back.
- Leave needle in place, detach syringe and place syringe containing drug onto end of needle.
- Pull back syringe plunger again before injecting—to ensure not in vein etc.
- Introduction of steroid should be effortless. Resistance implies wrong space.
- On completion remove syringe and needle and throw away 'sharps'.
- Cover the injection site with clean gauze or elastoplast.
- Rest joint for 24h (consider up to 48h for a weight-bearing joint) and re-emphasize possible side-effects and benefits.

The glenohumeral joint

- The anterior route gives reliable access in patients with adhesive capsulitis. It is also better suited for aspiration of joint effusions.
- Palpate the coracoid process anteriorly and the acromion posteriorly. The injection is made just lateral to the coracoid with the needle pointing towards the acromion.
- The posterior route requires the clinician to palpate the spine of the scapula with the thumb to its lateral end where it bends forward as the acromion. With the forefinger then palpate the coracoid anteriorly. The line between finger and thumb then marks the position of the joint line. The needle is advanced from behind, 1 cm below the acromion, and towards the coracoid. There should be no resistance.
- A slight withdrawal of the needle and its advance upward at about 30° also allows this approach to reach the rotator cuff with the same needle!

Subacromial articulation and acromioclavicular joint

- The subacromial bursa is approached from the lateral side. To inject this space the arm is placed in a neutral position, hanging to the side, and the gap between the acromion and the humeral head is palpated. The needle is directed medially and slightly posterior and not too deep (see Plate 13).

- The ACJ is located by following the clavicle laterally. The joint is often tender to palpate. The patient lies supine and a small gauge needle with 0.5 ml of steroid is directed into the joint at about 45° anteriorly.

The elbow joint and periarticular elbow structures

- Lateral humeral epicondylitis is injected with the elbow resting on the examination table and flexed at 90°. This superficial injection is directed at 45° to the end of the common extensor tendon origin. A fair amount of pressure is required for this injection. It is often painful (see Plate 14).
- Medial humeral epicondylitis is managed similarly. The needle is directed to the flexor tendon origin. However, care should be taken to avoid the groove just behind the medial epicondyle—the site of the ulnar nerve.
- An olecranon bursa can be aspirated and injected superficially with minimal effort. Needle position is confirmed by the aspiration of fluid.
- The elbow joint is most easily reached by a posterior approach. Place the thumb on the lateral epicondyle and the third finger on the olecranon. The groove between the two fingers identifies the joint line. Inject at 90° to the skin, just above and lateral to the olecranon. Alternatively the radial head can be palpated (with forearm pronation/supination) and the needle sited tangentially just under the capsule (anterolateral approach).

Lesions of the wrist

- The radiocarpal joint is best felt with the patient's hand held palm down and the wrist in slight flexion. A triangular gap is felt between the radius and the carpal bones. The needle is pointed proximally and at 60°.
- The carpal tunnel is injected on the palmar surface of the wrist in the first crease. If the palmaris tendon is present the injection should be sited just medial (i.e. closer to the 'little finger') to the midline, by about 1 cm, and towards the palm at 45°. There should be no resistance on injection or nerve pain (see Plate 15).
- De Quervain's tenosynovitis should be injected at the point of maximal tenderness, tangentially along the line of the tendon sheath.

The hand

- The small joints of the hand will normally only accept 0.5–1 ml of injected fluid.
- It is important to remember that the joint line of an MCPJ is about 1 cm distal to the crest of the knuckle. The approach to a PIPJ is from the lateral side.
- PIPJs and DIPJs are often difficult to inject. Accuracy of needle placement within a joint space might be improved by using US guidance.
- Efficacy may be greater using US-guided injection though as yet this is unproved.
- US guidance is mandatory when MCPJs/PIPJs are injected with intra-articular erbium-169 colloid (radiation synovectomy).

Hip joint and periarticular hip lesions

- Hip injection is not a routine outpatient procedure and aspiration and injection under US or fluoroscopic guidance is recommended.
- Meralgia paraesthetica occurs as a consequence of lateral cutaneous nerve entrapment (see p.101) as it traverses the fascia 10cm below and medial to the anterior superior iliac spine. If this spot can be clearly demarcated because of localized tenderness, steroid injection has a greater chance of success.
- The ischial tuberosities are located deep in the medial side of the buttocks. The overlying bursae can become inflamed, causing pain on sitting. These tender points can be injected. The differential diagnosis is enthesitis or possibly coccydinia.
- The coccyx can be palpated centrally (with the patient prone or lying on their side). This site is also amenable to local anaesthetic and steroid injections.
- Adductor apophysitis occurring from a sports injury can be injected simply although it can be difficult to access. An inflamed symphysis pubis is best injected under US guidance.
- Trochanteric bursitis or enthesitis at the greater trochanter can be injected with the patient lying on their good side. The injection site can be very deep and to reduce the risk of fat atrophy from a 'blind approach', it is reasonable to try using hydrocortisone first. Injection failure should raise the possibility of poor needle position or a different diagnosis, e.g. gluteus medius muscle tear at its insertion or pain referred from a lumbosacral disorder.

The knee joint and periarticular lesions

- The most common technique for injection of the knee joint is either the lateral or medial retropatellar approach.
- From the lateral side, the joint line is marked between the upper and middle third of the patella. Access to the joint space may be improved by depressing the medial aspect of the patella, tipping it up laterally. The needle is advanced tangentially between the patella and the femoral condyle.
- The entry site for the medial approach is below the midline of the patella, with the needle advanced tangentially towards the suprapatellar pouch.
- In both techniques, aspiration as the needle is inserted will reveal fluid as soon as the capsule is entered, so reducing the risk of forcing the needle too far forward causing cartilage damage.
- Prepatellar bursitis, painful ligaments, and trigger points around the knee may all respond to local steroid and anaesthetic.
- Popliteal cysts can be directly aspirated and injected but owing to the risk of damaging superficial neurovascular structures, should be done under US guidance.

Ankle and foot disorders

- The ankle joint is located most easily with the patient supine on a couch. The joint line can be palpated just lateral to the extensor digitorum tendon as it crosses the ankle crease. The needle is initially advanced downwards over the talus.

- Tendon sheaths and the tarsal tunnel can all be injected; the latter is injected under the flexor retinaculum between the calcaneum and the medial malleolus.
- Painful points under the heel should be injected from the medial side after carefully localizing the position of maximal pain. Never inject through the sole of the foot. Some clinicians will numb the area by local anaesthetic to the posterior tibial nerve, in the tarsal tunnel.
- The MTPJs are injected from the lateral side. Care should be taken as these joints have a greater than normal risk of infection after the procedure.

Principles of rehabilitation

Adulthood

It is beyond the scope of this book to address the many techniques employed in rehabilitation. The reader is encouraged to discuss and observe the management of patients with arthritis with the rehabilitation 'team'.

- In the last decade the development of a multiprofessional approach to rehabilitation has transformed the way most rheumatologists think about disability.
- Two main types of measurement exist for assessing outcome in rehabilitation (beyond the various scoring systems for particular 'diseases).
- 'Generic' measures take a global view of disability and afford later comparison. Generic measures also help in assessing different programmes, populations, and practices. 'Specific' measures deal with the individual patient and their function in their own environment.
- No one instrument will suffice and there are now many, some well-validated, disability scores:
  - Ritchie index—impairment
  - Health Assessment Qustionnaire—disability
  - SF36
  - General Health Questionnaire—quality of life
  - Nottingham Health Profile
  - Beck depression score—depression
  - Spielberg score—anxiety
  - Sickness Impact Profile (SIP)
  - Multi-dimensional pain inventory—psychological response to pain and disability.
- Important components of rehabilitation for patients with arthritis include:
  - a coordinated team
  - problem-solving approach
  - functionally relevant programme
  - education
  - community orientated
  - cognitive and psychological behavioral therapy
  - addressing social factors e.g. work, housing etc.
  - access to support services
  - commitment to long-term follow-up and reassessment.
- As such the team will consist of doctors, specialist nurses, physiotherapists, occupational therapists, counsellors, psychologists, orthotists, chiropodists, dieticians, rehabilitation engineers, and social workers.

Childhood

There are important additional issues to consider in the management of children:

- A child's rheumatic disease always has an impact on their family. Many normal activities are impossible or time-consuming, and financial hardship is common.
- Siblings may feel neglected and parents are often overburdened with tasks and worries to focus completely on the family. The 'team' aims to share out that burden and assist the whole family.

- The child should be integrated in school ('mainstream' preferably) and social life as much as possible. It is important to achieve the highest level of integration, hopefully ceasing a child's perception of sickness and difference, acquiring a sense of belonging and purpose.
- The therapist will spend as much time preventing deformity in early disease as dealing with chronic disability, the aim being to maintain or restore function.
- For a child with chronic progressive disease a regular, often daily, therapy programme is necessary. The best way to guarantee this is to involve the parents or carer. With education on the role of splints/exercise and the impact of rehabilitation on disease progression, most parents are eager and capable participants in the therapy.
- Joint protection training is important—proper positioning, use of several joints in a task, safe transfer of loads, avoidance of prolonged position, planning of rest breaks, and adapted aids and devices should all be addressed.
- Chronic diseases may elicit different emotions in different children—often frustration with lack of mobility in the young, and peer group issues and psychosexual anxieties in the adolescent. Positive adjustment, focusing on strengths not weakness, is important, as is the constant awareness of such issues in those that make up the support structure. Competence comes in many forms, not simply physical ability, and should be praised at every level, building a child's self-esteem.
- Many children who have learned to cope with their disease develop a more mature personality earlier than others in their age group. As such the adolescent may be earlier and better qualified to bid for an independent life despite physical limitations. It is important to ensure they are not 'held back'.

Adolescence

At some point in a patient's development from childhood to adulthood, the paediatric physician must start to relinquish care to the adult physician. This phase of patient management, the 'transition', should be handled carefully. Some important principles to consider are stated below.

- Transfer should only occur when a young person feels ready to function in an adult clinic.
- From an early stage adolescents should be encouraged to take responsibility for medications.
- The whole concept of independence should be introduced well ahead of an anticipated 'transfer time'. This could be introduced at about the age of 11 years and encouraged by trying to see the adolescent by themselves for part of their consultation by the time they are 13–14 years of age.
- A schedule of events leading to 'transition' and finally to transfer of care should be drawn up.
- Adolescents should be given information on health care rights and taught how to recognize changes in their disease (good or bad) and how to seek help from health professionals.

Patterns of disease presentation: making a working diagnosis

Oligoarticular pains in adults

Background

The assessment of an inflamed joint

- The clinical features of inflammation and pain at any given synovial joint and the differential diagnosis in the context of other possible regional musculoskeletal diagnoses are discussed in Chapter 2.
- Synovitis is the term given to inflammation of the synovial lining. Inflammation may be a consequence of a range of cellular processes but there are no clinical features that are both frequent and specific enough to allow a reliable diagnosis to be made of its cause in any single joint. Joint effusions (of variable size) invariably accompany synovitis.
- In any given joint, synovitis may not be the only inflamed tissue. Enthesitis of insertions of joint capsules, intra-articular and periarticular ligaments/tendons may be the 1° site of inflammation in some disorders. Subtle differentiating clinical and radiological signs may exist.
- The differential diagnosis of synovitis includes haemarthrosis and other synovial processes, e.g. pigmented villonodular synovitis (PVNS).

Table 3.1 lists the commonest causes of oligoarticular joint pain.

History: general points

- Pain and stiffness are typical though not invariable features of synovitis and enthesitis. Pain and stiffness are often worse during or after a period of immobility. The presence or absence of stiffness does not discriminate between diagnoses. Pain is often severe in acute joint inflammation. In chronic situations, pain may be less severe (e.g. owing to mechanisms which increase physical and psychological tolerance). There are no specific descriptors that discriminate pain from synovitis or enthesitis, although descriptions of 'aching' and 'tightness' are common.
- Swelling, either due to synovial thickening or effusion, often but not always, accompanies synovitis. Enthesitis may be associated with periarticular soft tissue swelling. A patient's report of swelling is not always reliable.
- Reduced mobility in a joint affected by enthesitis/synovitis is almost universal regardless of its cause.

Examination: general points

- Swelling may be observed or detected by palpation. Its absence does not rule out synovitis or enthesitis. Synovial swelling needs to be discriminated from bony swelling, fat, and other connective tissue swellings (e.g. ganglia, nodules, etc.). Without imaging or attempting to aspirate joint fluid, it is often difficult to discriminate synovial thickening from effusion. It is perhaps easiest in the knee.
- Skin erythema (implying periarticular inflammation) and heat do not always accompany joint inflammation but are common with crystal and septic arthritis. Erythema can also occur in reactive arthritis, rheumatic fever and with early Heberden's/Bouchard's nodes in OA.

Table 3.1 The commonest causes of oligoarticular (including monoarticular) joint pain and typical patterns of presentation

Disease	Typical pattern
Gout (Chapter 15)	Age >40 years. Initially acute monoarthritis. Strong association with hyperuricaemia, renal impairment, and diuretics. Possible general symptoms mimicking sepsis. Possible family history. Acute phase often high. Neutrophilia occurs. Joint fluid urate crystals seen by PLM. Joint erosions (radiographically typical) and tophi occur in chronic disease
Spondylarthritis (Chapter 8)	Age <40 years, ♂ > ♀. Mostly oligoarticular lower limb joint enthesitis/synovitis. May occur with sacroiliitis, urethritis or cervicitis, uveitis, gut inflammation, psoriasis (scaly or pustular). Possible family history. ESR/CRP may be normal. More severe course in HLA B27 positive people
CPPD arthritis (Chapter 15)	Mean age 72 years. Oligoarticular, acute monoarticular (25%) and occasionally polyarticular patterns of synovitis
Haemarthrosis	Obvious trauma does not always occur. Swelling usually considerable. Causes include trauma (e.g. cruciate rupture or intra-articular fracture), pigmented villonodular synovitis, bleeding diatheses, and chondrocalcinosis
Osteoarthritis (Chapter 6)	Soft tissue swelling is usually not as obvious as bony swelling (osteophytes). Typical distribution (e.g. first carpometacarpal and knee joints)
Rheumatoid arthritis (Chapter 5)	Unusual presentation in a single joint. Can present with just a few (usually symmetrical) joints
Septic arthritis (excluding *N. gonorrhae*) (Chapter 17)	Commonest cause *Staphylococcus aureus*. Associated with chronic arthritis, joint prostheses, and reduced host immunity. Peak incidence in elderly. Systemic symptoms common and sometimes overt, though may not occur. Synovial fluid is Gram stain positive in 50% of cases and culture positive in 90% of cases
Gonococcal arthritis (Chapter 17)	Age 15–30 in urban populations and with inherited deficiency of complements C5 to C9. One form presents as an acute septic monoarthritis. Organism detected by Gram stain of joint fluid in 25% and by culture in 50% in the second group

- Tenderness of thickened synovium is common but is not always present. Severely tender swelling suggests joint infection, haemarthrosis or an acute inflammatory reaction to crystals. Inflammation of entheses results in 'bony' tenderness at joint margins and sites of tendon or ligament insertion.
- Decreased range of movement is almost always demonstrable in a joint affected by synovitis or enthesitis. The degree to which passive and active joint mobility is reduced depends on a number of often interdependent factors (e.g. pain, size of effusion, periarticular muscle weakness or pain).

- Symptoms elicited by movement of a joint affected by synovitis or enthesitis include pain and stiffness, though neither may be specific. Reaching the end of (reduced) joint range, whether elicited passively or actively, invariably causes pain (though it should be noted that if any normal joint is forced through the end of range, pain can result).

Taking a history

Age, sex, and occupation

The age, sex, and occupation of the patient give non-specific but important clues in many cases:

- Oligoarthritis is uncommon in young adults. SpA, especially reactive arthritis, is likely to be the main cause.
- 75% of patients who develop reactive arthritis are <40 years old.
- Gout typically occurs in those >40 and is the commonest cause of inflammatory arthritis in men (self-reported in 1 in 74 men and 1 in 156 women).
- The mean age of patients with calcium pyrophosphate dihydrate (CPPD) arthritis is about 72 years (range 63–93 years).
- Forestry workers in areas endemic for tick infection with *Borrelia* are at risk of Lyme arthritis.

Which joints are affected?

Some processes are more common in certain joints than others:

- Shoulder synovitis is typical in hydroxyapatite arthritis (Milwaukee shoulder/knee syndrome) and AL amyloidosis.
- Involvement of a shoulder or hip is extremely unusual in gout.
- CPPD arthritis (as pseudogout) occurs rarely in the small finger joints.
- The knee is the commonest site of acute CPPD arthritis and is the site of about 50% of septic and the majority of gonococcal arthritis cases.
- Acute massive swelling of the knee is typical in Lyme arthritis and can occur with septic arthritis. Massive swelling of the knee can also occur in psoriatic arthritis but the history is usually chronic.
- There are many theoretical causes of synovitis in a single first MTPJ but the majority of cases are due to gout (50–70% of first attacks occur in this joint).

Preceding factors

Factors preceding swelling of a single joint or oligoarthritis may be highly relevant. These importantly include infection and trauma:

- Acute non-traumatic monoarticular synovitis is most commonly due to crystal-induced synovitis or associated with SpA.
- A preceding history of trauma typically suggests intra-articular fracture (?haemarthrosis), a meniscus tear (knee), or an intrarticular loose body such as an osteochondral fragment (?locking).
- Twinges of joint pain often precede an acute attack of gout (petit attacks). Acute arthritis occurs in 25% of patients with CPPD arthritis.
- In hydroxyapatite arthritis, synovitis is usually mild-to-moderate, gradual in onset and typically worse at night.
- An acute monoarthritis with fever in familial Mediterranean fever (FMF) is a mimic of septic arthritis. Such joint manifestations are a common (75% of cases) but not invariable feature of the disease.
- ⚠ Septic arthritis should always be considered (and promptly ruled out) as a cause of acute joint swelling (see Chapter 21).

Crystal arthritides

Crystal arthritides are associated with non-musculoskeletal conditions:

- Hyperuricaemia, causes of which include obesity, renal insufficiency, tumour lysis syndrome, myeloproliferative diseases, and haemolytic anaemia, is associated with gout.
- Hypertension and hypertriglyceridaemia are associated with gout.
- A history of renal stones (urate) may be a clue to hyperuricaemia and associated gout.
- Attacks of gout and CPPD arthritis can be precipitated by any non-specific illness, trauma and surgery. The commonest associated metabolic disorder is hyperparathyroidism (10% of cases).
- Though uncommon, hypomagnesaemia, hypophosphatasia (low ALP activity), haemochromatosis, Wilson's disease, and ochronosis are all associated with CPPD arthritis. The commonest cause of calcium oxalate crystal arthritis (rare) is dialysis-managed end-stage renal disease.

Link with infection

Many types of infection are linked to oligoarticular arthritis. Often a high index of suspicion is needed to make a link:

- Specific infections are directly (joint invasion) and indirectly ('autoimmune reaction') associated with joint synovitis.
- Viruses, bacteria, protozoa, helminthes, and fungi can all directly invade joints. The range of systemic features is wide and pathogens can cause both polyarticular and oligoarticular patterns of joint involvement.
- The infections recognized to trigger reactive arthritis are salmonella, *Yersinia*, *Shigella*, *Campylobacter* and *Chlamydia*. The development of reactive arthritis in those who acquire chlamydial (nongonococcal) urethritis is relatively uncommon (about 1 in 30).
- Acute HIV infection is associated with a subacute oligoarticular arthritis commonly involving knees and ankles.
- Chronic arthritis of any type, diabetes, immunodeficiency, and joint prostheses are risks for septic arthritis.
- Lyme disease should be considered a cause of oligoarthritis in patients with a history (weeks to years ago) of erythema chronicum migrans (macule/papule initially, expanding 0.5–1 cm/day to a mean diameter of 15 cm (range 3–68 cm) fading often without treatment in 3–4 weeks).
- Migratory arthritis is typical in untreated rheumatic fever; however, persistent monoarthritis is a common finding in treated patients.
- A history of circumcorneal eye redness with pain, photophobia, and blurred vision may be due to anterior uveitis most commonly associated with SpA but also sarcoid, Behçet's, and Whipple's disease.

Family and social history

There may be important clues from the family and social history:

- Both gout and SpA may be familial. Between 6–18% of patients with gout have a family history. There may be a family history of SpA or uveitis in patients who have reactive, psoriatic, or enteropathic arthritis or AS.
- Gout in young adults suggests an inherited abnormality (usually ↑ urate production from ↑ 5-phosphoribosyl-1-pyrophosphate synthetase activity, because the other enzyme deficiencies present in childhood).

- Excessive alcohol consumption is associated with gout. Alcohol can also contribute to lactic acidosis that inhibits urate breakdown.
- Consider Lyme disease if patients live, work, or visit endemic areas for infected ticks (within the northeast rural United States, Europe, Russia, China, and Japan). Peak incidence of infection is June/July.
- Brucellar arthritis is generally monoarticular and occurs primarily in areas where domesticated animals are infected and poor methods of animal husbandry, feeding habits, and hygiene standards coexist.

Ask about other (associated) features

Associated extra-articular features include previous eye, gastrointestinal, cardiac, and genitourinary symptoms:

- Low-grade fever, malaise, and anorexia occur commonly in both septic arthritis and gout. Marked fever can occur in gout and only occurs in about a third of patients with septic arthritis.
- Marked fever, hypotension and delirium can occur (rarely) in acute flares of CPPD arthritis.
- Ask about any current or previous features which might suggest SpA: back or buttock pain (enthesitis or sacoiliitis); swelling of a digit (dactylitis); plantar heel pain (plantar fasciitis); red eye with irritation (anterior uveitis); urethritis, balanitis, cervicitis or acute diarrhoea (reactive arthritis); psoriasis; symptoms of inflammatory bowel disease.
- Behçet's disease (see Chapter 18) is a cause of oligoarticular synovitis. Other features include painful oral and genital ulcers and uveitis.
- The involvement of > one joint does not rule out septic arthritis. In up to 20% of cases, multiple joints can become infected.

Examination

General

Review the features (see the beginning of this section) for which you're looking to confirm synovitis in a joint. Always compare sides.

- It is important to establish from the examination whether there is true synovial swelling. A history of swelling is not always reliable and other, non-synovial, pathology can present with single or oligoarticular joint pain. An example might be enthesial inflammation in SpA (though a joint effusion may coexist).

Examine the affected joints

Examine the affected joints for tenderness. Check the range of (passive) movement, for locking and instability:

- Acute processes such as crystal arthritis, infection and post-traumatic effusion often lead to a painful swelling, marked tenderness of swollen soft-tissues, and painfully restricted active and passive movement of the joint. These features are usually less overt with chronic arthritis.
- Instability of an acutely inflamed joint or tests for cartilage damage in the knee may be difficult to demonstrate. Further examination will be necessary after drainage of joint fluid/haemarthrosis.
- Detection of enthesis tenderness around the affected joints or at other sites is a useful clue to the underlying diagnosis of SpA.

Examine other musculoskeletal structures

- Examine the low back and typical sites of bony tenderness—sacroiliitis and enthesitis are common features of SpA.
- Tendonitis is not specific and can often occur in gout, CPPD arthritis, SpA, and gonococcal infection.
- Infection is not always monoarticular.

Look for skin rashes and any inflammation

Oligoarthritis may be part of a systemic inflammatory/infective condition.

- Temperature and tachycardia can occur with some non-infective causes of acute arthritis (e.g. crystal arthritis) though their presence in the context of oligoarticular joint swelling requires exclusion of joint infection.
- Gouty tophi may be seen in the pinnae but also anywhere peripherally. They can be difficult to discriminate clinically from rheumatoid nodules. PLM of material obtained by needle aspiration will be diagnostic for tophi.
- The hallmark of relapsing polychondritis is lobe-sparing, full thickness inflammation of the pinna.
- Mouth ulcers are a typical association of any illness; however, crops or large painful tongue and buccal lesions associated with oligoarticular arthritis suggest Behçet's disease.
- A typical site for the osteitis (tender swelling of bone) of SAPHO syndrome is around the sternum and clavicle.
- Skin erythema over a joint suggests crystal arthritis or infection.
- Associated skin rashes may include erythema nodosum (associated with ankle/knee synovitis in acute sarcoid), the purpuric pustular rashes of Behçet's, gonococcal infection (single pustules), and SAPHO syndrome, erythema marginatum (rheumatic fever), or the rare keratoderma blenhorragica (aggressive-looking rash of the sole of the foot in Reiter's disease).
- Psoriasis may be associated with both synovitis and enthesitis.

Investigations

Doubt about the presence of synovitis can be addressed by obtaining US or MR of the joint(s) in question. At larger joints, both are sensitive investigations for the detection of effusion and synovial thickening. Inflammation at periarticular or capsular entheses can be seen.

Joint aspiration

The most important investigation of a patient with monoarticular synovitis is joint aspiration and prompt examination of fluid. Fluid should be sent in sterile bottles for microscopy and culture:

- Synovial fluid appearances are not specific; however, blood or bloodstaining suggests haemarthrosis from trauma (including the aspiration attempt), a haemorrhagic diathesis, haemangioma, PVNS, synovioma, or occasionally CPPD arthritis.
- Turbidity (↓ clarity) of fluid relates to cellular, crystal, lipid, and fibrinous content and is typical in septic arthritis and acute crystal arthritis mainly owing to the number of polymorphonuclear (PMN) leucocytes.

- Cell counts give some diagnostic guidance but are non-specific (see Table 3.2). There is a high probability of infection or gout if the PMN differential is >90%.
- Joint fluid eosinophilia is not specific.
- Compensated PLM of fluid can discriminate urate (3–20μm in length, needle-shaped and negatively birefringent—blue and then yellow as the red plate compensator is rotated through 90°) and calcium-containing crystals such as calcium pyrophosphate (positively birefringent crystals, typically small and rectangular or rhomboid in shape).
- Lipid and cholesterol crystals are not uncommon in joint fluid samples but their significance is unknown.
- Crystals appearing in synovium less commonly but in typical settings include hydroxyapatite associated with Milwaukee shoulder (and knee) syndrome (alizarin red-S stain positive), calcium oxalate in end-stage renal failure on dialysis (may need scanning electron microscopy), cystine in cystinosis, and xanthine in xanthinosis.
- The presence of crystals in joint fluid does not exclude infection.
- The commonest causes of non-GC septic arthritis in Europe and North America are *Stapylococcus aureus* (40–50%), *Stapylococcus epidermidis* (10–15%), *Streptococcal* species (20%), and Gram-negative bacteria (15%).

Radiographs
Radiographs can confirm an effusion, show characteristic patterns of chondral and bone destruction (e.g. in infection or erosive gout) and can reveal intra-articular calcification associated with CPPD or hydroxapatite arthritis:

- If septic arthritis is suspected radiographs are essential. Patchy osteopenia and loss of bone cortex are cardinal signs.
- 'Punched-out' erosions (within joints or around metaphyses), soft tissue swellings (tophi), and patchy calcification are hallmarks of chronic gout.
- Intra-articular calcification may commonly be either chondrocalcinosis (fine linear or punctate fibrocartilage calcification) or larger loose bodies (often with prolific osteophytes)—both are associated with CPPD arthritis.
- Numerous regularly-shaped calcific masses in a joint may be due to synovial chondromatosis (commonest in middle-aged men, 50% of cases affecting the knee).
- The presence of erosions does not implicate RA. The arthritis may be 2° to an enthesitis associated with SpA.

Further imaging
Further imaging should be discussed with your radiologists:

- MR confirmation of traumatized structures such as meniscus damage in the knee and labral damage in the shoulder should be sought if suspected.
- MR can confirm synovitis, although appearances are usually nonspecific. Characteristic MR appearances of enthesitis and PVNS are recognized.

Table 3.2 Characteristics of joint fluid

Characteristic	Normal	Group I (non-inflammatory)	Group II (inflammatory)	Group III (septic)
Viscosity	Very high	High	Low	Variable
Colour	None	Straw	Straw or opalescent	Variable with organisms
Clarity	Clear	Clear	Translucent or opaque	Opaque
Leucocytes (cells/mm³)	200	200–2000	2000–50 000	>50 000
PMNs (%)	<25	25	Often >50	>75

Laboratory investigations to consider

- FBC/CBC, acute phase response (ESR, CRP). Neutrophilia is not specific for infection and can occur in crystal arthritis.
- Blood urea, electrolytes, creatinine and urate (e.g. hyperuricaemia and renal impairment associated with gout).
- Blood calcium, phosphate, albumin, ALP (±PTH), thyroid function tests and ferritin to screen for hyperparathyroid or thyroid disease or haemochromatosis associated with CPPD arthritis.
- Autoantibodies: RF may help to characterize an autoimmune process where synovitis is chronic. It is not specific for RA.
- Serum angiotensin converting enzyme (sACE) (i.e. sarcoid), IgM *Borellia burgdorferi* serology (?acute arthropathy or patients with history of migratory arthritis in Lyme disease).
- Antibodies to the streptococcal antigens streptolysin O (ASOT) DNAase B, hyaluronidase, and streptozyme in patients who have had sore throat, migratory arthritis, or features of rheumatic fever.

Synovial biopsy

- If there is a haemarthrosis or suspicion of PVNS, MR of the joint is wise before undertaking a biopsy to characterize the vascularity of a lesion.
- Consider a biopsy in the following situations: undiagnosed monoarthritis, suspicion of: sarcoid arthropathy, infection despite negative synovial fluid microscopy and cultures, gout despite failure to detect crystals in synovial fluid and amyloid (see below).
- Formalin fixation of samples is sufficient in most cases. Samples for PLM are best fixed in alcohol (urate is dissolved out by formalin). Snap freezing in nitrogen is essential if immunohistochemistry is required.
- Arthroscopic biopsy will yield more tissue than needle biopsy, it may add diagnostic information and joint irrigation can be undertaken.
- Congo red staining of synovium, ideally with PLM, should be requested if AA, AL, or β₂-microglobulin amyloid is a possibility. Typical situations are in myeloma (AL) and long-term dialysis patients (β₂-microglobulin). AA amyloid (in long-standing RA, AS, FMF, and Crohn's disease) is a rare though recognized complication of each condition.

Oligoarticular pains in children and adolescents

Background

Disease classification

There has been considerable debate as to the best way of classifying the autoimmune (non-infective, non-reactive) articular disorders in children. The following section aims to help you evaluate conditions that present with one or just a few inflamed joints. In 2001 a working group under the auspices of The International League of Associations for Rheumatology (ILAR) met to establish a consensus regarding classification criteria for paediatric and adolescent arthritides (see below). For a review of these new and old autoimmune arthritis classifications see below and Table 3.4 and under the relevant diagnostic headings in Chapter 7.

Important issues pertinent to children and adolescents

- Compared with the process with adults, it may be quite difficult to establish whether there is synovitis in a child's joint (see Table 3.3).
- An awareness of injurious and mechanical conditions that present at or around specific joints, notably at epiphyseal or apophyseal growth plates, is essential. Prompt investigation in hospital is essential.
- In very young children a history from both the child and parent or main carer is important. It is important to note that monoarticular or oligoarticular synovitis:
  - may present with limb pain
  - may not necessarily present with joint pain and stiffness
  - may result in non-use, altered use, or irritability, any of which may be the main or only complaint.
- Systemic juvenile idiopathic arthritis (JIA) (previously systemic onset juvenile chronic arthritis (JCA)) is proposed to be classified as arthritis preceded by or with daily recurring fever of >2 weeks' duration (documented for >3 days) plus one or more of: an evanescent, non-fixed, erythematous rash; generalized lymphadenopathy; enlarged liver or spleen; serositis.
- Persistent oligoarthritis is proposed to be defined by the involvement of no more than four joints throughout the disease course. Extended oligoarthritis affects a cumulative total of five joints or more after the first 6 months of disease. Excluded from each group will be those with: a family history of psoriasis (first- or second degree relative); a positive RF; HLA B27 (males >8 years old); systemic arthritis.

Table 3.3 The major causes of monoarticular/oligoarticular joint synovitis or swelling in children

Condition	Distinguishing features
Septic arthritis	Systemically unwell child. With TB—pulmonary disease, lower limb, insidious onset, and rapid joint destruction
Trauma	Direct blow/forced hyperextension, haemorrhage into joint
Foreign body synovitis	History of injury
PVNS	Recurrent joint haemarthrosis
Thalassaemia	Episodic and migratory arthritis
Malignancy	Acute monoarticular joint swelling, associated with leukaemia and neuroblastoma
Viral arthritis	Associated with rash or immunization
Lyme disease	Exposure in endemic area, rash, positive serology
Post-streptococcal	Sore throat, migratory arthritis, signs of rheumatic fever
FMF	Ethnic grouping and familial aggregation, acute febrile episode with chest/abdominal pain
Behçet's disease	Rare. Orogenital ulceration and skin rashes
Oligoarticular JIA	Monoarticular in 60% of cases and involves two joints in 31% of cases. Diagnosis of exclusion, associated with asymptomatic uveitis
Enthesitis-related arthritis	Usually age 8 or over, boys > girls, iritis, most have enthesitis, HLA B27. Sacroiliac joint involvement, low back stiffness
Psoriatic arthritis*	Rash, nail pitting, or other changes
Sarcoid	Usually associated with rash and ocular symptoms
Vasculitis	Rash, high ESR/CRP
SLE	UV-sensitive skin rash, ANA

* In the new ILAR classifications, psoriatic arthritis is distinguished from enthesitis-related arthritis (see below).

- It is proposed that, enthesitis be adopted to have a key-classifying role in the group of conditions previously classified as spondylarthropathy (SpA), now to be termed enthesitis-related arthritis (ERA).
- The definition of psoriatic arthritis will be broadened under the new ILAR classification (Table 3.4). Enthesitis, iritis and HLA B27 are absent from its proposed classification criteria: arthritis beginning before 16 years of age and either typical psoriasis or at least three of dactylitis, nail pitting, psoriasis-like rash, family history of psoriasis (first- and second-degree relatives). The definitions may be altered further.

Table 3.4 Proposed ILAR classification of arthritis in childhood (juvenile idiopathic arthritis)

ILAR classification of juvenile idiopathic arthritis (JIA)	Previous classification
Systemic arthritis*	Systemic onset JCA
Oligoarthritis* which is either: persistent (always 4 joints or less) extended (after 6 months >4 four joints affected)	Oligoarticular JRA Pauciarticular JCA
Polyarthritis (RF+)* 5 or more joints affected	Polyarticular JRA Polyarticular JCA (RF+)
Polyarthritis (RF−)	Polyarticular JCA (RF−)
Psoriatic arthritis*	Psoriatic arthritis
Enthesitis-related arthritis (ERA)*	SpA

JCA = juvenile chronic arthritis; JRA = juvenile rheumatoid arthritis; RF = rheumatoid factor.
* See text for notes.

Taking a history
Epidemiology
Recall epidemiological features associated with different groups and ages:
- The peak incidence of oligoarticular JIA (or pauciarticular JCA) is between the ages of 1 and 3. It is relatively very rare after 12 years of age.
- Enthesitis-related arthritis (ERA or SpA) is more common in boys (ratio up to 10:1) and typically occurs after the age of 8.
- Familial Mediterranean fever (FMF) can manifest in children as young as 1 year old. There is restriction to ethnic groups in Iraq, Turkey, Libya, Algeria, Morocco, and Tunisia and in Sephardic Jews, and familial aggregation. Acute or chronic oligoarthritis can occur.

Trauma?
Monoarticular synovitis may be associated with trauma:
- Time to onset of joint swelling after trauma (<2 h) and intensity of pain (severe) may help discriminate whether a haemarthrosis is present. Intra-articular fracture should then be suspected.
- An absence of a history of trauma does not rule out the possibility of osteochondritis dissecans (only 10% are associated with trauma).
- Be aware that non-accidental trauma can present with traumatic joint swelling.

Infection/malignancy
Infection and malignancy should be considered as it is a priority that they are ruled out in all cases of atraumatic monoarthritis:
- An insidious onset does not rule out infection. This pattern is well recognized in TB. Joint destruction, however, may not be insidious, therefore don't delay investigation.
- *Haemophilus influenzae* is the commonest cause of septic arthritis in children <5 years and *Staphylococcus aureus* in those >5 years.

- The commonest neoplastic causes of monoarticular joint swelling in children are leukaemia and neuroblastoma.

Rare causes of symptoms

The rarer causes of monoarticular synovitis, joint swelling, or pain, and joint-specific causes of pain in a single joint should be recalled at an early stage:

- Intra-articular haemangiomas, osteoid osteomas, synovial chondromatosis and lipomatosis arborescens can occur in most joints.
- Anterior knee pain in growing adolescents, commonly girls.
- Isolated hip pain conditions such as Perthes'.
- Oligoarticular JIA (Pauci-JCA) of the hip is very rare.
- Osteochondritides/avulsion fractures, e.g. Osgood–Schlatter's.
- Osteonecrosis at typical sites, e.g. tarsal navicular, carpal lunate.

Preceding symptoms

Ask about preceding symptoms of infection and rashes. Consider viral (including vaccinations), streptococcal and enteric infections, and Lyme disease:

- Oligoarthritis (or monoarthritis) may be a reaction to an infection and may be short-lived usually lasting 3–6 weeks, but occasionally up to 8 weeks.
- A streptococcal sore throat can lead on to a migratory arthritis. The differential diagnosis would include rheumatic fever and Lyme disease.
- The most distinctive features of acute rheumatic fever should be sought in patients with oligoarthritis, especially if it has been partially treated with aspirin or NSAIDs which can mask its migratory nature: carditis with prolonged PR interval, chorea, skin nodules, erythema marginatum.
- Salmonella, shigella, yersinia, and campylobacter enteric infections are associated with reactive arthritis.
- *Eschericia coli* and *Clostridium difficile* infections have the potential for triggering reactive arthritis.
- A facial rash occurs in rubella—coalescing erythema that clears as the limbs become affected, and with parvovirus B19 infection (erythema infectiosum—'slapped cheeks').
- Pink or faintly red erythema on the trunk or limbs but not the face is typical of erythema marginatum (rheumatic fever). The outer rash margin is often distinct and continuous. Firm, non-tender skin nodules, which may have regressed, may also suggest rheumatic fever.
- Lyme disease causes erythema chronicum migrans, a spreading erythema from a tick bite.
- Live attenuated rubella vaccines are associated, in up to 15% people, with subsequent joint/muscle symptoms. Arthritis may occur 2 weeks after the injection and clears in a week, but symptoms can remain for a year or so.

Family history

Ask about a history of illness in the family or a family history of enthesitis-related (SpA) features:

- In children suspected of having septic arthritis due to TB, establishing a history of contact with sources may be important.
- Owing to a link with HLA B27, there may be a history of similar musculoskeletal features in family members.

Examination

General principles of paediatric musculoskeletal examination

- Ensure that the child is comfortable in the environment, whilst changing, and with the people present at the time of examination.
- Reassure the child that the examination will not persist if it is painful.
- Observe small children playing at first.
- Try to leave the painful area until last.

Confirmation of synovitis/enthesitis in a joint

Review the features that help to confirm synovitis/enthesitis in a joint:

- It is important to establish from the examination whether there is true synovial swelling. Remember, a history of swelling is not always reliable and other, non-synovial, pathology can present with single or oligoarticular joint pain, e.g. enthesitis.
- Always compare sides. Even subtle differences in joint range may be important and denote synovial thickening.
- Doubt about synovial swelling can be addressed by obtaining US or MR.

Additional musculoskeletal examination

Additional musculoskeletal examination must include a search for muscle atrophy, tenosynovitis, enthesitis tenderness elsewhere, and spinal limitation:

- Adjacent muscle wasting may be a clue to the severity or chronicity of joint inflammation.
- Tenosynovitis is unusual in oligoarticular JIA but can occur in sarcoid, occasionally in ERA/SpA and in the polyarticular conditions.
- Enthesitis should discriminate between oligoarticular JIA and ERA/SpA. Commonly involved sites include Achilles, patellar tendon, and plantar fascia insertions.
- Clinical detection of spinal disease in patients who develop AS or ERA/SpA is not always possible at the time of presentation of the first musculoskeletal manifestations of the disease, i.e. enthesitis, although spinal examination assessing localized pain and impaired mobility should be done.

Look for skin rashes and any inflammation

Oligoarthritis may be part of a systemic inflammatory/infective condition. Look closely for skin rashes:

- Skin erythema overlying a joint suggests infection.
- Associated skin rashes may include erythema nodosum the purpuric pustular rashes of Henoch–Schönlein purpura (HSP) (extensive lower limb) or Behçet's (less florid than HSP), gonococcal infection (single pustules), SAPHO syndrome, erythema marginatum (rheumatic fever) and psoriasis.

Investigations

Although synovitis may be obvious clinically, its presence in any joint needs to be confirmed if there is doubt:

- The soft tissue appearances of joint radiographs are sufficient in confirming effusion and synovial thickening in many instances.
- US and MR can identify effusion and synovial thickening.

Joint aspiration

The most important investigation of a child with monoarticular synovitis is joint aspiration and prompt examination of fluid. Fluid should be sent in sterile bottles for microscopy and culture. This procedure may be psychologically traumatic. Discussion of the case with paediatric colleagues is wise. Consider using sedation (at least) in older children and a light general anaesthetic in younger ones:

- Synovial fluid appearances are not specific. Blood or bloodstaining suggests haemarthrosis from: trauma (including the aspiration), haemorrhagic diathesis, PVNS, synovioma, or haemangioma.
- Turbidity (↓clarity) of fluid relates to cellular, crystal, lipid, and fibrinous content and is typical in septic arthritis and acute crystal arthritis mainly owing to the number of PMNs.
- Crystals in synovial fluid in children are rare.
- The commonest causes of non-gonococcal septic arthritis in Europe and North America are *Staphylococcus aureus* (40–50%), *Staphylococcus epidermidis* (10–15%), streptococcal species (20%), and Gram-negative bacteria (15%). In children <5ys it is *Haemophilus influenzae*. Gonococcal infection should be considered a possibility in teenagers.

Radiographs

Radiographs can confirm an effusion and show characteristic patterns of chondral epiphyseal and bone destruction (e.g. in infection or malignancy):

- In septic arthritis osteopenia and loss of bone cortex are cardinal signs. The main differential diagnosis is malignancy.
- If calcified, loose bodies due to osteochondritis dissecans may be visible.
- The characteristics of tumours/tumour-like lesions can be determined and help decide whether further intervention is necessary.
- Erosions can occur in oligoarticular JIA or in ERA/SpA (enthesial).
- Discriminating erosions from ossifying cartilagenous epiphyses in normal joints (which can appear irregular) is sometimes difficult. Bilateral views are sometimes helpful in this respect.
- Joint space narrowing is difficult to confirm from radiographs because of normal changes in epiphyseal cartilage thickness, projectional errors, and difficulty in weight bearing on painful joints.
- Marked joint destruction is thought to occur primarily in those extending from oligoarticular to polyarticular JIA.

Further imaging

Further imaging should be discussed with your radiologist. US and scintigraphy can confirm synovitis and its pattern of joint involvement. CT and MR are useful in discriminating against the causes of synovitis:

- US is a very sensitive investigation for detection of synovitis and is particularly useful in evaluating the hip.
- US and MR can detect erosions earlier than radiographs.
- Where malignancy and infection are suspected bone scintigraphy is essential for identifying or ruling out additional osseous lesions.

- Because of its high sensitivity, bone scintigraphy can be useful in establishing whether significant bone/joint pathology is present in children with joint symptoms but few clinical findings.
- Bone scintigraphy has a low spatial resolution, thus abnormalities may need further investigation with CT or MR. Therefore, consideration should initially be given to whether the answer to all diagnostic questions can be achieved by proceeding directly to these investigations.
- In a normal joint MR differentiates all the major joint structures including epiphyses. Sedation may be needed in young children.
- MR is an accurate and sensitive tool for identifying joint and epiphyseal damage at an early stage of a disease process. This may be invaluable for example if there is any doubt about the status of oligoarticular JIA or peripheral joint involvement in ERA/SpA as early treatment can then be directed to prevent permanent deformities and disability.

Laboratory tests

Laboratory tests should provide or exclude evidence of infection, give discriminatory diagnostic information, and exclude non-rheumatic diseases:

- FBC/CBC, acute phase response (ESR, CRP). Neutrophilia is compatible with, but not specific for, infection. Monoarticular JIA can be associated with normal indices, however.
- A low platelet or white cell count but ↑ acute phase indices may be suggestive of an underlying malignancy.
- Antibodies to streptolysin O (ASOT) in patients who have had sore throat, migratory arthritis, or features of rheumatic fever. If there is persistent clinical suspicion despite a normal ASOT, antibodies to streptococcal DNAase B, hyaluronidase, and streptozyme may be positive.
- Autoantibodies: a single positive test for RF has little value. Repeatedly positive tests might suggest (RF+) JIA. ANAs are present in 40–75% of children with oligoarticular JIA (JCA). They are not disease-specific but identify a subset within it at particular risk of (often asymptomatic) ureitis.
- Other tests: sACE, Lyme serology (acute arthropathy or patients with history of migratory arthritis).

Synovial biopsy

- If there is a haemarthrosis or suspicion of PVNS, MR of the joint is wise before undertaking biopsy to characterize the vascularity of a lesion.
- Consider a biopsy in the following situations: undiagnosed monoarthritis, suspicion of: sarcoid arthropathy, infection despite negative synovial fluid microscopy and cultures, malignancy.
- Arthroscopic biopsy will yield more tissue than 'blind' needle biopsy. Direct viewing may add diagnostic information and joint irrigation can be undertaken.

Widespread pain in adults

Widespread (musculoskeletal) pain is a common reason for adults to seek medical advice (see Table 3.5). Many conditions are characterized by musculoskeletal symptoms, some of which may be diffuse or multicentric. In addition, the interpretation and reporting of symptoms varies considerably and can be a source of confusion.

Such patients are often referred to rheumatologists in health systems where there is 'gate-keeping' of referral to specialists by primary care physicians. A referral may be made with a working diagnosis in place: 'multiple joint pains, ?rheumatoid arthritis', for example, is a typical comment on such a letter.

In the following section we have aimed to review important aspects of the history, examination, and initial investigations in the diagnostic work-up of patients who present with non-localized, multicentric pains.

Background
Initial impressions
- Think broadly about possible diagnoses from reading any referral letter and whilst meeting the patient.
- Assimilate what you know about the epidemiology of likely conditions. For example, you might reason that the man you are about to see ('age 25 with joint pains') is more likely to have SpA rather than systemic lupus erythematosus (SLE), which occurs mostly in women age 14–50, or PMR which is a condition of the elderly, though joint pains can occur in all.

Age, sex, and racial background
What clues can be drawn from the age, sex, and racial background?
The degree to which these factors influence the likelihood of disease varies according to the background disease occurrence in the (local) population.
- Review what you know about the epidemiology of the major diseases and an appreciation of the limitations of the value of epidemiological data will help you avoid making poor judgements in your diagnostic work-up. Such simple information may prompt the recall of useful data. For example:
  - there is a very low incidence of ankylosing spondylitis (AS) in patients aged >65y with back and joint pains.
  - generalized OA is rare in young men.
  - with an incidence of <1 in a million autoimmune PM is rare compared with PMR which has an incidence of about 1 in 10 000 (age >50 years).
  - SLE is up to five times more common in Black than in White people.
  - osteomalacia occurring in temperate zone 'Western' populations is more likely in economically deprived than in affluent areas, in the institutionalized elderly than in young adults, and in some Asian ethnic groups rather than Caucasians.

Table 3.5 Broad categories of conditions that may present with widespread musculoskeletal pain

Common	Inflammatory polyarthritis (e.g. RA—see Chapter 5, SpA—see Chapter 8)
	Generalized (nodal) OA (see Chapter 6)
	Fibromyalgia/chronic pain syndromes (see Chapter 18)
	Non-specific myoarthralgia* associated with infection (e.g. viruses)
Less common	Myoarthralgia* 2° to autoimmune connective tissue disease
	Myalgia 2° muscle inflammation (e.g. polymyositis) (see Chapter 13)
	Myoarthralgia* associated with neoplasia (e.g. lymphoma)
	Skeletal metastases
	Polyostotic Paget's disease (see Chapter 16)
Rare	Metabolic bone diseases (e.g. osteomalacia, renal osteodystrophy) (see Chapter 16)
	Metabolic myopathies (e.g. hypokalaemia)
	Neurological disease (Parkinson's disease)

* In certain situations/conditions patients may complain of both muscle and joint pains. This is easily appreciated if you've ever had influenza! The combination of myalgia and arthralgia is summarized as myoarthralgia.

Previous diagnoses

Presenting features may be put in context early if you have knowledge of musculoskeletal associations of diagnoses that have already been made. For example:

- Synovitis in patients with (radiological) chondrocalcinosis.
- Arthropathy in patients with hyperparathyroidism and hypercalcaemia (see Chapter 16).
- Enthesitis/synovitis in patients with Crohn's disease or ulcerative colitis (see Chapter 8).
- Polyarticular synovitis and myalgia in patients with lymphoma.
- Crystal-induced or β_2-microglobulin deposition arthritis and osteodystrophy in chronic renal disease.

Taking a history

Firstly, establish whether pains arise from joints or tendons/entheses, muscles, bone, or are neurological (see Table 3.5).

- Though the patient or referral letter may report pains as 'joint pains', take care and time to establish where exactly you think the pains arise.
- Listen carefully to the description of the pains that may help discriminate whether the patient has a single condition or a number of causes for pains.

Obtain a detailed history of the pain at different sites

- A good history should give you the anatomical site of pains and should be able to reveal the tissue of origin in the majority of cases. For example, a 70-year-old man referred with 'widespread joint pains mostly in his legs', could have multiple weight-bearing joint OA or, perhaps, lumbosacral nerve root claudication symptoms. In a middle-aged woman with 'hand and neck pain', could the pain be radicular pain associated with cervical spondylosis, or does she have an arthropathy?
- Widespread pain due to bone pathology alone should always be considered and ruled out owing to the possibility of skeletal metastases. Bony pain is often unremitting, day and night. It changes little with changes in posture and movement.
- One pitfall is to assume that all pains arise from a single pathological process. For example, in a retired manual labourer is there PMR or RA causing shoulder, neck, and knee pain or are there different but common causes of the pains such as bilateral subacromial impingement, mechanical neck and upper limb radicular pain, and anterior knee pain owing to patellofemoral OA?

Joint pain at rest, after rest, or with joint use?

How do you establish whether pains arise from joints or tendons/entheses, and are likely to reflect a single process?

- Pain occurring with inflammation is conventionally regarded as being associated with stiffness and worse with immobility, e.g. on waking. It tends to be prominent in conditions such as RA, SpA, PMR, and myositis; however, mild degrees of immobility-associated pain and stiffness occur in some other conditions such as OA and fibromyalgia. Note that stiffness may be a feature of muscle spasm and soft-tissue oedema.
- Mechanical joint damage is also painful. This is typified in OA. Pain may be due to a number of changes in the joint but is usually prominent on weight bearing or use of the joint and rest often eases it.

Ask, and document in detail, which joints are affected

- A symmetrical polyarticular pattern of small joint synovitis is typical of, but not specific for, RA. RA can also present with carpal tunnel syndrome, tenosynovitis, tennis elbow, or an asymmetrical pattern of joint involvement, and can be preceded by a palindromic pattern of joint pain (see below).
- Chronic arthritis from parvovirus B19 infection may also be polyarticular and symmetrical.
- Small hand joint pain occurs in nodal generalized OA. DIPJs and PIPJs and thumb joints are usually affected. Patients often have pain in the spine, hips, and knees owing to changes of OA.
- The combination of sacroiliac (low back and buttock) pelvic, and lower limb joint/enthesis pain, typically in an asymmetrical oligoarticular pattern, is suggestive of SpA. Typical sites include anterior knee, posterior heel and inferior foot (plantar fascia).
- Enthesitis (as the hallmark of SpA) can affect the wrists and small joints of the hand and feet (plantar fascia origin and ?insertion at metatarsal heads) and may be difficult to distinguish from RA on clinical grounds alone.

- Large and medium-sized joints are typically affected in an inflammatory condition 2° to CPPD crystals, but a picture of multiple joint involvement similar to that in RA is possible (including tenosynovitis). CPPD arthritis primarily occurs in old age.
- Widespread arthralgia/arthritis occurs in patients with leukaemias, lymphoma and myeloma and with certain infections.

Ask about the pattern of joint symptoms over time

- A short, striking history of marked, acute polyarticular symptoms often occurs with systemic infection (see Table 3.6). Prominent malaise and fever should raise suspicion of infection.
- There might be a longer history than is first volunteered. Autoimmune rheumatic and connective tissue diseases may evolve over a period of time and often naturally relapse and remit, thus the distribution and severity of joint/tendon/muscle involvement may vary over time.
- Conventionally, persistent inflammatory joint symptoms should be present for at least 6 weeks before RA is diagnosed.
- Migratory arthralgia occurs in 10% of RA patients initially: a single joint becomes inflamed for a few days then improves and a different joint becomes affected for a few days and so on. A similar pattern can occur in post-streptococcal arthritis, occasionally in acute sarcoid, is not unusual before frank oligoarthritis develops in Lyme disease (see Chapter 17), and occurs in >60% of patients with Whipple's disease.
- The onset of enthesopathy may be insidious or acute—when it can be associated with marked extremity swelling.
- Recurrent pains from various musculoskeletal lesions, which have occurred either from injury or developed insidiously, are typical in patients with underlying hypermobility (benign joint hyper-mobility syndrome or other heritable diseases of connective tissue such as Ehlers–Danlos, see Chapter 16).

Is there widespread muscle pain?

If you think there is widespread muscle pain, remember to consider that:
- The myalgia may be fibromyalgia or enthesitis.
- Pain locating to muscle group areas may be ischaemic in origin or 2° to neurological disease and not necessarily due to inherent muscle pathology.
- The differential diagnosis of PM and dermatomyositis (DM) is wide though many conditions are rare (see Table 3.7 and Chapter 13).

Ask about the distribution and description of myalgia and weakness

- PMR (rare <50 years), myositis and endocrine/metabolic myopathies typically affect proximal limb and truncal musculature but PMR is also associated with inflammatory polyarthritis and giant cell arteritis (GCA) and therefore may present with headache (for example). In PMR, muscles may characteristically be described as 'stiff ' on waking (see Chapter 14).
- Though rare, truncal muscle pain and stiffness can be a presenting feature of Parkinson's disease.
- Cramp-like pains may be a presenting feature of any myopathy (e.g. hypokalaemic) or even motor neuron disease. However, some

patients may interpret radicular (nerve root) pains as 'cramp-like' and therefore explain their presence in a muscular distribution.

- Inflammatory and endocrine/metabolic myopathies are not always painful.
- True weakness may denote either myopathy or a neurological condition. However, patients may report a feeling of weakness if muscles are painful, therefore, rely more on your examination before deciding muscles are weak.
- Occasionally some genetic muscle diseases (e.g. myophosphorylase, acid maltase deficiency), can present atypically late (in adults) with progressive weakness which may be mistaken for PM.

Ask about the pattern of muscle pains over time

- Severe, acute muscle pain occurs in a variety of conditions. The commonest causes are viral, neoplastic, and drugs. Some toxic causes may result in rhabdomyolysis, myoglobinaemia, and renal failure.
- Usually PM/DM is characterized by slowly evolving but progressive muscle pain and weakness (weeks to months).
- In severe, acute presentations consider also the rare eosinophilic fasciitis or eosinophilic-myalgia syndrome (toxic reaction to L-tryptophan).
- Low-grade episodic muscle pains may denote a previously undisclosed hereditary metabolic myopathy.
- Fibromyalgia is chiefly a chronic pain syndrome and symptoms may have been present for a considerable time at presentation.

Are the pains ischaemic?

- Lay persons may have little concept of ischaemia and might describe their symptoms in the context of muscles and in a muscular distribution.
- Ischaemic muscle pain often occurs predictably in association with repeated activity and eases or resolves on rest. Consider this especially if pains are confined to a single limb or both legs.
- The distribution of pains may give clues as to sites of underlying pathology, e.g. upper limbs in subclavian artery stenosis or thoracic outlet syndrome or, typically, thighs and calves in atherosclerotic vascular disease or lumbosacral spine/lumbar nerve root stenosis. Sitting forward may relieve the latter.
- Ischaemic pains in the context of a rash may suggest systemic vasculitis.

Table 3.6 Common infections that can present with acute polyarthritis and a raised acute phase response

Infection	Common extra-articular clinical features	Key laboratory diagnostic tests in acute infection
Rheumatic fever (group A β-haemolytic streptococci)	Acute infection 1–2 weeks earlier, fever, rash, carditis	Positive throat swab culture. High ASOT (in 80%). Anti-DNAaseB IgM
Post-streptococcal (?rheumatic fever)	Acute infection 3–4 weeks earlier, tenosynovitis	As above
Parvovirus B19 (adults[†])	Severe flu-like illness at onset, various rashes	Anti-B19 IgM
Rubella (also post-vaccine)	Fever, coryza, malaise, brief rash	Culture. Anti-rubella IgM
Hepatitis B	Fever, myalgia, malaise, urticaria, abnormal liver function	Bilirubin+, ALT+, AST+, anti-HBsAg, anti-HBcAg
Lyme disease (Borrelia burgdorferi)	Tick bites, fever, headache, myalgias, fatigue, nerve palsies	Anti-Bb IgM (ELISA + immunofluorescence)
Toxoplasma gondii	Myositis, parasthesias	Anti-Toxo IgM

Even if serological tests have high sensitivity and specificity, the positive predictive value of the test is low if the clinical likelihood of the infection is low. Therefore, do not use serological tests indiscriminately.

ASOT = anti-streptolysin O titre.

[†] The presentation of parvovirus B19 illness may be quite different in children.

Widespread pain may be due to bone pathology

- Bone pains are unremitting and disturb sleep. They could denote serious pathology—radiographic and laboratory investigations will be important.
- The major diagnoses to consider include disseminated malignancy, multiple myeloma, metabolic bone disease (e.g. renal osteodystrophy, hyperparathyroidism, osteomalacia) and polyostotic Paget's disease.

Past medical history

Specific questions are often required because previous problems may not be regarded as relevant by the patient. For example:

- For those with joint pains a history of the following may be of help: other autoimmune disease (↑ risk of RA, SLE, etc.); Raynaud's phenomenon (association with scleroderma, RA, and SLE); dry eyes (possible Sjögren's syndrome); uveitis or acute 'red eye' (association with SpA); recurrent injuries/joint dislocations (association with hypermobility); genital, urine, or severe gut infection (link with SpA); psoriasis (association with SpA); diabetes (cheirarthropathy).
- For those in whom myalgia/myositis seems likely: preceding viral illness (possible viral myositis); foreign travel (?tropical myositis); other auto-immune disease (associated with PM/DM); previous erythema nodosum, i.e. previous sarcoid (cause of myositis); drugs and substance abuse (see below).
- For all patients: weight loss or anorexia (association with malignancy); temperatures or night sweats (association with infection); sore throat (possible post-streptococcal condition); persistent spinal pain (association with fibromyalgia); rashes (association with Lyme disease, SLE, DM, vasculitis).
- For those with widespread bony pain: history of rickets (association with privational osteomalacia); chronic renal disease (will precede renal osteodystrophy and may predispose to osteoarticular deposition of β_2-microglobulin and crystal arthritides).

Psychosocial and sexual history

- Preceding sexual contact and genital infection is important primarily because of an association of *Chlamydia trachomatis* infection with reactive arthritis and enthesitis/SpA (see Chapter 8).
- Reactive arthritis has an association with seropositivity of HIV. HIV can itself cause acute PM and is a risk factor for pyomyositis.
- There is an association of anxiety and depression with fibromyalgia (see Chapter 18).

Ask about travel

- Residence in, or travel to, rural areas populated by deer might be important in indicating a risk of exposure to *Borrelia burgdorferi* and contracting Lyme disease (the spirochaete is carried by ticks which colonize deer, boar, and other animals and bite other mammals).
- *Plasmodium falciparum* (intertropical areas), trypanosoma (mainly South America), trichinella, and cystercerciae infections are associated with myalgia/myositis.

Table 3.7 The major causes of myopathies and conditions associated with diffuse myalgia (see also Chapter 13.)

Infectious myositis	Viruses (e.g. influenza, hepatitis B or C, coxsackie, HIV, HTLV-I)
	Bacteria (e.g. *Borrelia burgdorferi* (Lyme))
	Other (e.g. malaria toxoplasmosis)
Endocrine and metabolic	Hypo/hyperthyroidism, hypercortisolism, Hyperparathyroidism
	Hypocalcaemic, hypokalaemic
Autoimmune diseases	Polymyositis, dermatomyositis, SLE, scleroderma, Sjögren's, RA, PMR
	Vasculitis (e.g. PAN, Wegener's granulomatosis, rheumatoid)
	Myasthenia gravis
	Eosinophilic fasciitis
Carcinomatous myopathy	
Idiopathic	Fibromyalgia (muscles should not be weak)
	Inclusion body myositis
	Sarcoid myositis
	Eosinophilic-myalgia (L-tryptophan-induced)
Drugs	Lipid-lowering drugs (e.g. lovastatin, clofibrate, gemfibrozil, niacin)
	Anti-immune (e.g. colchicine, CyA, D-Pca*)
	Rhabdomyolysis (e.g. alcohol, opiates)
	Others (e.g. AZT chloroquine*)
Muscular dystrophies	Limb girdle, fascioscapulohumeral
Congenital myopathies†	Mitochondrial myopathy
	Myophosphorylase deficiency Lipid storage diseases

*Drugs most likely to cause painful myopathy.

†Owing to variable severity, some conditions may not present until adulthood.

Note: Guillain–Barré and motor neuron disease may be considered in the differential diagnosis of non-painful muscle weakness.

Family history

Ask about family with arthritis or autoimmune diseases:

- There is an hereditary component to large joint and generalized nodal OA and hyperuricaemia/gout.
- The risk of developing any autoimmune condition is higher in families of patients with autoimmune diseases than generally.

Drug history
- The following drugs have been reported, amongst others, to cause a myopathy (those marked * are more likely to be painful): lithium, chloroquine*, clofibrate, statins, salbutamol, penicillin, colchicine, D-penicillamine*, sulphonamides, hydralazine, cyclosporin, phenytoin, cimetidine* (muscle cramps), zidovudine, carbimazole, and tamoxifen.
- The myositis occurring with D-penicillamine is not dose- or cumulative dose-dependent. It can be life threatening.
- Drug-induced SLE, which is characterized commonly by arthralgia, aching, and malaise, and less commonly by polyarthritis, can occur with a number of drugs including hydralazine, procainamide, isoniazid, and minocycline. Quinidine, labetalol, captopril, phenytoin, methyldopa, and sulphasalazine are among others that probably cause the condition.
- L-tryptophan, which has been available as a health food supplement in some countries, has been implicated in causing eosinophilia-myalgia syndrome.
- Mild myoarthralgia may be caused by a number of commonly used drugs, e.g. proton pump inhibitors and quinolone antibiotics.
- Alcohol in excess and some illegal drugs are associated with severe toxic myopathy occasionally resulting in rhabdomyolysis (see Table 3.7).

Ask about chest pain, dyspnoea, palpitations, cough, and haemoptysis
- Cardiac abnormalities are features of autoimmune rheumatic and connective tissue diseases, though infrequent at initial presentation. Cardiac infection is associated with widespread aches and pains (e.g. rheumatic fever/post-streptococcal myoarthralgia, infective endocarditis).
- Chronic effort-related dyspnoea 2° to interstitial lung disease occurs in many patients with autoimmune connective tissue and rheumatic diseases. Up to 40% of RA patients may have CT evidence of lung fibrosis. In the majority of fairly sedentary patients, however, symptoms are not prominent. Dyspnoea may be present at presentation.
- Ventilatory failure and aspiration pneumonia (?postural/nocturnal cough) can occur as a result of a combination of truncal striated, diaphragmatic, and smooth muscle weakness in PM.
- There is an association between bronchiectasis and RA.
- The commonest neoplasm in patients diagnosed with carcinomatous myositis is of the lung.

Ask specifically about dysphagia, abdominal pain, and diarrhoea
- Patients may have overlooked volunteering abdominal and gut symptoms especially if symptoms have resolved. There are many links between bowel disease and polyarthralgia/polyarthritis.
- Ask specifically about previous severe diarrhoeal or dysenteric illnesses, which due to *Campylobacter, Yersinia, Shigella,* or *Salmonella,* may be relevant to diagnosing reactive arthritis/SpA.
- Gut smooth muscle may be affected in PM and give rise to dysphagia and abdominal pain.

Examination

In patients with widespread pain a full medical examination is always necessary.

Skin and nails (see Chapter 4)

In all patients look carefully at the skin and nails:

- Nails may show prominent ridges or pits in psoriatic arthropathy (be suspicious of a previous diagnosis of fungal disease), splinter haemorrhages in infective endocarditis, rheumatoid vasculitis or antiphopholipid syndrome (APS), or periungual erythema.
- Skin rashes in conditions characterized by widespread pain. For example:
  - erythema migrans in Lyme disease
  - erythema marginatum in rheumatic fever
  - UV sensitive rash on face/arms in SLE
  - violacious rash on knuckles/around eyes/base of neck in DM
  - livedo reticularis in SLE and APS
  - purpuric rash in vasculitis (e.g. HSP)
  - erythema nodosum in sarcoidosis.
- Lymphadenopathy may be present with either infection or inflammation and is non-specific. However, if prominent it may denote lymphoma.
- Signs of anaemia are a non-specific finding in many chronic systemic autoimmune diseases.
- Clubbing of the digits may be present in Crohn's disease and ulcerative colitis (associated with SpA) and bronchiectasis (associated with RA).
- Oedema can occur in both upper and lower limb peripheries in a subset of patients presenting with inflammatory polyarthritis/ tenosynovitis. The condition has been termed RS$_3$PE (remitting seronegative symmetrical synovitis with pitting edema). This condition is striking in that it occurs suddenly, often in patients between 60–80 years old and is very disabling. It may be associated with other conditions e.g. haematologic, malignancy.

Examination of the joints

Important points to note when examining joints (detailed examination techniques that help discriminate synovitis from other pathology at specific joints are included in sections in Chapter 2).

- Each joint should be examined in comparison with its symmetrical partner, firstly by observation, then palpation, then by its active and passive range.
- Useful examination tools include a tape measure for recording swelling (circumferential) and a goniometer (protractor with arms) for measuring the range of joint movement.

Patterns of abnormality

Note the specific cause of joint swelling and site of tenderness, distribution of affected sites, and hypermobility

- In nodal generalized OA, osteophytes (bony swelling—may be tender) can be noted at DIPJs (Heberden's nodes) and PIPJs (Bouchard's nodes). Periosteal new bone at sites of chronic enthesitis may be palpable and tender.

- Nodules may occur in nodal OA, RA, polyarticular gout, multicentric reticulohistiocytosis (see Plate 16) or hyperlipidaemia (xanthomata).
- Soft tissue swelling with tenderness and painful restriction of the joint on movement suggests inflammatory arthritis. There is often adjacent muscle wasting. This is most easily appreciated in the interossei in small hand joint arthritis or quadriceps in knee arthritis.
- The 'painful joints' may be inflamed tendons or entheses. Tender tendon insertions and periarticular bone tenderness, often without any joint swelling, may denote enthesis inflammation associated with SpA.
- Tendonitis may be part of many autoimmune rheumatic or connective tissue diseases. Look specifically for thickening of the digital flexors and swelling of the dorsal extensor tendon sheath in the hand, and tenderness/swelling of both peroneal and posterior tibial tendons in the foot.
- Gross swelling with painful restriction of small joints is unusual in SLE. Often there is little to find on examination of joints.
- General joint hypermobility may account for, or contribute to, joint and other soft tissue lesions. An examination screen for hypermobility (see Chapter 16) may be helpful (see Table 3.8). Check also for associated features.

Examination of patients with widespread myalgia

- Check for muscle tenderness and weakness. Document the distribution. Is there evidence of neurological or vascular disease?
- As it is common, the characteristic sites of tenderness in fibromyalgia should be confidently recognized (see Fig. 3.1). Despite discomfort, muscles should be strong.
- Examine the strength of both truncal and limb muscle groups (see Fig. 3.2). In the presence of pain it may be difficult to demonstrate subtle degrees of muscle weakness.
- Patterns of muscle weakness are not disease specific; however, there are some characteristic patterns: symmetrical proximal limb and truncal in PM/DM; quadriceps and forearm/finger flexors in inclusion body myositis; limb muscles in mitochondrial myopathy. (Note: using specific apparatus metrologists or physiotherapists can help document isometric muscle strength in certain muscle groups.)
- Muscles in PMR are not intrinsically weak.
- Muscle wasting is not specific. It does not occur in fibromyalgia alone. If wasting is profound and associated with a short duration consider neoplasia. Wasting will occur in most long-standing myopathies.
- Check for ↑ limb tone and rigidity—most evident by passive movement at a joint—consistent with extrapyramidal disease. There may be resting tremor in the hand, facial impassivity, and 'stiff' gait. Muscular tone in the limbs may also be ↑ in motor neuron disease (MND); however, if presenting with muscle pains, the patient with MND is more likely to have a lower motor neuron pattern of neuronal loss (progressive muscular atrophy) with muscular weakness/wasting, flaccidity, and fasciculation.
- Diagnostic testing for fatiguability in myasthenia (strictly) requires an examination before and after a placebo-controlled, double-blind injection of an anticholinesterase.

Table 3.8 Features of the benign joint hypermobility syndrome (BJHS). See also p.486, for new 'Brighton' criteria.

Examination screen (scored out of 9)	Ability to extend fifth finger >90° at MCPJ (score 1 + 1 for R + L)
	Ability to abduct thumb (with wrist flexion) to touch forearm (score 1 + 1)
	Extension of elbows >10°(1 + 1)
	Extension of knees >10°(1 + 1)
	Ability to place hands flat on floor when standing with knees extended (1)
Associated features	Prolonged arthralgia
	Skin striae, hyperextensibility, and abnormal scarring
	Recurrent joint dislocations
	Varicose veins
	Uterine/rectal prolapse
	Recurrent soft-tissue lesions
	Marfanoid habitus (span > height)
	Eye signs: drooping eyelids, myopia, down-slanting eyes

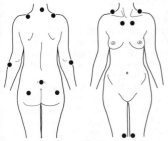

- Tenderness of skin overlaying trapezius
- Low cervical spine
- Midpoint of trapezius
- Supraspinatus
- Pectoralis, maximal lateral to the second costochondral junction
- Lateral epicondyle of the elbow
- Upper gluteal area
- Low lumbar spine
- Medial fat pad of the knee

Fig. 3.1 Typical sites of tenderness in fibromyalgia (see also p.486)

- Muscle pains/cramps owing to large-vessel ischaemia are likely to be non-tender at rest and strong. Demonstrate absent pulses and bruits and substantiate findings with US Doppler examination.
- In suspected cases of PM/DM examine carefully for cardiorespiratory abnormalities. Other associated signs in DM include periungual erythema/telangiectasias, erythematous violacious rash and skin calcinosis; include dysphonia and swallowing abnormalities in both PM and DM.
- Because of its associations (see Table 3.7), patients with myositis should be carefully examined for the following signs: dry eyes/mouth (Sjögren's—see Chapter 11), skin thickening/tenderness or discoloration (scleroderma—see Chapter 12), skin rashes (SLE—see Chapter 9), thyroid tenderness/enlargement (endocrine myopathy).

Investigations

General points

- ESR and CRP may be raised in either infection or autoimmune connective tissue or rheumatic diseases. A slightly ↑ ESR is a common finding in healthy elderly people.
- ANA may occur in association with many autoimmune conditions, in other diseases (see Table 3.9) and in some healthy people. It is, therefore, not diagnostic for SLE or any single condition; however, high-titre ANA is often significant and, from a converse perspective, SLE without ANA is rare (immunofluorescence on Hep2 cells).
- RF is not specific for RA. Testing for it will result in little helpful diagnostic information as 1 in 6 people with any infection or an inflammatory condition produce detectable RFs.
- Controversy exists about the diagnosis of fibromyalgia. It is prudent only to make a diagnosis of fibromyalgia in the presence of normal ESR/CRP, FBC (CBC), urea, electrolytes, liver function, and thyroid function tests and if enthesitis can be confidently excluded. Blood calcium, phosphate, serum immunoglobulins and protein electrophoresis may reasonably be added to this list.

Basic tests in patients with polyarthropathy

- Urinalysis (dipstick) may show proteinuria or haematuria. Both glomerular and tubular damage are possible. Glomerulonephritis (in SLE, vasculitis, or endocarditis for example) is usually associated with significant proteinuria (quantified from a 24h urine collection). These patients will need urgent specialist attention.
- ESR and CRP are often raised in autoimmune rheumatic/connective tissue diseases though are non-specific and may be normal in the early stages of these conditions. If very high (e.g. ESR >100) be suspicious of infection or malignancy. ESR >50 is one diagnostic criterion of giant cell arteritis. ESR ↑ slightly in OA but is usually normal. There is often no evidence of an acute phase response in patients with enthesitis (even though pain and bony tenderness may be widespread). FBC (CBC): a mild normochromic normocytic anaemia often accompanies autoimmune connective tissue or rheumatic diseases (e.g. RA, SLE, PMR) infections and malignancy.
- Throat swab, ASOT, anti-DNAaseB antibodies (post-streptococcal condition).

(a) **Functional**

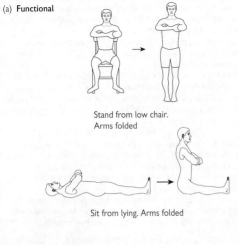

Stand from low chair.
Arms folded

Sit from lying. Arms folded

(b) **Specific resisted**

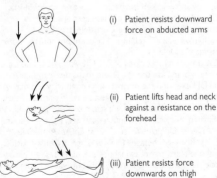

(i) Patient resists downward
force on abducted arms

(ii) Patient lifts head and neck
against a resistance on the
forehead

(iii) Patient resists force
downwards on thigh

Fig. 3.2 Screening examination for proximal myopathy. (a) Functional movements
requiring truncal and proximal lower limb muscle strength. (b) Resisted movement
testing of deltoid (i), longitudinal flexors of the neck (ii), and iliopsoas/quadriceps
(iii) strength

- Other simple blood tests which should be considered given appropriate clinical evidence for the relevant disease: random blood sugar (diabetes); TFTs/thyroid antibodies (hyper/hypothyroidism); LFTs, prostatic specific antigen (malignancy).
- Joint fluid aspiration and culture is mandatory for patients in whom sepsis is a possibility. Fluid should be examined by PLM in suspected cases of crystal-induced synovitis.
- Testing serum for extractable nuclear antigens (ENAs) may be useful for characterizing the type of autoimmune process. None should be considered alone to be diagnostic or specific for any disease, although diagnostic information is available from certain positive or negative associations.
- Radiographs. In many patients presenting with a short history of widespread joint pains, radiographs may be normal. An early sign of joint inflammation is periarticular osteopenia, though this will not be specific, for example, for RA. Recognized types of erosions and their distribution can be noted by experienced radiologists in specific conditions (e.g. RA, psoriatic arthritis, gout).
- Referral to a sexual health clinic for further detailed investigations if there is a suggestion of recent or recurrent genital infection may help to strengthen the evidence for a diagnosis of reactive arthritis.

Basic laboratory tests in patients with widespread muscle pain/weakness

- Dipstick urinalysis: to screen for haematuria or myoglobinuria.
- FBC (CBC) and measures of acute-phase response.
- An endocrine and metabolic screen: urea/electrolytes, creatinine, thyroxine, TSH, blood calcium, phosphate and 25-hydroxyvitamin D, LFTs.
- Elevated CK occurs in most cases of PM. CK, ALT, AST, LDH, are non-specific markers of muscle damage. Note that specific muscle isoenzymes of CK and LDH exist and the normal range of all enzymes may vary in different populations probably mainly as a function of muscle bulk (e.g. Afro-Caribbean > Caucasian). Muscle enzymes may be elevated after non-inflammatory causes of muscle damage, e.g. exercise/trauma.
- Check for ANA and, if positive, screen for ENAs. Antibodies to certain (cytoplasmic) tRNA synthetases (e.g. Jo-1) are myositis-specific.
- All of the above tests may reasonably be done in cases where you think muscle pains are due to fibromyalgia but want to rule out other pathology.
- Think of checking for urinary myoglobin in cases where acute widespread muscle pain may be associated with excessive alcohol or ingestion of certain drugs (cocaine, amphetamines, ecstasy, heroin), exercise, or trauma. Patients will be at risk of renal failure.
- PM can be the presenting feature of HIV disease thus consider testing HIV serology. In HIV-positive patients, infections causing muscle disease include TB and microsporidia.
- Viral myositis is often clinically indistinguishable from PM. On occasions serology and PCR of muscle tissue/inflammatory cells may reveal diagnostic clues.

Table 3.9 Examples of the prevalence of antinuclear antibodies (ANA) in some diseases using Hep2 cells as substrate

Population group		Prevalence of ANA
Normal population		8%
SLE		95%
Other autoimmune rheumatic diseases	Systemic sclerosis	90%
	Sjögren's syndrome	80%
	Rheumatoid arthritis	60%
	Polymyositis	40%
	Polarteritis nodosa	18%
Other diseases	Chronic active hepatitis	100%
	Drug-induced lupus	100%
	Myasthenia gravis	50%
	Waldenstrom's macroglobulinaemia	20%
	Diabetes	25%

Electrophysiology and imaging in patients with muscle conditions

- Electromyographic abnormalities occur in two-thirds of patients with muscle inflammation. More information is likely if studied in the acute rather than the chronic phase of the illness. In the acute condition denervation and muscle degeneration give rise to fibrillation potentials in 74% of PM and 33% of DM patients. Other features include: low-amplitude short-duration motor unit and polyphasic potentials.
- Electromyography is poor at discriminating on-going muscle inflammation in myositis from steroid-induced myopathy.
- There are characteristic MR patterns of abnormality in PM/DM. Images can be used to identify potential muscle biopsy sites to avoid false-negative results associated with patchy muscle inflammation.

Muscle biopsy

- With sizeable tissue samples from affected muscle and the judicious application of a range of laboratory techniques, important diagnostic information can be provided. Differential diagnosis needs to be discussed with the pathologist whilst planning the biopsy.
- Myositis may be patchy and biopsy may miss affected muscle. MR is sensitive in identifying areas of muscle inflammation.
- In PM inflammatory infiltrates predominate in the endomysial area around muscle fibres without perifascicular atrophy. In DM inflammation is more prominent in the perimysial area and around small blood vessels and there is typically perifascicular atrophy.
- Routine tests do not reliably distinguish PM from cases of viral myositis. Some of the glycogenoses will become obviously apparent from light microscopy of biopsy material.

Investigations for malignancy

Investigations in adults with widespread bony pain should aim to rule out malignancy, particularly myeloma and 2° malignancies from breast, renal and prostate cancers:

- Investigations may include: breast US/mammography/MR, urine cytology, PSA, renal US, serum and urinary protein electrophoresis.
- Hypercalcaemia may accompany these conditions, thus check blood calcium, phosphate and albumin (also PTH).
- PTH should also be checked in suspected cases of osteomalacia (raised 2° to calcium/vitamin D deficiency) together with 25-hydroxyvitamin D levels (low or low/normal), ALP (high/normal), and 24h urinary calcium (low).
- Radiographs of affected sites are important. Include a CXR.
- Bone scintigraphy can identify sites of neoplasia, Paget's disease, polyostotic osteoporosis or osteomalacia (see Plate 17), but although characteristic patterns exist, it is generally not specific for any condition.
- Bone biopsy (maintained undecalcified by placing sample in 70% alcohol) of affected sites will be diagnostic in some, but not all, cases of osteomalacia, osteoporosis, renal osteodystrophy, malignancy, and Paget's disease as good samples are hard to obtain. The best samples are obtained from a transiliac biopsy. Bone marrow can be aspirated for examination at the same time.

Widespread pain in children and adolescents

Background

Disease classification

A working party, under the auspices of The International League of Associations for Rheumatology (ILAR) met in 2001 to establish a consensus about a unifying classification of arthritis in childhood termed juvenile idiopathic arthritis (JIA). A comparison of old and new classification is shown in Table 3.10. For a details of each condition see relevant diagnostic headings in Chapter 7.

- Systemic JIA (previously systemic onset JCA) is proposed to be classified as arthritis preceded by or with daily recurring fever of >2 days (documented for >3 days) plus one or more of: an evanescent, non-fixed, erythematous rash; generalized lymphadenopathy; enlarged liver or spleen; serositis.
- Persistent oligoarthritis is defined by the involvement of no more than four joints throughout the disease course. Extended oligoarthritis affects a cumulative total of five joints or more after the first 6 months of disease. Excluded from each group will be those with: a family history of psoriasis (first- or second-degree relative); a positive RF; HLA B27 (male >8 years of age); systemic arthritis.
- The definition of psoriatic arthritis will be broadened under the new ILAR classification. The definitions may be altered further.
- It is proposed that enthesitis be adopted to have a key-classifying role in the group of conditions previously classified as SpA.

Assess the distribution of the pain(s)

Are the pains in a joint distribution? What is their pattern?

- Arthralgias may accompany any infection. In this (common) scenario they are short-lived. Persistent (>6 weeks) joint pains raise the possibility of many other diseases (see Table 3.11).
- Post-streptococcal arthralgias are often migratory. Skin overlying joints often appears red in acute rheumatic fever but not in systemic JIA (systemic onset JCA).
- The presentation of polyarticular JIA (RF+ or RF−) is often profound with several weeks' history of worsening joint stiffness and swelling.
- Stiffening is a prominent associated feature of the joint pain in both (RF+) and (RF−) polyarticular JIA.

Table 3.10 Proposed ILAR classification of arthritis in childhood (juvenile idiopathic arthritis)

ILAR classification of JIA	Previous classifications
Systemic arthritis*	Systemic onset JCA
Oligoarthritis* which is either: persistent (always 4 joints or less) extended (after 6 months >4 four joints affected)	Oligoarticular JRA Pauciarticular JCA
Polyarthritis (RF+)* 5 or more joints affected	Polyarticular JRA Polyarticular JCA (RF+)
Polyarthritis (RF–)	Polyarticular JCA (RF–)
Psoriatic arthritis*	Psoriatic arthritis
Enthesitis-related arthritis*	SpA

JCA = juvenile chronic arthritis; JRA = juvenile rheumatoid arthritis; RF = rheumatoid factor.
* See text for notes.

Table 3.11 The differential diagnosis of (RF–) JIA

Infection (multiple sites in immunodeficiency)	*Staphylococcus* septic arthritis
	Haemophilus influenzae septic arthritis
Reactive to an infectious agent	Parvovirus B19, hepatitis, rubella, rubella vaccination
	Post-streptococcal, rheumatic fever
Autoimmune connective tissue disorders	SLE
	MCTD, overlap syndromes
	Poly/dermatomyositis
Systemic vasculitis syndromes	Kawasaki disease (young child, high fever, desquamating extremity rash)
	Polyarteritis nodosa
	Wegener's granulomatosis
	HSP, Behçet's disease, Familial Mediterranean fever
Sarcoid arthritis (polyarthritis, rash, uveitis)	
Haematological disorders	Sickle cell disease
	Constitutional bleeding disorders
	Acute leukaemia (bone and joint pain)
Other causes	Chronic recurrent multifocal osteomyelitis
	Diabetic cheiroarthropathy

Taking a history

Are the pains myalgic or are they in a muscle distribution?

Differential diagnosis is wide (see Table 3.12):

- Acute viral myositis is distinguished from chronic myositis by its localization to calf muscles, severe pain, and its resolution within 4 weeks.
- Chronic muscle weakness suggests an autoimmune connective tissue disease such as PM/DM. Myalgia and muscle cramps occur in hypothyroidism, uraemia, and electrolyte imbalance. Myalgia is common in paediatric SLE but myopathy occurs rarely (10%).
- Episodic cramping or muscle pain related to exercise in early childhood might reflect muscular dystrophy, congenital myopathy, myotonic disorders, or genetic defects in glycogen or glucose metabolism.
- A pain syndrome (e.g. fibromyalgia) is a diagnosis of exclusion. Enthesitis (ERA) should be carefully excluded.

Is there bone pain?

Do the pains represent bone pain—persistent, deep-seated pains which change little with posture or movement?

- Night-time pain is typical of bony involvement in malignancy or osteomyelitis. Acute lymphoblastic leukaemia, lymphoma, and neuroblastoma are the commonest malignant lesions.
- Achy 'bony' pain around joints may be due to enthesitis. Patients with ERA/SpA can present with enthesitis alone.
- Migratory bone pains are typical in multifocal osteomyelitis.

Is the child with arthritis systemically unwell?

- Malignancy should be ruled out and vasculitis and autoimmune connective tissue diseases considered in all children with persistent polyarthritis or widespread pains who have systemic symptoms.
- Fever is non-specific though is essential to making a diagnosis of systemic JIA (see Fig. 3.3). It is spiking with chills and sweats. Anorexia and weight loss are common. Vasculitis (see Chapter 14) and FMF (see Chapter 18) should be considered in appropriate patients.
- There may be several years between the onset of systemic features and the arthritis of systemic JIA.
- Low-grade fever can often be present in patients with (RF−) JIA but is rare in (RF+) JIA.
- Serositis is typical in systemic JIA but also occurs in SLE.
- In children <1 year, fever and arthralgia raise the possibility of chronic infantile neurological cutaneous and articular (CINCA) syndrome (see Chapter 7) and hyperimmunoglobulin D syndrome.

Table 3.12 Classification of childhood disorders characterized by myalgia and muscle weakness

Muscular dystrophies	X-linked, e.g. Duchenne
	Autosomal dominant, e.g. fascioscapulohumeral
	Autosomal recessive: limb girdle
Congenital myopathies	e.g. myopathic arthrogryposis
Myotonic dystrophy	
Metabolic disorders	Glycogen storage disease, e.g. acid maltase/phosphorylase/phosphofructokinase deficiency
	Familial periodic paralyses
	2° to endocrinopathies, e.g. Addison's disease, Cushing's disease
Inflammatory diseases	Post-infectious, e.g. viruses—influenza B, coxsackie B, echo, polio
	Autoimmune, e.g. juvenile RA, dermatomyositis, SLE
Genetic abnormalities	Osteogenesis imperfecta
	Ehlers–Danlos
	Mucopolysaccharidoses
Trauma	Physical, e.g. rhabdomyolysis
	Toxic, e.g. snakebite
	Drugs, e.g. steroids, hydroxychloroquine, diuretics
Neurogenic atrophies	Spinal muscular and anterior horn cell dysfunction
	Peripheral nerve, e.g. peroneal muscular atrophy
	Neuromuscular, e.g. congenital myasthenia

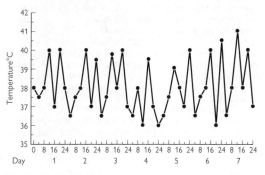

Fig. 3.3 Double-daily fever spikes with rapid return to below 37°C in systemic JIA (systemic-onset JCA)

- A catastrophic illness can occur in children with systemic JIA. It is termed macrophage-activation or haemaphagocytic syndrome and is characterized by haemacytopenias, hepatic dysfunction, encephalopathy, and disseminated intravascular coagulation with bleeding.
- A history of recurrent infections and arthritis may suggest immunodeficiency. The commonest is X-linked humoral deficiency.

Is there a rash?

Does the child have a rash or did one precede the onset of pains?

- Rashes raise the possibility of preceding infection: EBV, rubella, and adenovirus are common and are associated with myoarthralgia and fever.
- The rash of systemic JIA is a salmon-pink macular rash. Lesions may either persist or come and go and may exhibit Köebner phenomenon—the exaggeration of the rash at sites of trauma.
- UV skin sensitivity may denote SLE or dermatomyositis.
- Check for a vasculitic rash (e.g. HSP, cutaneous PAN). Systemic vasculitis can be associated with recurrent fevers and joint pains.

Are there ophthalmic symptoms?

Eye symptoms are an important indicator of underlying autoimmunity in the context of persistent joint or muscle pains:

- Uveitis is associated with most forms of JIA (particularly in association with ANA), but also may indicate an ERA/SpA (uveitis = pain/discomfort, blurring of vision, photophobia and a 'red eye').
- Impairment of visual fields suggests a retinal abnormality—a typical manifestation in juvenile DM (due to occlusive vasculopathy).

Examination

Full medical examination

A full medical examination is essential:

- Pharyngeal erythema is non-specific and swabs should be cultured for streptococci. Sterile pharyngitis is a known feature of systemic JIA.
- Lymphadenopathy is common but non-specific.
- For skin examination in detail see pp.204–8. UV sensitivity occurs in DM and SLE; healing psoriasis may mimic Gottron's lesions; calcinosis and pretibial hypopigmentation are signs of DM.
- Cardiovascular examination is important. Pericarditis is common in systemic and other forms of JIA but is infrequently detected clinically. Myocarditis and heart failure also occur (rarely) in systemic JIA. Persistent tachycardia without anaemia/fever raises the possibility of myocarditis. Cardiac conduction defects are common in juvenile DM.
- A variety of cardiac conditions occur in (RF+) JIA including aortic valve insufficiency. The latter also occurs in ERA/SpA (8–30%).
- Respiratory examination may be abnormal if the arthralgia/arthritis is associated with respiratory tract infection; however, fixed crackles may indicate fibrosis (e.g. (RF+) JIA, PM) and a simultaneous reduction in expansion, breath sounds, and vocal fremitus suggests pleural effusion (e.g. (RF+) JIA).

- Bedside eye examination may be unrevealing even in those with ophthalmic symptoms. Retinal vascular changes and field defects might suggest PM/DM. Thrombosis of dilated blood vessels at the margin of the upper lid is characteristic in PM/DM. Eyes may be dry (Shirmer's tear test <5 mm after 5 min) non-specifically in association with autoimmunity.
- As with all chronic conditions of childhood, growth and maturation (skeletal, endocrine/pubertal, and psychological) assessments should be considered at regular intervals.

Musculoskeletal examination—general principles

- Synovitis of a joint is characterized by soft-tissue swelling, effusion, and a reduced range of joint movement.
- Enthesitis around or within joints may coexist with effusion but alone may be represented by tenderness at bony insertions of ligaments/tendons with joint stiffness but without swelling.
- Tendonitis can be difficult to distinguish from synovitis. Its diagnosis requires a precise knowledge of anatomy. The inflamed tendon may be painful on: passive stretch, movement against (an examiner's) directional resistance, and during its normal function.
- If the condition is chronic an assessment of limb growth should be done, e.g. measuring leg length discrepancy (see Plate 18).

Musculoskeletal examination—patterns of joint, tendon, and enthesis involvement

A full examination should be undertaken:

- Ligament/tendon insertion tenderness, not necessarily associated with swelling, may denote enthesitis. Enthesitis, which is probably more common, or at least more commonly recognized in lower limbs, raises the possibility of ERA/SpA.
- Within 2 years of onset of symptoms most cases of systemic JIA would be termed oligoarticular because few joints are typically affected initially though often the disease extends to involve more joints. Almost any joint can be involved, including those in the cervical spine. Hip joint involvement is almost always symmetrical.
- There is no consistent pattern of joint or tendon involvement that distinguishes polyarticular (RF+) JIA from the majority of conditions associated with, or characterized by, polyarticular (RF−) JIA.
- Subsets of polyarticular (RF−) arthritis have been suggested on the basis of features such as 'painful' or 'dry' synovitis, stiffness, and other laboratory and genetic indices.
- Muscle tenderness is not specific. If confined to the calves consider viral myositis. Weakness can accompany metabolic and endocrine myopathies and is not specific for PM/DM.
- Muscle weakness at rest may be present in children with severe forms of inherited metabolic muscle diseases. Often weakness only becomes apparent after exercise in these conditions (see Table 3.13).

Laboratory investigations

- Laboratory abnormalities are non-specific in polyarticular (RF–) JIA.
- Not unreasonably because of the appearance of RF in association with infections, ILAR criteria propose that significant titres of RF should be demonstrated on two occasions at least 3 months apart to enable a diagnosis of polyarticular (RF+) JIA to be made.
- A range of laboratory investigations is suggested when considering a diagnosis of systemic JIA (Table 3.14).
- Lymphopenia is a hallmark of DM and SLE and makes a diagnosis of any 1° autoimmune arthritis less likely.
- Neutrophilia and thrombocytosis are invariably present and can be marked in systemic JIA whereas leucopenia and thrombocytopenia are uncommon.
- Urinalysis is important in all children with widespread pains and may detect blood or haemoglobinuria in some muscle diseases (actually is myoglobin). Protein and blood may be a sign of underlying kidney inflammation in connective tissue diseases.
- Conventional acute phase markers can be normal in PM/DM. A sensitive indicator (though non-specific) of active disease is von Willebrand factor.
- A raised CK, ALT/AST, or aldolase is a sensitive but not specific sign of autoimmune myositis.
- ANA is not diagnostic but is associated with all autoimmune connective tissue diseases and some JIA subsets. ANA (speckled) is positive in 60–70% of children with PM/DM.
- Additional initial investigations in those suspected of having myopathic pains include bone biochemistry and TFTs.

Imaging investigations: radiographs

- Employ specialist paediatric radiographers/radiologists if possible.
- Proper X-ray beam coning, high-speed intensifying screens, gonadal shielding, and digital radiography all importantly reduce radiation dose.
- Soft tissue swelling and joint-space widening are important, but non-specific, early signs in all the arthritides in young children.
- The most easily recognized early sign of polyarthritis in an older child will be periarticular osteopenia.
- At joints also look for joint space narrowing, erosions, growth abnormalities, subluxation, and ankylosis. All occur at multiple joints in systemic JIA and polyarticular JIA.
- In children with abnormalities in stature/skeletal morphology look for diffuse (?subtle) changes in bone quality and epiphyses.
- Destruction of bone cortex at sites of pain in patients with myalgia, arthralgia, or polysynovitis may suggest malignancy.

Table 3.13 Characteristics of rare inherited causes of muscle pain and/or weakness

Condition	Musculoskeletal features	Other features
Malignant hyperpyrexia (muscle sensitivity to severe physical or metabolic stress)	Acute rigidity and subsequent rhabdo-myolysis	Acute—fever. Hyperkalaemia
McArdle's disease (myophosphorylase deficiency)	Painful (temporary) muscle contractures triggered by exercise	Autosomal recessive. Genotypic and phenotypic heterogeneity
Tauri's disease (phosphofructokinase deficiency)	Similar to McArdle's	Haemolytic anaemia (reticulocytosis)
Von Gierke's disease (glucose 6 phosphatase deficiency)	Skeletal myopathy	Hepatomegaly. Growth retardation. Hypoglycaemia. Lactic acidosis
Pompe's disease (acid maltase deficiency)	Severe skeletal muscle weakness and cardiomyopathy	Death in first year
Cori–Forbes disease (debrancher enzyme deficiency)	Variation from severe childhood myopathic to symptomless adult forms	
Mitochondrial myopathies	Severely limited exercise capacity	Dyspnoea. Lactic acidosis

Imaging investigations: US, skeletal MR, and bone scintigraphy

- The role of US is expanding. It is non-invasive, non-ionizing, can be done at the bedside, and is generally accepted well by children.
- With US, cartilagenous forms of bones can be visualized in comparison to radiographs. This is especially advantageous in the hip where femoral head position and abnormal movement can be seen in young children.
- US is very useful in identifying effusion, notably in the hip and discriminating effusion from synovial thickening.
- Bone scintigraphy provides critical information in musculoskeletal pain when radiographs are unrevealing. Though of less use when joints are involved, bone scintigraphy should be considered when pain originates in bone or infection is a possibility.
- CT is a reliable way of documenting sacroiliac disease in children suspected of having ERA (SpA).
- MR has become the imaging of choice, especially where the diagnosis of JIA is not straightforward. It is more sensitive than radiographs in detecting soft-tissue and most bone lesions, particularly those of the bone marrow.
- MR is more sensitive for detecting changes in joints associated with chronic arthritis compared with radiographs. MR should provide diagnostic information if there is doubt about the presence of arthritis in a joint after clinical examination and radiographs.
- The discrimination of synovitis and enthesitis by MR may have implications for the diagnosis of ERA (SpA) compared with JIA.

Investigations of muscle pains

- EMG patterns of abnormality occur in muscular dystrophy, myasthenia gravis, and autoimmune myositis but each is not specific.
- Evidence of an inflammatory myopathy on EMG is not specific to juvenile DM and may be due to a myositic component of another autoimmune connective tissue disease.
- MR can confirm myositis and reveal potential sites of biopsy in what can be a patchy process.

Table 3.14 Useful tests in investigating suspected systemic JIA

In all patients:	FBC (CBC), ESR, CRP
	Renal and liver biochemistry, serum albumin
	Serum immunoglobulins
	Clotting screen
	Blood cultures
	ECG, CXR, abdominal/pelvic US
	ANA
	Bone marrow aspiration and biopsy
	Ocular slit-lamp examination
	Joint aspirate (single joint)
	Radiographs of selected affected joints
In selected patients:	Muscle enzymes (CK, ALT/AST, and aldolase)
	RF
	Isotope bone/gallium scan
	Upper GI series/small bowel follow-through
	Tissue biopsies
	Viral serology—parvovirus, adenovirus, others
	Echocardiogram
	ASO/antihyaluronidase antibodies
	Urinary homovanillic/vanillylmandelic acid
	Serum IgD

The spectrum of presentation of rheumatic disease

Skin disorders and rheumatic disease

The importance of examining the skin
- The skin is the most accessible organ to examine.
- Pattern recognition of skin symptoms and lesions is valuable in aiding diagnosis (e.g. acute or chronic sarcoid) and prognosis of rheumatic diseases (e.g. nodules and vasculitis in RA).
- Musculoskeletal abnormalities may be mirrored by skin abnormalities, e.g. joint hypermobility and skin laxity with bruising, scarring, and striae.
- Some anti-rheumatic drugs produce highly specific and potentially serious reactions that require prompt diagnosis and management.

Regional abnormalities
The scalp

Scalp symptoms and lesions may be subtle:
- Scalp tenderness and the description of scalp 'lumps' is recognized in giant cell arteritis.
- C2 root/occipital neuropathy (e.g. in RA) or shingles may be associated with dysaesthesiae over the scalp and occipital neuralgia.
- Alopecia may be localized (areata) or diffuse (e.g. in SLE or iron deficiency). Scarring alopecia is typical of discoid lupus.
- Scalp psoriasis may be patchy and discrete.

Face and ears

Face and ears are in sun-exposed areas. Consider UV skin sensitivity:
- A variety of patterns of SLE-associated, UV-sensitive rashes may occur. The rash is often diffuse. Shaded areas (e.g. nasolabial folds) may not be affected (see Chapter 9).
- As in SLE, rosacea can present with telangiectatic papules. Distinction is sometimes difficult without biopsy.
- Periorbital oedema occurs in dermatomyositis (?heliotrope rash), angioedema (may be a presenting feature of SLE), and in nephrotic syndrome.
- Heliotrope rash refers to violaceous oedema/erythema of eyelids in dermatomyositis (see Chapter 13).
- The cutaneous infiltration of chronic sarcoid (lupus pernio) (see Chapter 18) across the nose and cheeks may be overt (papular) but also may be quite subtle (see Plate 19).
- Saddle nose deformity/nasal cartilage destruction has a number of causes: Wegener's granulomatosis (WG) (see Chapter 14), relapsing polychondritis (see Chapter 18), or hereditary connective tissue disease (e.g. Stickler's syndrome see Chapter 16).
- Oral aphthous ulcers are common. Oral ulceration may follow disease activity (e.g. in SLE). Ulcers in sexually acquired reactive arthritis are typically painless.
- Large punched-out and numerous tongue and buccal ulcers which scar are a hallmark of Behçet's disease (see Chapter 18). They may remain for several weeks.

- The strawberry erythema of tongue and lips should not be missed in children. It may denote self-limiting streptococcal infections but may also herald the desquamating palmar (and sole) rash of Kawasaki disease (see Chapter 14).
- Lacy white streaks on the buccal mucosa suggest lichen planus.
- The pinna is a common site for gouty tophi and discoid lupus. Relapsing polychondritis typically causes softening and distortion of cartilage.
- Lipid skin deposits around the eye occur in hyperlipidaemia and multicentric reticulohistiocytosis

Hands and nails

Hands and nails should be examined closely:

- A photosensitive eruption spares the finger webs and palms.
- Erythema on the back of fingers may help distinguish dermatomyositis from SLE.
- In patients with Raynaud's phenomenon (RP), finger ulceration, finger pulp atrophy, induration and tethering of skin indicates scleroderma (see Chapter 12).
- Onycholysis, pitting, salmon patches, and subungual hyperkeratosis are typical of psoriasis (see Chapter 8).
- Subungual splinter haemorrhages may be associated with trauma, infective endocarditis, systemic vasculitis, or thromboangiitis obliterans.
- Nailfold vasculopathy is non-specific and changes may range from erythema to infarcts. Consider systemic vasculitis, dermatomyositis, and infective endocarditis.
- Nailfold capillaries can be examined with an ophthalmoscope at 40 dioptres applying a drop of oil to the cuticle. Enlarged (dilated) capillary loops and capillary 'dropout' suggests an underlying autoimmune connective tissue disease, particularly SScl.

Types of eruption

Macular rashes

Macular rashes are flat, impalpable areas of altered skin colour. Papules are lumps <1 cm in diameter:

- Maculopapular rashes are typical of viral infections.
- A short-lived pinkish, maculopapular eruption occurs on the trunk and limbs in Still's disease. It is often marked in the late afternoon coinciding with fever. If scratched the rash may blanch ('Koebner phenomenon').
- Erythema that enlarges to form large figurative patches in hours suggests rheumatic fever.
- A spreading area of erythema from an original bite may be erythema chronicum migrans—Lyme disease.
- Maculopapular eruptions can occur from NSAIDs, gold, D-penicillamine, sulphasalazine, azathioprine hypersensitivity, and leflunomide (see Chapter 5).

Pustules and blisters

Blisters may be vesicles (<0.5 cm diameter) or bullae (>0.5 cm diameter):
- The commonest pustular rash is due to folliculitis.
- Pustules confined to the hands and feet suggest Reiter's, though local forms of psoriasis may be indistinguishable. Psoriasis can also occur as 'raindrop' erythematous lesions (guttate lesions).
- Generalized pustular rashes can occur in vasculitis, intestinal bypass syndromes, Behçet's disease, and gonococcal bacteraemia.
- Bullous eruptions are most likely to be due to SLE and drug reactions in rheumatological practice.

Plaques

Plaques are slightly raised, circumscribed areas of skin, often disc shaped:
- Plaques are the hallmark of psoriasis. Skin may be scaly and flake off easily. Lesions are often red.
- Psoriatic plaque lesions can occur anywhere on the skin but typical sites are over the extensor surfaces of joints, in the natal cleft, and the umbilicus.
- Scaling may be a feature of discoid lupus. The flakiness tends to be at the periphery of the lesion.

Bleeding into the skin

Bleeding into the skin, which does not blanch is termed purpura. It may sometimes be palpable. Telangiectasias are dilated small vascular lesions that blanch on pressure:
- Impalpable purpura may be due to thrombocytopenia, platelet function disorders, trauma (± capillary/skin fragility, e.g. chronic steroid use), haemophilia and hereditary connective tissue diseases (e.g. Ehlers-Danlos—see Chapter 16).
- Palpable purpura suggests vasculitis including drug-induced (see Chapter 14).
- Widespread telangiectasias occur in limited cutaneous SScl (lcSScl) (see Chapter 12), hereditary haemorrhagic telangiectasia, and DM.

Ulcers and ulcerating rashes

Ulcers are defined as a loss or defect of dermis and epidermis produced by sloughing of necrotic tissue:
- Cutaneous ulceration may have more than one cause in autoimmune diseases. Vasculitis, venous hypertension in an immobile patient, and ulceration over nodules or pressure points where trauma may be relevant, may all be important.
- An indurated, expanding plum-coloured plaque or acneiform pustule, which then ulcerates, suggests pyoderma gangrenosum. The crater has irregular, bluish margins.
- Neurotropic ulceration occurs rarely in RA (see Chapter 5). More commonly it occurs in mononeuritis multiplex in association with vasculitis, autoimmune connective tissue disease, or syringomyelia.
- Severe widespread ulceration developing rapidly in a child may suggest dermatomyositis.
- Vasculitic ulcers in the context of livedo reticularis and antibodies to phospholipids (e.g. cardiolipin) may denote antiphospholipid syndrome (APS) (see Chapter 10).

Textural abnormalities

Abnormalities of the texture of the skin may be difficult to discern. Atrophy and thinning, laxity, thickening, and induration may all be associated with disease:

- Generalized skin atrophy and thinning is an age-related process though may be marked at any age in association with chronic steroid use (or at injection sites) and with some heritable diseases of connective tissue.
- Skin laxity can best be demonstrated over elbow and knee extensor surfaces. Generalized laxity of connective tissue may result in varicose veins and internal organ prolapse.
- True acral and digital puffiness in a patient with Raynaud's is suggestive of SScl. Skin thickening has a variety of causes (see below). SScl and scleroderma-like skin may be localized or in a limited or a generalized distribution—distinction is important (see Table 4.1).

Diagnostic issues in patients with skin thickening

- Raynaud's phenomenon (RP) invariably precedes the onset of SScl but is not typical in morphoea or linear scleroderma.
- In patients with RP, abnormal nailfold capillaries on capillaroscopy are a predictive sign of progression to SScl (see Plate 4).
- The specificities of autoantibodies are often predictive of SScl subtype. In patients with RP, ANA has predictive value for identifying patients who may progress to SScl; anti-centromere antibody can predict progression to lcSScl; anti-topoisomerase I (Scl-70) and anti-RNA polymerase antibodies are linked to progression to diffuse cutaneous SScl (dcSScl).
- Patients with dcSScl have a preponderance of visceral organ involvement in the first 5 years of disease and screening investigations are usually useful (barium studies of gut, echocardiography, lung function tests, biochemical assessment of liver and renal function).
- Eosinophilic fasciitis is a recognized paraneoplastic syndrome. Haematological malignancies are over-represented.
- Linear scleroderma in children can produce lifelong deformities owing to failure of limbs to develop correct length and bulk.
- Scleroderma-like syndromes may occur secondarily to exposure to some industrial chemicals: vinyl chloride, chlorinated organic solvents, and silicon and epoxy resins.

Table 4.1 Pattern recognition in patients with skin thickening

Classification	Skin features
Morphoea may be localized (guttate) or generalized	Early small skin areas affected (itchy). Progression to hidebound skin, typically on trunk (areola spared) and legs. Lesions become waxy and hypo/hyperpigmented. Guttate (small <10 mm papules) usually on neck and anterior chest
Linear scleroderma	Linear band-like pattern often in dermatomal distribution. Atrophy of muscles is common. Fixed joint deformities and growth abnormalities can occur
'Coup de sabre'	Linear scleroderma on the face/scalp can be depressed; ivory in appearance. Hemiatrophy can occur
Systemic sclerosis (early)	Early morning 'puffiness' in hands and feet, facial 'tightness'. Non-pitting oedema of intact dermal and epidermal appendages. High degree of suspicion needed
Systemic sclerosis (classic)	Firm, taut, hidebound skin proximal to MCP joints. Skin may be coarse, pigmented, and dry. Epidermal thinning, loss of hair, and sweating can occur. Telangiectasias and skin calcinosis become obvious. Skin creases disappear. Such change proximal to elbows or knees in the limbs or below the clavicles (in those with face and neck involvement) classifies disease as diffuse as opposed to limited systemic sclerosis
Systemic sclerosis (late)	2–15 years after onset of classical phase, skin softens but pigmentation changes remain. Skin becomes atrophic and can ulcerate
Eosinophilic fasciitis	Phases: early—pitting oedema; progressive—*peau d'orange*; late—induration ('woody feel') with venous guttering when limb elevated. Arms and legs most commonly affected but fingers mainly spared. Synovitis and low-grade myositis may occur. Eosinophilia is usually striking but not always present
Lipodermatosclerosis	Fibrotic induration of lower legs associated with venous stasis ('champagne-bottle legs')
Diabetes	Waxy thickening of extremities. Insidious progression. Joints of the hands become stiff, the tendons can thicken. Skin changes proximal to wrist and on the face very unlikely but stiffening of elbow and shoulder joints not uncommon
Dependent lymphoedema	Feet/ankles/lower legs. Often pitting. Chronic presence may give hyperkeratosis. Main causes: R- or L-sided heart failure, renal failure, nephrotic syndrome, and low-protein states

Skin vasculitis in adults

Background

There is a variety of ways in which systemic vasculitis may present, including pyrexia of unknown origin, organ infarction, gastrointestinal bleeding, and high acute phase response in a generally unwell patient. However, a vasculitic skin rash is a relatively common presenting feature of systemic vasculitis and therefore its recognition is important.

When to consider a diagnosis of vasculitis
(see also Chapters 14 and 21)

- Systemic vasculitis is rare. Overall the annual incidence is about 40 per million (UK rural population).
- Vasculitis can follow viral or bacterial illness, can be triggered by drugs, and is associated with malignancy. Such vasculitis is often found to be leucocytoclastic on biopsy. The list of causes is long (see Table 4.2); however, in about 50% of cases no cause may be found.
- Vasculitis may be part of another autoimmune disease as in SLE or RA or a disease may be defined by it, e.g. WG, Churg–Strauss, microscopic polyangiitis.
- The commonest systemic vasculitis is WG (12.5 per million average annual incidence) and skin involvement occurs in up to 50% of patients, but the cumulative incidence of other skin vasculitides implies that WG will not be the commonest cause of most skin vasculitis seen.

Important considerations

The following important points of clinical assessment should be followed in patients with possible vasculitic rashes. Vasculitis may be confined to the skin or may be systemic:

- Take a history to include possible triggering causes such as starting a new drug or having had a recent infection. Is there a risk the patient may have hepatitis B/C or HIV?
- Other autoimmune rheumatic or connective tissue, bowel, or hepatic disease may be relevant.
- Ultimately, malignancy will have to be ruled out as a cause.
- The wheals of urticarial vasculitis last 24–72h and tend to have a burning or painful quality. Patients are at risk of glomerulonephritis and chronic lung disease (recurrent cough and haemoptysis). Lymphadenopathy, uveitis, benign intracranial hypertension, low complement and IgM macroglobulin are associated findings.
- Arthritis occurs in many different conditions and is not specific.
- Oral ulceration is common with vasculitis. Severe orogenital lesions are a hallmark of Behçet's syndrome. Eye lesions, thrombophlebitis and arthritis are frequent. The condition is common in Mediterranean populations.
- Dry eyes and mouth are features common to many conditions. If present with vasculitis consider Sjögren's syndrome, which is associated with RP (21%) and cheek (parotid) swelling (24%).

Table 4.2 Precipitants and associations of hypersensitivity (allergic) small vessel vasculitis

Drugs	Sulphonamides and penicillins, for example—there are many
Infections	Hepatitis B, hepatitis C, HIV
	β haemolytic streptococcus
Foreign protein	e.g. serum sickness
Autoimmune disease	Rheumatoid arthritis
	Sjögren's syndrome (anti-Ro positive)
	Systemic lupus erythematosus
Inflammatory diseases	Sarcoid
	Crohn's disease, ulcerative colitis
	Chronic active hepatitis
Malignancy	Myelo- and lymphoproliferative disorders
	Solid tumours
Cryoglobulinaemia	

- Systemic symptoms are common in the 'systemic vasculitides' (WG, Churg–Strauss, polyarteritis nodosa, and microscopic polyangiitis). The diagnosis relies heavily on the results of investigations in all cases.
- In WG there is often a long history of recurrent symptomology, which may include nasal stuffiness, epistaxis, sinus symptoms, middle ear, or inflammatory eye symptoms.
- Churg–Strauss vasculitis occurs in asthmatics. Often patients have had childhood asthma that has resolved to recur severely. There may be allergic rhinitis.

Systemic vasculitis

⚠ Systemic vasculitis is a life-threatening condition (see Chapter 21). Two essential initial tasks are firstly to recognize a rash as vasculitic and secondly to determine whether there is multisystem or internal organ involvement:

- The commonest type of vasculitic skin rash is palpable purpura. Lesions may also be impalpable purpura, urticarial, or livedoid.
- Localized vasculitis such as granuloma faciale or erythema elevatum diutinum rarely present to rheumatologists.
- Aggressive panniculitis and neutrophilic dermatoses can sometime present diagnostic difficulties.
- Panniculitis (e.g. erythema nodosum) is usually regional and is due to subepidermal vasculopathy. There may be atrophy and scarring. A migratory panniculitis is recognized.

- Panniculitis is associated with infections: streptococcus, TB, psittacosis, *Yersinia*, *Salmonella*, leprosy, histoplasmosis, blastomycosis, cat scratch fever, and coccidiomycosis; also with oral contraceptives, pregnancy, IBD, pancreatitis, and sarcoid.
- Sweet's syndrome is a combination of painful erythematous plaques, fever, arthralgia, and leucocytosis. The lesions appear in crops, may be initiated by a variety of traumatic injuries (pathergy) and heal without scars. The condition has reported to be para-neoplastic and associated with pregnancy.

Investigations

Skin biopsy

- Try to discuss the case with the pathologist first.
- Take an elliptical biopsy (10 x 5 mm) unless it is undesirable cosmetically. Punch biopsy is simple to do and is often sufficient.
- Include subcutaneous fat in the biopsy, especially if panniculitis is suspected. It allows easier wound closure too.
- Use a needle to lift the skin sample—this avoids forceps-induced damage.
- Fixing in formalin is appropriate for routine histological staining and diagnosis in most cases.
- Immunofluorescence (IF) is important in suspected SLE and in blistering disorders. The lupus band test is positive in clinically uninvolved skin in 70% of cases (sun-exposed sites best).
- Samples for IF should be snap frozen in liquid N_2 or dry ice or transported immediately to the laboratory, ideally in PBS.

Key examination and investigation steps to determine whether there is internal organ or nerve involvement

- Dipstick urinalysis to check for protein or blood, and urine microscopy to look for cellular casts is important. Blood urea, creatinine and electrolytes should be checked. If there is protein, quantify it with a 24hr collection and obtain nephrological advice.
- Pulmonary evaluation and CXR. Cough, dyspnoea, and haemoptysis may suggest WG or pulmonary vasculitis. If lung nodules or infiltrates are seen on the radiograph obtain lung function tests, a high-resolution CT and advice from a chest physician.
- Abdominal pain, diarrhoea and abdominal tenderness may be common findings and due to a number of causes: in some forms of allergic vasculitis, endothelial lesions can lead to gut bleeding (e.g. HSP); gut infarction (in PAN) and mesenteric panniculitis can lead to an acute abdomen; allergic vasculitis may be triggered by hepatitis B and is associated with chronic active hepatitis and inflammatory bowel disease.
- Parasthesiae and numbness may reflect mononeuritis multiplex due to vasculitis. Symptoms may seem trivial. Obtain nerve conduction tests.
- Laboratory investigations should be thorough (see Table 4.3).
- Further investigations which warrant consideration: CT of upper respiratory tract to show the distribution of disease in WG; angiography in suspected cases of PAN; kidney biopsy in cases where renal inflammation is suggested by investigations. Endoscopy and inflammation scintigraphy in suspected cases of bowel vasculitis.

Table 4.3 Laboratory investigations in patients with suspected vasculitis

Haematology	FBC (CBC), ESR
Biochemistry	Urea, electrolytes, creatinine
	Liver function enzymes, serum ACE
	CRP
	Serum and urine protein electrophoresis
Microbiology	Blood cultures
	Hepatitis B and C serology. Consider HIV
	Streptococcal antibodies
Immunology	Immunoglobulins, cryoglobulins, complement
	ANA (ENAs), rheumatoid factor
	ANCA

Skin vasculitis in children and adolescents

Epidemiology

- Classification of childhood vasculitis is difficult. A system that has clinical utility is shown in Table 4.4.
- Statistically the commonest type of vasculitis is likely to be HSP then hypersensitivity angiitis (both leucocytoclastic vasculitides). On a worldwide basis, giant cell arteritis is the third commonest.
- Kawasaki disease (KD) affects primarily the under 5s.
- Though commonest in Japan (150/100 000 under 5s), KD occurs worldwide (3–10/100 000 under 5s in Europe and N America).

Clues from the history

- All vasculitides may be associated with features such as fatigue, fever, gastrointestinal symptoms, lymphadenopathy, and myoarthralgia.
- Drugs or infection are often identified as a precipitant of a small vessel leucocytoclastic vasculitis, although links to an infective trigger have also been made in cutaneous polyarteritis (URTI), KD (numerous but lately staphylococcus), giant cell arteritis (TB).
- WG is rare. As in adults, it may be characterized by a limited localized form involving the respiratory tract. Subglottic stenosis, nasal septum disease, and respiratory infections may all have occurred.
- Testicular pain is a rare though fairly specific feature for PAN.
- Abdominal pain is not specific. Gut bleeding can occur in HSP and DM especially.
- Vasculitis associated with FMF is not unknown.

Examination

Characteristic examination features of the rash

- Erythematous rash with swelling progressing to desquamation of palms and soles of the feet is typical of KD.
- Lower limb and buttock palpable purpura is typical of, but not specific for, HSP and hypersensitivity angiitis.
- Skin nodules are not specific but are common in cutaneous polyarteritis and frequently occur in hypersensitivity vasculitis. A nodular, painful rash on the medial sides of the feet is frequent in cutaneous polyarteritis.
- Extensive necrotic and ulcerative rash with notable muscle pains suggests DM. Periungual erythema and both eyelid and nail bed telangiectasias are typical.
- Livedo reticularis is a feature of cutaneous polyarteritis (often with painful skin nodules) but also SLE and antiphospholipid syndrome (see Chapters 9 and 10 respectively).

Other typical or specific examination features

- Bilateral conjunctival injection, lip/oral/buccal inflammation, and acute non-purulent cervical lymphadenopathy are typical features of KD.
- The incidence of cardiovascular manifestations is 35% in KD. Murmurs, gallop rhythm, and coronary artery aneurysms (30%) can occur.

Table 4.4 A classification of childhood vasculitis

Polyarteritis	Macroscopic
	Microscopic
Kawasaki disease (mucocutaneous lymph node syndrome)	
Granulomatous vasculitis	Wegener's granulomatosis
	Churg–Strauss vasculitis
Leucocytoclastic vasculitis	Henoch–Schönlein purpura
	Hypersensitivity angiitis
Cutaneous polyarteritis	
Vasculitis and autoimmune connective tissue disease	SLE
	JIA
	Mixed connective tissue disease
	Dermatomyositis
	Scleroderma
Large vessel vasculitis	Giant cell arteritis
	Takayasu's disease
Miscellaneous vasculitides	

- Pulselessness may suggest major vessel vasculitis. The most likely is giant cell arteritis.
- Severe oral aphthous ulceration raises the possibility of Behçet's syndrome. It is rare but does occur in children.

Investigations

- Leucocytosis, thrombocytosis, anaemia, and an acute phase response are typical in all forms of vasculitis and are not specific.
- ECG, echocardiography, and usually coronary angiography are essential in suspected KD.
- Glomerulonephritis is not specific and should be ruled out in all cases (urinalysis, urine microscopy, 24-h urinary protein estimation, and in some cases ^{51}Cr EDTA GFR).
- ANCA is not specific but c-ANCA with antibodies to proteinase 3 in appropriate patients suggests that WG should be suspected.
- Biopsy of the skin rash is a key investigation in all patients though in mild typical cases without gut or renal involvement it may not be necessary in HSP.
- Impaired renal function with nephrotic range proteinuria is an indication for renal biopsy in patients with suspected HSP.
- Renal biopsy may be necessary in polyarteritis and WG. The distinction of microscopic polyarteritis from macroscopic disease relies on the extensive glomerular involvement in the former (focal segmental). Aggressive crescentic glomerulonephritis is a feature of WG.
- The most valuable investigation in patients with suspected macroscopic polyarteritis is hepatic and renal angiography.

Endocrine conditions

Well-characterized musculoskeletal conditions occur in many endocrine disorders. Some are specific, others occur with greater frequency than in the general population. Musculoskeletal manifestations occur either as a result of metabolic disturbances or are influenced by a common link through their autoimmune pathophysiology.

Diabetes

- Dupuytren's contracture, trigger finger, carpal tunnel syndrome (about 15% of diabetics), diffuse idiopathic skeletal hyperostosis (DISH), and adhesive capsulitis are more frequent than in the normal population.
- Some form of tissue or joint hypomobility/stiffness is common (see Table 4.5) and can appear similar to scleroderma. However, histopathological differences are recognized. Thus to avoid misdiagnosis, do a skin biopsy.

Table 4.5 Patterns of joint and tissue hypomobility or stiffness in diabetes by reported series. Tissue changes are thought to occur from excessive hydration (a consequence of an excessive local production of sugar alcohols)

Patient series	Major abnormalities	Associations
Diabetics overall	In about 30–40% mainly in long-standing disease: slow decrease in hand mobility; waxy skin thickening ('scleroderma-like')	Occasional lung fibrosis. Microvascular diabetic complications
Adults	55–76% prevalence of joint hypomobility in type 1/type 2 diabetes respectively	Not associated with diabetic complications
Mature onset diabetes (mean 61 years)	Stiffening of connective tissue (assessed in hands)	Diabetic nephropathy
Children with type 1 diabetes	31% had limited joint mobility	None with glycaemic control, retinopathy, or proteinuria
Juvenile and young adult onset (age 1–24 years) diabetes	34% had skin thickening. Changes rarely proximal to MCPJs and never proximal to wrists. Joint contractures in >50%, often third or fourth fingers	No flexor tendon rubs (as seen in scleroderma)

- Hand weakness may be due to diabetic neuropathy and may be mistaken for carpal tunnel syndrome. Neurophysiology tests help discriminate.
- Calcification of soft tissues around the shoulder is common (about 20% of diabetics) but is associated with variable symptoms and disability.
- Amyotrophy is rare. It presents acutely with pain, weakness, and wasting of the proximal lower limb muscles. It may be unilateral. Differential diagnosis includes myositis (see Chapter 13) and polymyalgia rheumatica (PMR—see Chapter 14). It is associated with uncontrolled hyperglycaemia. Aetiology is unknown but it is probably a neuromyopathy.
- Though rare (1:500 diabetics), neuropathic arthritis can occur in advanced disease. Most patients are aged 40–60 years and have poor glycaemic control. Tarsal and metatarsal joints are most frequently affected (60%). The usual presentation is of swelling of the foot with no or little pain. Trauma may have occurred. Early radiographic changes can resemble OA (see Chapter 6).
- Asymptomatic osteolysis can occur at the distal metatarsals and proximal phalanges with relative joint sparing. The aetiology is unknown.
- Osteomyelitis is not uncommon and needs to be discriminated from cellulitis and neuropathic arthritis. A three-phase bone scan should be helpful. Osteomyelitis is usually disclosed by prominent blood flow in the dynamic (first) phase and increased uptake of tracer by soft tissue and bone in later stages. Cellulitis is associated with minimal uptake of tracer in bone in the delayed (third) phase. Neuropathic joints display minimal first-phase abnormality but prominent tracer uptake in the third phase.
- Muscle infarction can present as a painful muscle mass and is a result of arterial narrowing. Often mistaken for thrombophlebitis, myositis or vasculitis this is a late complication of diabetes. Biopsy may be needed.
- Insulin resistance is associated with features of autoimmune connective tissue disease such as arthralgia, alopecia, glandular enlargement, ↓WCC, ↑Igs and antinuclear antibodies.

Hypothyroid disease

- Over 25% of patients may have an arthropathy. The arthropathy can be mistaken for RA (see Chapter 5).
- The commonest arthritis usually involves large joints, especially knees. It is characterized by pain, stiffness, effusions, and synovial thickening. It is not clear whether this inflammatory arthropathy can be ascribed entirely to synovitis caused by calcium pyrophosphate dihydrate deposition (CPPD arthritis— 'pseudogout' (see Chapter 15)).
- Also a small joint arthropathy occurs. Symptoms are more obvious than signs. A third have flexor tenosynovitis and acroparasthesiae are common.
- Carpal tunnel syndrome is frequent (7%). Up to 10% of patients with carpal tunnel syndrome may have hypothyroidism.

- Chondrocalcinosis (radiographically defined) is only marginally increased compared with controls (17% vs 10%). About 1/10 patients with pseudogout (p.444) are hypothyroid.
- Hyperuricaemia is common but gout attacks are rare. However, screening for hypothyroidism in patients with gout is recommended. Treated hypothyroidism then requires review of the need for uric acid-lowering therapy.
- Musculoskeletal symptoms are otherwise common with patterns of pain similar to PMR (normal or slightly ↑ESR) or fibromyalgia. Improvement occurs after the thyroid is treated.
- Consequences of hypothyroidism in children included retarded bone age, short stature, and epiphyseal dysgenesis with premature epiphyseal plate closure and chance of slipped femoral epiphyses.
- Myopathy is relatively common. About 1 in 20 cases of acquired myopathy are due to hypothyroidism. Presentation can mimic polymyositis with elevation of muscle enzymes though muscle biopsy typically shows no inflammatory cell infiltrate. Improvement with thyroxine replacement is sometimes complicated by muscle cramps but takes only a few weeks.
- The combination of weakness, muscular stiffness, and an increase in muscle mass in an adult with myxoedema is termed Hoffman's syndrome. Muscle mass increase is sometimes striking and can take many months to resolve on treatment. The same condition occurs in children (Kocher–Debre–Semelaigne syndrome).
- Lymphocytic thyroiditis (Hashimoto's) is an autoimmune condition characterized by hypothyroidism and autoantibodies to thyroglobulin and thyroid microsomes. These antibodies are found in 40% of patients with primary Sjögren's disease but only about 10% are or have been overtly hypothyroid.

Hyperparathyroidism (see also Chapter 16)

Unless stated, points refer to both primary and secondary disease:
- Musculoskeletal symptoms are the initial manifestation in up to 16% of patients with primary hyperparathyroidism.
- Hyperparathyroidism, chondrocalcinosis, and pseudogout frequently coexist. Pseudogout (CPPD) can be triggered by parathyroidectomy.
- A polyarthropathy can occur which can mimic RA. It differs in that synovial proliferation is absent. Radiographically, erosions have a predilection for the ulna side of distal upper limb joints (radial in RA), joint space is preserved, pericapsular calcification is often present, and reactive bone formation ultimately occurs.
- A polyarthropathy can occur with renal osteodystrophy in about 20% of patients with chronic renal failure on dialysis. It does not appear to be related to CPPD.
- Hyperparathyroidism is associated with a specific shoulder arthropathy characterized by intra/periarticular erosions of the humeral head. Calcification may be absent and damage subclinical.

- Subjective muscle weakness is common, objective weakness less so. Fatiguability is a common complaint. Muscle enzymes are normal. Biopsy shows type II fibre atrophy and features of an inflammatory myopathy are absent.
- The hallmark of radiographic changes is bone resorption: subperiosteal (typically on the radial side of second and third phalanges), intracortical, subchondral, trabecular, subligamentous, and localized (Brown's tumours). Bone sclerosis, periostitis, and chondrocalcinosis also occur.
- Fragility fracture is common and often precedes a diagnosis of primary hyperparathyroidism. Although significant and fast accretion of bone occurs after surgery, long-term relatively low bone mass often remains.

Thyrotoxicosis

- Hyperthyroidism can cause a proximal myopathy (70%), shoulder periarthritis (7%), acropachy (thickening of extremities), and osteoporosis.
- Acropachy is rare (<2% of patients with thyrotoxicosis) and most often occurs in treated patients who are hypo/euthyroid. It consists of clubbing, painful soft tissue swelling of hands and feet, and periosteal new bone on the radial aspect of the second and third metacarpals.
- Graves' disease is frequently associated with fatiguability and muscular weakness. It is associated with autoimmune rheumatic and connective tissue diseases.

Acromegalic arthropathy

- Over-stimulation of bone and connective tissue cells from excessive growth hormone can result in a multiplicity of features: bursal and cartilage hyperplasia, synovial and bony proliferation, an OA-like picture, backache, and hypermobility.
- Joint complaints usually manifest about 10 years after the onset of clinical acromegaly. Knees are frequently affected.
- Joint symptoms are not typical of an inflammatory arthritis—morning stiffness is not prominent and joint swelling is present in <50% of patients.
- Carpal tunnel syndrome (see Chapter 2) affects >50% of patients and is frequently bilateral.
- Back and neck pain and radicular symptoms from nerve root compression or spinal stenosis are not uncommon and are related to axial bony proliferation.
- A painless proximal myopathy occurs infrequently.
- Radiographs characteristically show widened joint spaces (e.g. >2.5 mm in adult MCPJs) and a thickened heel pad (>23 mm in men and >21.5 mm in women).
- Diagnosis relies on demonstration of a failure of growth hormone to be suppressed by a glucose tolerance test but a lateral skull radiograph is a good screening test as 90% have enlargement of the pituitary fossa.

Gut and hepatobiliary conditions

Musculoskeletal features frequently occur in patients with gut or hepatobiliary disease (see Table 4.6)

- Data on the frequency of rheumatological features are largely based on studies of hospital patients with clinically overt gut or biliary disease. This may lead to an underestimate of the frequency of association.
- The most frequent associations are: sacroiliitis, arthritis and enthesitis in patients with inflammatory bowel disease; inflammatory arthritis in coeliac disease and viral hepatitis; and degenerative arthritis in haemochromatosis and Wilson's disease, for example.
- The frequency of enthesitis in patients with inflammatory bowel disease may be underestimated. Be aware of the easiest sites where inflammation (tenderness) may be detected: medial/lateral humeral epicondyles, Achilles tendon insertion, calcaneal plantar fascia origin and insertion, patellar tendon origin and its insertion at the tibial tubercle.
- Radiological studies in patients with inflammatory bowel disease suggest that sacroiliitis is under-recognized by clinicians.

Severity of rheumatological manifestations

- Optimal surveillance strategies for the musculoskeletal manifestations of gut or biliary disease are not known in many instances.
- Life-threatening vasculitis is associated with hepatitis B or C.
- In most patients who develop joint inflammation or enthesitis after bacterial dysentery, the condition is self-limiting. Chronicity and severity may be linked to HLA B27 prevalence. Progressive spondylitis is rare.

Characteristic gut and hepatobiliary conditions in patients with rheumatological diseases (see Table 4.7)

- The commonest problem in RA patients is dyspepsia associated with gastroduodenal erosions or ulcers due to NSAIDs. Peptic lesions may be clinically silent and may present with dropping haemoglobin levels or an acute bleed.

Table 4.6 Rheumatological features in patients with gut or hepatic disease

Gastrointestinal disorder	Rheumatic manifestation	Association
Enteric infection	Reactive arthritis: self-limiting in most	Arthritis in 2% who get shigella, salmonella, yersinia, campylobacter or C. difficile overall but in 20% of infected who are HLA B27+
Crohn's disease	Arthritis 20%. AS 10%. Sacroiliitis in 26%	60% of spondylarthropathy patients have histological evidence of bowel inflammation. See also below
Ulcerative colitis	Arthritis 20%. AS 7%. Sacroiliitis 15%	See also above. Severity of gut and joint inflammation varies in its association but SIJ/spine inflammation does not
Whipple's disease	Migratory arthritis in >60%	T. whippelii identified in small bowel. Diarrhoea occurs in >75% ultimately
Intestinal by-pass surgery (blind loop syndrome)	Polyarticular symptoms 50% in scleroderma	Intestinal bacterial overgrowth in small bowel. ?Associated with joint symptoms
Coeliac disease	Arthritis is rare	?Increased intestinal permeability
Viral enteritis	Rare (<0.5%)	Most common: coxsackie or echo
Hepatitis A	Arthralgia 15%. Vasculitis rare	Causal association
Hepatitis B	Arthralgia 10–25%. PAN	Aetiological. Vasculitis in 50% HBsAg carriers
Hepatitis C	Sialadenitis in >50%. Vasculitis (cryoglobulinaemic)	?Aetiological in Sjögren's. Hepatitis C identified in 27–96% of patients with cryoglobulinaemia
Primary biliary cirrhosis	Polyarthritis 19%. Scleroderma 18%. Sjögren's 50%	Autoimmune 'overlap'. Features may be subclinical
Chronic active hepatitis	Polyarthralgia or arthritis in 25–50%	Autoimmunity
Hemochromatosis	OA 50%	Iron storage disease
Wilson's disease	OA in 50% adults. Chondrocalcinosis	Copper storage disease

Table 4.7 Gut and hepatobiliary manifestations in rheumatological diseases (I: General)

Disease	Abnormalities	Presentation with
Rheumatoid arthritis (Chapter 5)	TMJ arthritis	Impaired mastication
	Oesophageal dysmotility	Dysphagia, reflux
	GI vasculitis (0.1%)	Ulcers, pain, infarction
	Portal hypertension	Splenomegaly (Felty's)
	Liver involvement (Felty's)	Enzyme abnormalities
	Hepatosplenomegaly	Palpable viscera
Systemic lupus erythematosus (Chapter 9)	Oesophageal dysmotility	Dysphagia, reflux
	GI vasculitis	Ulcers, pain, perforation
	Protein-losing enteropathy	Hypoalbuminaemia
	Peritonitis	Ascites (10%), serositis
	Hepatosplenomegaly (30%)	Palpable viscera
Scleroderma (Chapter 12)	Oesophageal dysmotility	Heartburn/dysphagia
	Delayed gastric emptying	Aggravated reflux
	Intestinal dysmotility and fibrosis (80%)	Malabsorption, pseudo-obstruction (<1%)
	Pseudo and wide mouth diverticulae	Haemorrhage, stasis, bacterial overgrowth
Polymyositis and dermatomyositis (Chapter 13)	Muscle weakness	Aspiration, dysphagia
	Disordered motility	Dysphagia, constipation
	Vasculitis (rare)	Ulcers, perforation
MCTD	Hypomotility	Dysphagia, reflux, pseudo-obstruction
Sjögren's syndrome (Chapter 11)	Membrane dessication	Xerostomia, dysphagia
	Oesophageal webs (10%)	Dysphagia (>60%)
	Gastric infiltrates/atrophy	Masses, dyspepsia
	Pancreatitis	Pain, amylasaemia
	Hepatic dysfunction	Hepatomegaly ($\cong$ 25%)
	Hepatic cirrhosis	Primary biliary cirrhosis
Spondylarthritis (Chapter 8)	Ileocolonic inflammation	May be asymptomatic
Adult onset Still's	Hepatitis, peritonitis, hepatosplenomegaly	Pain or abnormal enzymes ($\cong$75%)
Systemic JIA (Chapter 7)	Serositis	Abdominal pain
	Hepatomegaly	Abnormal enzymes
Marfan, Ehlers-Danlos (Chapter 16)	Defective collagen	Hypomotility, Malabsorption, visceral rupture/laxity

- Gut amyloid is present in 21% of RA patients (autopsy study). In some, (non-gut) amyloid was considered the cause of death.
- The rate of deaths from amyloid in JIA has ↓ from 42 to 17% since the 1970s due to aggressive treatment.
- Amyloid can be diagnosed from rectal (75% diagnostic yield), lip (86% yield) or subcutaneous fat biopsy. Characteristic patterns of deposition are recognized with ^{111}In-labelled serum amyloid-P scintigraphy.
- Quite severe GI disturbances can coexist with relatively stable limited cutaneous scleroderma, i.e. skin and gut disease does not necessarily correlate. Overall GI problems are extremely frequent.
- In SLE serious gut and hepatobiliary manifestations are relatively uncommon (5%) though nausea, anorexia, vomiting, and diarrhoea are quite frequent.
- GI vasculitis is associated with virtually all the autoimmune connective tissue diseases and is part of systemic vasculitides (see Table 4.8). It can present in a variety of ways such as with non-specific features such as abdominal pain, anorexia, and anaemia or with an 'acute abdomen' in patients with established disease. It can also be the disease-presenting feature.

Gut and hepatobiliary side-effects from drugs used in treating rheumatological and bone diseases

Such side-effects are common:
- NSAIDs should be considered as potentially toxic as some other drugs used for rheumatological diseases including immunosuppressive drugs.
- Peptic ulcers and gastroduodenal erosions appear to occur less frequently with selective cyclo-oxygenase II (COX II)-inhibiting NSAIDs such as celecoxib, etoricoxib, valdecoxib and meloxicam than with NSAIDs that inhibit COX II less selectively.
- Vioxx, one of the initial COX II NSAIDs, has been withdrawn over its proved role in ↑risk of IHD. Some data to suggest celecoxib has similar effects. As yet it is unknown if this is a class effect of all COX II NSAIDs. It may be.
- Glucocorticoids are (rarely) associated with peptic ulceration, perforation and pancreatitis. The latter two are unusual at doses <12.5 mg/day.
- Methotrexate gut and hepatobiliary side effects are relatively common. Abdominal pain, nausea, vomiting, diarrhoea, stomati-tis/mouth, ulcers and altered taste occur. All may respond to dose reduction. Liver enzyme elevation occurs in up to 88% at some time during treatment. Serious hepatic disease is unusual, though cirrhosis is a risk. Children typically tolerate higher doses than adults (even up to 40–50 mg/week).
- IM gold can cause mouth ulcers (5–20%). Diarrhoea is rare (1%) with IM but common with oral gold (40%). Significant liver disease and enterocolitis occur with both forms but are rare.

Table 4.8 Gut and hepatobiliary manifestations in rheumatological diseases (II Vasculitis (see also Chapter 14))

Disease	Frequency of GI vasculitis and features
Polyarteritis nodosa	80% (mesenteric). Buccal ulcers, cholecystitis (15%), bowel infarction, perforation, appendicitis, pancreatitis, strictures, chronic wasting syndrome
Henoch–Schönlein Purpura	44–68%. Abdominal pain, meleana, haematemesis, ulcers, intussusception, cholecystitis, infarction, perforation, appendicitis
Churg–Strauss Syndrome	≅40%. Haemorrhage, ulceration, infarction, perforation
Behçet's syndrome	Buccal and intestinal ulcers, haemorrhage, perforation, pyloric stenosis, rectal ulcers
Systemic lupus erythematosus	2%. Buccal ulcers, ileocolitis, gastritis, ulceration, perforation, intussusception, volvulus (1%), pneumatosis
Kawasaki disease	Abdominal pain, intestinal obstruction, non-infective diarrhoea
Wegener's granulomatosis	<5%. Cholecystitis, appendicitis, ileocolitis, infarction
Juvenile dermatomyositis	Well recognized. Perforation, pneumatosis
MCTD	Rare. Ulceration, perforation, pancreatitis
RA (including RF+ JIA)	0.1%. Buccal ulcers, abdominal pain, peptic ulcers, acalculus cholecystitis, gut infarction, and perforation
Polymyositis and dermatomyositis	Very rare. Mucosal ulcers, perforation and pneumatosis
Cryoglobulinaemia	Rare. Ischaemia and infarction

- Sulphasalazine gut and hepatobiliary side-effects are common and may occur in up to 20% of patients. The most frequent are mostly mild: indigestion, nausea, vomiting, anorexia, and abdominal pain. Gut ulceration, bloody diarrhoea, and serious liver problems are rare. In about 65% of side-effects occur in the first 3 months of treatment.
- Azathioprine can cause nausea (15%), vomiting (10%), and abdominal pain (8%). Diarrhoea is rare (5%). Liver enzyme abnormalities are often mild and may remit on lowering the dose. The GI side effects are not always dependent on TPMT status.
- D-penicillamine causes altered taste (25% within the first 3–6 months), nausea or vomiting (18%), and stomatitis/mouth ulcers (5%). Hepatotoxicity and haemorrhagic colitis are rare.

- Chloroquine and hydroxychloroquine, used in mild SLE particularly, can cause non-specific GI intolerance (10%). The onset is often insidious.
- Ciclosporin causes gingival hyperplasia, nausea, diarrhoea, and elevation in hepatic enzymes.
- Effects of cyclophosphamide on the gut are frequent and include nausea, vomiting, diarrhoea, and stomatitis. Serious hepatotoxicity is rare.
- Chlorambucil has a low incidence of GI side-effects.
- Leflunomide can cause nausea (8–13%), diarrhoea (up to 25%), and abnormal liver enzymes. In studies to date, most rises in transaminases have been mild (< two-fold) and are reversible on drug withdrawal.
- Oral bisphosphonates, given for osteoporosis, such as alendronate and risedronate can cause nausea, dyspepsia, and diarrhoea. Oesophageal ulceration has occasionally been noted with alendronate though it is thought this occurs only in people who do not follow the instructions for taking them. Myoarthralgias can also occur.
- Strontium ranelate is as well-tolerated as placebo in all studies but can cause GI side-effects. Extensive post-marketing data on side-effects are not yet available.
- Calcitonin either given as s/c injection or as nasal spray can give abdominal pains and diarrhoea.

Malignancy

Rheumatic features may be clues to the existence of cancer and may be caused either by direct invasion or indirectly as a paraneoplastic syndrome.

Primary and secondary neoplastic diseases of bone and joints

- Synovial tumours are rare. Sarcoma (synovioma) is commoner in men than women and unusual in those over 60. It usually occurs in the legs (70%) and can occur around tendon sheaths and bursae. At diagnosis, pulmonary metastases are common.
- Para-articular involvement by bone tumours may give a monoarticular effusion. Invasion of synovium may occur and malignant cells can be detected in joint fluid. Breast, bronchogenic carcinoma, GI tumours, and melanoma can all metastasize to joints.
- Lymphomas and leukaemias may simulate various conditions and cause synovitis in a single or in multiple joints.
- Arthritis complicating presentation of myeloma or an acute leukaemia is most likely to be polyarticular asymmetrical.
- In adults, arthritis complicating leukaemia is rare (5% of cases).
- Leukaemia is the most frequent malignancy in Caucasian children and the most frequent cause of neoplastic skeletal symptoms in childhood and adolescence (15% of leukaemia cases).
- Neuroblastomas are the most frequent cause of a solid tumour metastasizing to the skeleton in children.

Clues that may lead to a suspicion of malignancy directly causing musculoskeletal symptoms

- Constitutional symptoms.
- Migratory arthralgia/arthritis.
- The coexistence of bone pain (also consider metabolic bone diseases, sarcoid, and enthesitis-related conditions).
- Haemorrhagic joint fluid (also consider trauma, pigmented villonodular synovitis (PVNS), chondrocalcinosis).
- Radiographs that show adjacent bone destruction, perhaps with loss of cortex (also consider infection).
- Radiographic calcification in soft-tissue mass (?synovioma).

Paraneoplastic myopathies

Paraneoplastic myopathies may occur at the time of presentation of malignancy, precede it sometimes by months to years, follow its treatment, or occur as a complication of established disease:

- Myopathy is usually due to carcinomatous neuromyopathy. Poly/dermatomyositis, Eaton–Lambert myasthenic syndrome (ELMS) and hypophosphataemic (oncogenic) osteomalacia are associated with, though not specific for, malignancy (see Table 4.9).
- Carcinomatous neuromyopathy is a condition characterized by symmetrical muscle weakness and wasting. The myopathy can pre-date malignancy.

Table 4.9 Myopathy and links with malignancy

Condition	Typical pattern of weakness	Common cancer associations	Other features
Carcinomatous neuromyopathy	Pelvic girdle—symmetrical	Lung: 15% men, 12% women. Ovary: 16%. Stomach: 7% men, 13% women	Wasting, EMG abnormality, and increase in muscle enzymes are not invariable
Dermatomyositis (+?PM)	Proximal limb. Truncal	Reflects underlying cancer frequency in local population	Response to steroids is usual
Myasthenia gravis (MG)	Frequently ocular and bulbar muscles involved	Thymus. Any	Muscle strength fluctuates (fatiguability). Responds to anti-cholinesterases
Eaton–Lambert myasthenic syndrome (ELMS)	Pelvic girdle muscles. Altered gait. Ocular muscles not affected	Small cell lung. Can occur up to 2–3 years after ELMS	Autonomic disturbances. EMG + poor response to anticholinesterase distinguish from MG
Oncogenic osteomalacia	Generalized. Develops insidiously	Small, discrete mesenchymal tumours in bone, soft tissues, and sinuses. Neurofibromatosis	Bone pain and bone demineralization. Hypophosphataemia and low circulating 1,25 vitamin D

Investigations

The following investigations are recommended for patients presenting with a form of cancer-related myopathy:

- To confirm muscle disease consider: FBC/CBC; measures of acute phase; muscle enzymes; EMG; muscle biopsy; autoantibodies, e.g. ANA, anti-RNP and anti-Jo1 (PM) and anti-acetylcholine receptor antibodies in MG.
- Rapid relief of symptoms with IV injection of edrophonium (up to 10 mg) is typical in MG but unlikely in ELMS. Prior injection of atropine 0.2 mg protects against antimuscarinic effects.
- A search for malignancy is essential. Suspicious clinical features will guide the focus and extent of the search. Frequent associations are shown in Table 4.9.
- Imaging studies need to be thorough and include skeletal scintigraphy and usually thoracoabdominal cavity studies.
- Other investigations to consider: chest radiograph and skeletal survey, ovarian and bowel tumour markers, mammography, PSA, serum protein electrophoresis.
- Surveillance for the appearance of tumours if initial investigations are unrevealing is prudent. Tumour appearance may be a few years after the onset of myopathy in some cases.

Non-myopathic paraneoplastic syndromes

The non-myopathic paraneoplastic syndromes are rare:

- Hypertrophic osteoarthropathy (HO) consists of clubbing, periostitis of tubular bones, and an arthropathy (may range from arthralgia to diffuse polyarthritis). Suspicion of this should prompt a request for an isotope bone scan which typically shows abnormally ↑ bone turnover in the long bones. Radiographs often show periosteal elevation.
- HO complicates 20% of primary lung tumours (thus 'hypertrophic *pulmonary* osteoarthropathy') though it is associated with other malignancies.
- Polyarthritis may be the presenting feature of cancer. Most cases occur in those aged over 60. Nodules and deformities do not occur as in RA and it is less likely to be symmetrical though both occur in multicentric reticulohistiocytosis—which is malignancy-asso-ciated and might be mistaken for RA.
- Eosinophilic fasciitis, severe bilateral palmar fasciitis (often mistaken for scleroderma), and fasciitis associated with panniculitis have been associated with malignancy. Cases of 'shoulder–hand' syndrome with cancer probably reflect similar pathological processes.

Rheumatic diseases associated with an increased incidence of malignancy

There are a number of rheumatic diseases that are associated with an increased incidence of malignancy compared with healthy populations. These are dealt with briefly here and in more detail in Part 2 of this book. Data gathering in this area has been difficult. Only the strongest data are reflected here.

- The most highly associated cancer in RA is non-Hodgkin's lymphoma. Paraproteinaemia and myeloma are also associated.
- RA patients may be partially protected from colorectal cancer owing to the chronic effects of NSAIDs on bowel mucosa.
- Use of cyclophosphamide and chlorambucil is associated with an ↑ cancer risk but use of methotrexate and azathioprine is probably not.
- Non-Hodgkin's B-cell lymphoma develops in a subset of patients with Sjögren's syndrome (4%). Its onset may be indicated by rapid enlarge- ment of salivary glands, the appearance of a paraprotein, or decrease in circulating immunoglobulins or RF titre.
- The association between malignancy and SLE or scleroderma is controversial. Cases may relate to use of cyclophosphamide.
- DM is probably associated with malignancy in adults, though convincing evidence for an association of PM with malignancy is lacking. Neither is associated with malignancy in children.
- There are no specific clinical or laboratory features which discriminate DM associated with malignancy from the 'uncomplicated' disease, although weight loss and a negative ANA should raise the possibility of a malignancy-related condition. Close surveillance for a tumour in the first year after DM (+?PM) diagnosis in those >45 years of age is justified.

Part 2

The clinical features and management of rheumatic diseases

Rheumatoid arthritis (RA)

Disease criteria and epidemiology

There is no exact definition of rheumatoid arthritis (RA), nor a pathognomic test. The diagnosis rests on a composite of clinical and laboratory observations. It is a common systemic inflammatory disease characterized by the presence of a destructive polyarthritis with a predisposition for affecting the small joints of the hands and feet and the wrists (though can affect any synovial joint).

Attempts to delineate criteria are dominated by signs and symptoms from the locomotor system. It is important to remember however that there are a number of 'extra-articular' manifestations to the disease, with involvement of, for example, the eyes, lungs, skin, and nervous system. The criteria for the diagnosis of RA ranges from the original American Rheumatism Association (ARA) scheme of 1958, through the development of the simpler New York criteria, to the current American College of Rheumatology (ACR) scheme of 1987 (see Table 5.1) which replaced the 1958 ARA criteria. It is important to remember that criteria are often developed and needed for both epidemiological work and classification in the context of trials. As such there are inevitable shortcomings and it is often difficult to apply these criteria to the diagnosis of 'possible', 'early', or atypical RA. These criteria may perhaps best be used in clinical trials aimed at patients with well-established disease. However, by their very nature, they provide a diagnostic guideline for the physician.

Table 5.1 The 1987 American College of Rheumatology criteria for the diagnosis of rheumatoid arthritis

	Criterion	Comments
1	Morning stiffness	Duration >1 hour lasting >6 weeks
2	Arthritis of at least three joints*	Soft tissue swelling/exudation lasting >6 weeks
3	Arthritis of hand joints	Wrists, MCPs, or PIPs lasting >6 weeks
4	Symmetrical arthritis	At least one area, lasting >6 weeks
5	Rheumatoid nodules	
6	Positive rheumatoid factor	
7	Radiographic changes	Erosions, particularly wrists, hands, and feet

At least four criteria must be fulfilled and there are no exclusion criteria.

* Possible areas: metacarpophalangeal joints (MCPJ), proximal interphalangeal joints (PIPJ), wrist, elbow, knee, ankle, metatarsophalangeal joints (MTPJ).

Incidence, prevalence, and morbidity

- The disease has a worldwide prevalence, identified in all populations that have been examined. Figures for prevalence range from 0.2 to 5.3%, but the age distribution in developing countries may be a confounding factor and perhaps contribute to low figures in, for example, some parts of Africa.
- Accepting the difficulties involved in establishing an early diagnosis of RA, population studies on the incidence of the disease suggest figures of 3.4/10 000 in ♀ and 1.4/10 000 in ♂. The incidence in men ↑ with age from age 45. In ♀, it ↑ until age 45, then plateaus and falls after the age of 75.
- RA is extremely heterogeneous with regard to severity and progression. Permanent remission can occur but is rare once joint damage has started. Distinction is sometimes made between cyclical disease and relentless progression but in practice it is perhaps more useful to consider widespread and limited chronic joint involvement.
- Life expectancy is reduced by approximately 7 years in ♂ and 3 years in ♀. This is mainly due to cardiovascular disease, infections, renal disease, respiratory disease, and RA itself.

The clinical features of rheumatoid arthritis

- A typical onset of insidious pain, stiffness, and symmetrical swelling of small joints is only one of several presenting patterns. Up to one-third of patients may have a subacute onset with symptoms of fatigue, malaise, weight loss, myalgia, morning stiffness, and joint pain without overt signs of swelling or radiological evidence of joint erosions.
- Synovitis of the small joints of the hands and feet with symmetry and sparing of the distal interphalangeal joints is the most characteristic feature of RA. However, a mono- or bilateral arthropathy of the shoulder or wrist may account for up to 30–40% of initial presentations, and the knee, 5%.
- Any synovial joint can become involved in RA. The hands, wrists, elbows, shoulders, and knees are involved most commonly, followed by the hip and temporomandibular joints. RA also affects the clavicular joints and the cricoarytenoid.
- Patients may also present with a tenosynovitis or bursitis. The diagnosis and management of these conditions is covered in Chapter 2 of this book.
- Though presented often in textbooks as features of 'swan neck' and 'boutoniere', deformity of the digits appears late in disease and are features of chronic disease; they are not usually seen at initial presentation where signs of synovitis and jointdamage may be subtle.
- Though often suspected by lay persons, there is no absolute evidence that stress, whether physical or psychological, triggers the disease.
- There is overwhelming evidence that pregnancy has a beneficial effect on RA, especially during the last trimester. Arthritic symptoms usually return within 1–2 months postpartum and may be more severe than prior disease. Lactation has no effect and there is no evidence that RA patients have more medical complications during pregnancy per se. Therapeutics and pregnancy are discussed later in this chapter.

Organ disease in rheumatoid arthritis (Table 5.2)

Lymph nodes
Lymph nodes are often enlarged but rarely palpable. In a few cases RA may present with widespread nodes mimicking Hodgkin's disease.

Pulmonary disease
- Pleuritis (like pericarditis) is frequent but often mild. Like other pulmonary and cardiac manifestations, it is more common in older ♂. Pleural effusions may also occur.
- Rheumatoid pulmonary nodules are an asymptomatic finding in sero-positive RA. Radiographically they are coin-shaped lesions that can be difficult to distinguish from malignancy. In patients in whom malignancy is clinically suspected, further imaging or tissue biopsy may be required.
- ⚠ Diffuse interstitial fibrosis and fibrosing alveolitis are rare associations. Methotrexate is also associated with the development of fibrosis.

Cardiovascular system
There is increasing evidence that patients with RA suffer from increased cardiovascular disease, independent of the traditional risk factors. Inflammation is thought to play an important part in the development of atherosclerosis and the systemic inflammatory response in RA may explain the link. Epidemiological studies show that cardiovascular mortality is increased in patients with early and established disease and is worse in women, a group traditionally at lower risk. Standardized mortality ratios for cardiovascular disease in ♂ are approximately 1.3 and 1.9 in ♀.

Skin
- Palmar eythema is common.
- Raynaud's phenomenon may also be present with associated infarcts, skin ulceration, and superinfection.
- Rheumatoid nodules occur in up to 30% of patients, and are found principally on the extensor surface of the forearm and over pressure areas throughout the skin. Nodules are not specific for RA but are useful in diagnosis and prognosis, correlating with seropositivity, disease activity, and progression.
- Leucocytoclastic vasculitis also occurs and is seen as palpable purpura; most often this resolves spontaneously.

Ocular involvement
- ⚠ Rheumatoid vasculitis gives rise to a severe form of painful scleritis, leading to scleromalcia.
- Episcleritis is benign and resolves. Uveitis and conjunctivitis are not associated with RA.

Table 5.2 Some organ disease in rheumatoid arthritis

Organ	Manifestation	Frequency (%)
Lymph nodes	Enlargement	>50
Spleen	Enlargement	25
	Felty's syndrome	<1
Lungs	Pleuritis	>30
	Nodules	5
	Fibrosis	Rare
Heart	Pericarditis	>10
	Myocarditis	>5
	Nodules	5
	Cardiovascular disease (RA is an independent risk factor)	Standardized mortality ratio: ♂ ~ 1.3 ♀ ~ 1.9
Muscle	Atrophy	Common
	Myositis	Rare
Bone	Osteoporosis	Common
Skin	Nodules	>20
	Vasculitis	1
Eyes	Sicca syndrome	10
	Scleritis	1
	Nodules	<2
Nervous system	Nerve entrapment	Common
	Mononeuritis multiplex	<1
	Cord compression	Rare

Neurological involvement

- Entrapment neuropathy secondary to synovitis is common. Median nerve compression can occur early in the disease. Other rarer examples included the ulnar nerve at the elbow, and the posterior tibial nerve at the tarsal tunnel.
- Mononeuritis multiplex, a peripheral and often bilateral neuropathy, can present acutely. A sudden onset of motor neuropathy can signal the presence of aggressive vasculitis and poor prognosis.
- Cervical subluxation at the atlantoaxial level is present in one-third of RA patients but is usually asymptomatic. Subluxation at lower levels is rare, but is more likely to cause pain and neurological symptoms.
  ⚠ Cervical myelopathy due to cervical instability can be fatal. Symptoms include paraesthesia, weakness, paralysis, sensory loss, incontinence, and syncope.

Fractures
- Cytokines, generated in inflammation, encourage bone resorption by osteoclast induction leading to periarticular osteoporosis.
- Inactivity, nutritional deficiency, glucocorticoid, and methotrexate use, and pre-existing osteoporosis constitute additional risk factors for spontaneous fractures.

Tendons and ligaments
Spontaneous rupture is common, most often at the wrist, hand, and rotator cuff. More often, tenosynovitis and weakening of ligaments leads to joint instability and subluxation.

Infection
There is anecdotal evidence that infections may trigger flares in RA. More importantly, RA patients are more susceptible to septic arthritis, often compounded by the use of immunosuppressive drugs (see later in this chapter). In such a situation, the usual signs of sepsis may be absent, delaying the diagnosis.

Secondary amyloidosis
Renal involvement is the most common type of organ failure, though the skin, liver, and GI tract are often affected. Intensive antirheumatic therapy now gives a more favourable outlook, with 80% 5-year survival rates.

Felty's syndrome
This is the association of splenomegaly and neutropenia in typically rather destructive RA. Systemic disease, hepatomegaly, and lymphadenopathy are also common, and the occurrence of RA in relatives is higher than expected. In uncomplicated cases, treatment should be conservative, splenectomy remaining controversial and often only transient in effect.

The evaluation and treatment of rheumatoid arthritis

- A clearly documented assessment is invaluable for the ongoing monitoring of the disease and treatment (see Table 5.3).
- The ESR and CRP are useful measures periodically in the assessment of disease activity, and haematological and biochemical parameters will not only expose underlying organ disease but are important in the regular monitoring of a number of drug treatments.
- Early erosive changes on plain radiographs of the hands and feet can be of great value in the assessment of patients with minimal clinical signs.
- IgM rheumatoid factor (RF) is of value in establishing the diagnosis, however, a low positive result can be misleading and a negative result should not alter a diagnosis made on clinical grounds. Only 70–80% of patients with RA will be RF positive. The RF need not be repeated regularly. Perhaps the main indication to do so is in those patients whose initial result is negative or very low but clinically have signs suggestive of the disease. With time these cases may become strongly positive and their disease will require more aggressive management.
- Anti-cyclic citrullinated peptide (anti-CCP) antibodies are potentially important surrogate markers for diagnosis and prognosis in RA. In both early and established disease, anti-CCP antibodies are more sensitive and more specific than RF. Anti-CCP antibodies may be detected in roughly 50–60% of patients with early RA. They are also a marker of erosive disease and may predict the development of RA in patients with non-specific inflammatory symptoms.
- The ultimate goal would be the complete remission of disease but this is rarely possible and initial assessment and decisions about treatment need to take account of the relative degree of both inflammatory and mechanical disease as well as their psychological impact.
- Whilst a functional assessment is of value, particularly in respect to trial data, regular monitoring need not employ formal status questionnaires and often a global view from the patient, physician, or physiotherapist, is enough.
- The Disease Activity Score (DAS) is a composite score using tender and swollen joint count, ESR, and patient global assessment of disease activity using a 100 mm visual analogue scale. The DAS is used to assess suitability for biological therapies and response to treatment. It is easy to do and can be done by doctors or other health professionals. The DAS28 is calculated as follows:

$$DAS28 = 0.56\sqrt{(\text{number tender joints})}$$
$$+ 0.28\sqrt{(\text{number of swollen joints})} + 0.70 \ln(\text{ESR})$$
$$+ 0.014 \text{ Global assessment (in mm)}$$

- The management of RA requires a multidisciplinary approach. Regular liaison with physiotherapists, occupational therapists, podiatrists, social services, and surgeons is an important part of keeping up-to-date with patient progress and new developments in therapeutics and management (see Table 5.4).

Table 5.3 Documenting the initial evaluation of RA

1	The duration of morning stiffness
	The degree of pain
	Fatigue
	Function (utilizing a score system such as Health Assessment Questionnaire—HAQ)
	Patient global assessment of disease activity
2	The distribution and number of painful joints, and the distribution and number of swollen joints, including periodicity
	The distribution and nature of mechanical joint disease noting loss of function, instability, and modifying factors
	The presence or absence of extra-articular disease
3	Radiographs of affected joints looking for erosive disease and mechanical damage
4	Laboratory tests
	ESR and CRP
	FBC
	Renal and liver function tests
	Urinalysis
	Rheumatoid factor
	Anti-CCP antibodies

Which drugs, when, and what to monitor?
(Table 5.5)

- Most patients will either periodically or continuously be taking NSAIDs. These agents offer reliable, even if sometimes limited, relief of pain, swelling, and stiffness, improving quality of life in the majority of cases. Adverse effects are, however, common and sometimes life-threatening and awareness and patient education is essential; combinations of NSAIDs should be avoided. Selective Cox-2 NSAIDs are of similar efficacy to diclofenac or naproxen. NICE guidance recommended they only be used in patients requiring an NSAID over the age 65, intolerant of standard NSAIDs, or using medicines known to ↑ the likelihood of gastric problems. However, recent evidence has shown that rofecoxib use ↑ risk of myocardial infarction. Rofecoxib and valde-coxib have been withdrawn but celecoxib is still available. Of concern is a study showing that even standard NSAIDs such as ibuprofen, di-clofenac and naproxen are associated with ↑ risk of myocardial infarc-tion. It is therefore vital that these drugs are used appropriately and avoided for long-term use in patients with adverse cardiovascular or GI risk profiles (see table 5.6). Further research is needed in this area.

Table 5.4 The main components in the treatment of RA

Modality	Examples
Education and counselling	Specialist nurse practitioner
	Self-care groups
	National organizations
Physiotherapy	Exercise
	Joint protection
Occupational therapy	Adaptation
	Aids
	Splints
Podiatry and chiropody	Orthoses
	Surgical shoes
Medication	Pain control
	Disease control
Non-medical pain management	Transcutaneous nerve stimulation
	Acupuncture
	Psychotherapy
	Surgery
Surgery	Joint replacement
	Arthrodesis
	Tendon release/repair

- All patients with active disease should be offered a disease-modifying antirheumatic drug (DMARD) early. The rationale is to prevent or reduce joint destruction. Evidence from systematic reviews suggest that early introduction of DMARDs ↓ pain, swelling, and joint damage. Guidelines now recommend that the majority of patients with newly diagnosed RA should be started on DMARD therapy within 3 months of diagnosis. However, efficacy is unpredictable and variable in duration. Toxicity is an important concern and this should always be discussed with patients, These agents are also slow-acting, sometimes taking up to 6 months to have effect. The final choice of DMARD is influenced by a number of factors including, patient compliance, convenience of administration, severity of disease, presence of other medical conditions, pregnancy, monitoring requirements and frequency, and nature of adverse events.
- Fundamental to the decision process remains the confidence of the physician in administering familiar DMARDs. Most physicians would currently use methotrexate.

Table 5.5 Pharmacotherapy of rheumatoid arthritis

Drug type	Examples
Pain relief	Simple analgesia
	NSAIDs
Disease-modifying drugs	Glucocorticoids (oral, IM, intra-articular)
	Methotrexate
	Sulfasalazine
	Azathioprine
	Hydroxychloroquine
	D-Penicillamine
	Sodium aurothiomalate: gold by IM injection
	Auranofin: oral gold
	Leflunomide
	Ciclosporin A
Biological therapies	Anti-TNF: etanercept, infliximab, adalimumab
	Anti B-cell: rituximab
	IL-1 receptor antagonists: anakinra
For disease complications	Anaemia: iron, erythropoetin
	Osteoporosis: oestrogens, bisphosphonates, strontium ranelate, teriparatide
	Vasculitis: glucocorticoids, cyclophosphamide
	Amyloidosis: chlorambucil, anti-TNF therapies

Sulfasalazine and hydroxychloroquine

- Sulfasalazine (SSZ) and hydroxychloroquine (HCQ) are often used initially in mild RA, partly because of their relative safety and convenience. Both agents are generally well-tolerated and take effect within 1–3 months. Many clinicians would now, however, choose methotrexate first if there is evidence of early aggressive disease.
- Retinal toxicity and maculopathy are the main concern with HCQ, the risk increasing, with abnormal liver or kidney function, after a cumulative dose of 800 g, and in patients aged 70 years and over. The eyes should be checked formally by an ophthalmologist once and the patient informed to report any visual disturbances.
- There is potential for accumulation of HCQ in the fetus during pregnancy, and for chromosomal damage. Some workers report no significant risk to the fetus but the potential for chromosomal damage has led many to avoid HCQ in pregnancy.
- Sulfasalazine has been used successfully in pregnancy. There have been case reports of congenital malformations, although the overall risk is considered very small.

- Sulfasalazine may cause leucopenia, pancytopenia, haemolysis, and aplastic anaemia. Serious bone marrow toxicity is, however, uncommon. It also induces a hepatic transaminitis.
- Spermatogenesis can be affected by SSZ, but subfertility is reversible. There does not appear to be an adverse effect on female fertility.

Methotrexate

- Methotrexate (MTX) is given weekly by mouth or S/C or IM injection. Toxicity, particulary stomatitis, GI disturbance, and alopecia, may be reduced by the addition of folic acid weekly, without loss of therapeutic effect.
- Pneumonitis is uncommon and pulmonary fibrosis (a rare complication of MTX) should not deter the physician from using MTX in aggressive systemic and skeletal disease. Rare, life-threatening, pulmonary toxicity can occur at any time and is not necessarily related to dose or duration of treatment. A chest X-ray should be taken before MTX is commenced.
- Mild drug-induced hepatitis is relatively common and is often corrected by the addition of folic acid. Overt liver disease is rare. Routine liver biopsy is not necessary, being restricted to pretreatment assessment of patients with other liver disease and patients with persistent liver function abnormalities in spite of discontinuing treatment.
- Myelosuppression is rarely severe. Antifolate drugs such as trimethoprim, and folate deficiency increase the risk of toxicity. Renal impairment reduces methotrexate clearance and may lead to toxicity. Pregnancy and breast-feeding are contraindications to the use of MTX. Both ♂ and ♀ patients should wait 3 months after stopping treatment before trying to conceive a child. Subfertility caused by MTX is reversible.
- NSAID use is not contraindicated. There is the potential for interaction and hepatotoxicity and close monitoring remains a pre-requisite for commencing therapy.
- Patients having major operations are often advised to stop treatment for 1–2 weeks either side of surgery, although there is no evidence to suggest that this reduces the risk of postoperative complications such as wound healing or sepsis, and ↑ the risk of a disease flare.

Other DMARDs

- Other effective DMARDs include oral and IM gold, D-penicillamine, azathioprine, leflunomide, ciclosporin, and cyclophosphamide. Combined therapy such as MTX + HCQ, MTX + SSZ, or gold + HCQ are also used, often weaning off one drug as disease activity subsides. Currently there is no evidence that combination therapy at the start of treatment is better than monotherapy alone. Decisons should be based on discussion between the doctor and patient taking into account the risks and benefits. These agents, their side-effects and monitoring are detailed in Table 5.7.
- Gold and cyclophosphamide should be avoided in pregnancy. Azathioprine may be used with caution. There are insufficient data at present to make recommendations on the use of ciclosporin or leflunomide in pregnancy.

Table 5.6 Adverse reactions of NSAIDs

Organ/complication	Occurrence	Comments
GI tract	Common	Gastritis, bleeding, and perforation. High risk in elderly and those with ulcer history
Renal	Common	Fluid retention Papillary necrosis
Hypertension	Common	Interference with drugs such as thiazide diuretics
Myocardial infarction	Increased risk in those with cardiovascular risk factors	Cox-1 and Cox-2 drugs
Pulmonary	Not uncommon	Exacerbation of asthma Pneumonitis (naproxen)
Skin	Not uncommon	Hypersensitivity Erythema multiforme
CNS	Not uncommon	Tinnitus, fatigue, cognitive disturbance
	Rare	Aseptic meningitis
Hepatic	Uncommon	Drug-induced hepatitis
Haematological	Rare	Bone marrow dyscrasias
Pregnancy		Diclofenac and low-dose aspirin appear to be safe

Glucocorticoids

- IM and oral steroids are very effective in active RA, reducing active disease in an acute crisis or whilst waiting for a DMARD to take effect. Many patients are often on a combination of NSAID and DMARD with intermittent doses of systemic steroid.
- Local steroid injections are of value in symptom control both early in the disease and in an acute 'flare'. The effect on joint recovery may be dramatic, but short-lived, with little impact on the overall process of RA, and should not be repeated any more than once every 3 months. It is sometimes of value to combine injections with a joint 'washout' in refractory cases. Using correct aseptic technique there is no evidence to suggest an increased risk of joint infection per se.

Table 5.7 Monitoring guidelines for DMARDs in rheumatoid arthritis

Drug	Main toxicity	Other side-effects	Monitoring
Sulfasalazine	Myelosuppression	Stains body fluid, rash, hepatitis	FBC and LFT every 2 weeks until dose stable and thereafter every 3 months
Methotrexate	Myelosuppression	Hepatitis, pneumonitis, rash	FBC and LFT every 2 weeks until dose stable. Baseline CXR. FBC and LFT every 4–6 weeks. U&E every 6 months thereafter
Hydroxychloroquine	Macular damage	Visual disturbance	Ophthalmic review if visual disturbance
Intramuscular gold	Myelosuppression	Rash, reversible proteinuria	FBC and urinalysis before every dose
D-penicillamine	Myelosupression, drug-induced myasthenic syndrome	Rashes, proteinuria	FBC and urinalysis every 2 weeks until dose stable then monthly
Azathioprine	Myelosuppression	Hepatitis	FBC every 2 weeks until dose stable then every 8 weeks. LFT every 3 months
Leflunomide	Myelosuppression	Hepatitis, diarrhoea, alopecia, skin allergies	FBC every 2 weeks for 6 weeks then every 8 weeks. LFT and blood pressure every 12 weeks
Ciclosporin (Neoral®)	Hypertension, renal toxicity	Gum hyperplasia, hyperlipidaemia, hyperuricaemia	Serum creatinine and BP every 2 weeks until the dose has been stable for 3 months. Thereafter serum creatinine and BP monthly. FBC, LFTs monthly until dose stable for 3 months and then 3-monthly. Serum lipids 6-monthly

FBC = full blood count; CXR = chest radiograph; LFT = liver function tests; U+E = urea and electrolytes.

- High-dose systemic administration may reduce overall disease activity in the short-term but adverse effects preclude its uninhibited use and it is best preserved for refractory RA and severe extra-articular complications.
- There have been reports linking glucocorticoid therapy to fetal congenital malformations; however, prednisolone, dexamethasone, and betamethasone appear to be safe (there is little data on lactation), though should be administered only if absolutely necessary.

Anti-TNF α therapy

- TNFα is a potent proinflammatory cytokine whose levels are ↑ in RA.
- At present (in the UK) there are 3 agents available for the treatment of active RA, namely adalimumab (Humira®), etanercept (Enbrel®), and infliximab (Remicade®). Infliximab is a chimeric human–murine anti-TNFα monoclonal antibody, etanercept is a recombinant human TNF receptor fusion protein, and adalimumab is a fully humanized anti-TNF monoclonal antibody. Infliximab is administered by slow IV infusion at 0, 2, 4, and every 4–8 weeks thereafter depending on response. Etanercept is administered by S/C injection and can now be given once instead of twice weekly. Adalimumab is given by S/C injection every 2 weeks. The cost of these agents per annum per patient in the UK is approximately £10 000. The National Institute for Clinical Excellence (NICE) in the UK and the British Society for Rheumatology BSR have published guidelines for the use of these drugs (see Table 5.8)
- All these agents have been shown to improve clinical response. Etanercept or infliximab in combination with methotrexate have a synergistic effect and lead to a better clinical response and slowing of radiological progression. Methotrexate use with infliximab also reduces the production of anti-infliximab and antinuclear antibodies.

Table 5.8 UK NICE/BSR Guidelines for the use of anti-TNF therapy in RA

1	Patients must satisfy 1987 ACR criteria for diagnosis of RA
2	A disease activity score of >5.1 at 2 points, 1 month apart
3	Adequate trial of at least 2 standard DMARDs, one of which should be methotrexate. An adequate trial is defined as: —treatment for at least 6 months, with at least 2 months at standard target dose (unless toxicity) —treatment for <6 months where treatment was withdrawn due to intolerance or toxicity, normally after at least 2 months of therapeutic doses
4	Exclusion criteria: pregnancy or breast-feeding. Active infection or high risk of infection. Malignant or pre-malignant states
5	Criteria for withdrawal of therapy: adverse events or inefficacy.

- These therapies are not without their adverse events. Common reactions include headache, nausea, and injection-site reactions. Serious bacterial infections have been reported, and patients with active infection should have their treatment stopped. Patients at risk of recurrent infection should not use these drugs (e.g. indwelling urinary catheter, immunodeficiency states). Reactivation of tuberculsosis has been reported mainly in infliximab patients, and most commonly within 3 months of commencement of treatment. Patients should be assessed for TB risk, and guidelines for assessing risk and managing Mycobacterium tuberculosis infection in patients due to start anti-TNF therapy have been published by the British Thoracic Society (www.britthoracic.org.uk). Other reported side-effects include demyelination, worsening of heart failure, lupus-like syndromes, and bone marrow dyscrasias.

- There remains concern about the long-term safety of these drugs, especially with regard to malignancy. In the UK patients are registered on a Biologics Registry, which collects data on adverse events, response to treatment, and patient demographic details. Debate continues as to whether reports of lymphoma in RA patients on anti-TNFα therapy reflect a real drug effect or the known ↑ incidence of lymphoma in RA patients. No ↑ risk has been found with other types of malignancy.

- Pregnancy, breast-feeding, sepsis, and malignancy are exclusion criteria, although there have been case reports of successful pregnancies in patients on anti-TNFα therapy.

Interleukin-1 receptor antagonists: anakinra

Interleukin-1 (IL-1) is a proinflammatory cytokine. Anakinra is an IL-1 receptor antagonist that competes with Il-1 for binding. The agent is given by daily S/C injection. Randomized controlled trials have shown it is more effective than placebo. Side-effects include injection-site reactions, blood dyscrasias, and infection. Anti-TNFα therapies should not be used in conjunction, and clearance is reduced in renal impairment. Although licensed for use in RA, NICE have not approved the drug for use in the UK as they felt it was not cost effective. Its use in the UK is therefore limited.

B cell therapy

There is increasing evidence that B cells play an important role in the pathogenesis of RA. Rituximab, a chimeric monoclonal antibody against human CD20 has been used in trials. CD20 is present on developing B cells prior to the plasma cell stage. Administration of rituximab leads to rapid CD20 positive B cell depletion in the peripheral blood. Normal B cell repopulation occurs within the next 3 months. Rituximab was first used in non-Hodgkins lymphoma. A randomized controlled trial has shown that in RF positive patients who have failed several DMARDs, a course of rituximab (2 infusions 2 weeks apart with corticosteroid cover) achieve a significant improvement in disease activity at 6 months compared to methotrexate alone. There is concern about persistent hypogammaglobulinaemia and risk of respiratory tract infection.

Experimental therapies in RA
Experimental therapies are detailed in Table 5.9.

Pregnancy and lactation
The use of antirheumatic drugs in pregnancy and lactation is summarized in Table 5.10.

Surgery in RA

- Damage to joints, with associated pain and loss of function remains a familiar feature of chronic RA. Surgical intervention may have a place in such situations, though certain procedures (e.g. shoulder replacement) may only be effective in reducing pain and may not necessarily improve function.
- Synovectomy is less frequently performed now, although tenosynovectomy is common, and a quick and safe relief of nerve entrapment.
- Common surgical procedures include:
  - decompression of the carpal tunnel
  - reconstructive arthroplasty of hip and knee; less often the shoulder, elbow, and small joints of the hand
  - corrective arthrotomies of the metatarsals
  - stabilization of the cervical spine
  - tendon release and transfer
  - arthrodesis, particularly of the ankle joint.
- Patients should ideally be seen by a surgeon with expertise in dealing with patients with RA.

Table 5.9 Experimental therapies for the treatment of rheumatoid arthritis

Target	Principle
Co-stimulation inhibitors	CTLA4 Ig
Cell cycle inhibitor	Temsirolimus
Ion Channel blockers	Receptor anatagonists
Cytokine inhibition	Anti-IL-6 antibody
	Oral TNF inhibitor
	Anti-TNF antibody fragment (CDP 870)
	Anti-IL-15 monoclonal antibody
B cells	Humanized anti CD-20 agents
	Anti-B cell stimulator protein (belimumab)
Cell adhesion molecules	Humanized 4-1 and 4-7 monoclonal antibody (natalizumab)
Proinflammation	Fish/plant seed oils

Table 5.10 Antirheumatic drugs in pregnancy and lactation

Drug	Effects
Methotrexate	*Pregnancy:* teratogenic experiments, protection with leucovorin. No adverse effects in low dose clinically (7.5 mg/week); termination not mandatory. Long-term follow-up data lacking but drug better avoided or stopped
	Lactation: no data and probably safe if dose not >7.5 mg/week
Corticosteroids	*Pregnancy:* no convincing evidence of teratogenic effects; occasional neonatal adrenal suppression; better avoided but can be used or continued if indicated—prednisolone dose preferably not >10 mg/day
	Lactation: drug should be avoided on theoretical grounds, especially if dose >7.5 mg/day prednisolone or equivalent
Sulfasalazine	*Pregnancy:* isolated report of fetal abnormalities but limited data and no convincing reports of teratogenic effects; drug can be continued
	Lactation: inadequate data; probably safe if dose not >2 g/day
Azathioprine	*Pregnancy:* genotoxic experimentally. No proven adverse effects clinically but long-term follow-up data lacking; better avoided but continue if indicated
	Lactation: no known adverse effects; safe if dose not >2.5 mg/kg/day
Alkylating agents	*Pregnancy:* case report of teratogenic effects of cyclophosphamide in first trimester; best avoided but inadequate data to make termination mandatory. Experimental data indicate that there may be variation in protective repair capacity. Long-term follow-up data lacking
	Lactation: no data but best avoided on theoretical grounds

Table 5.10 (*Contd.*)

Drug	Effects
Ciclosporin A	*Pregnancy:* experimental teratogenesis and autoantibody formation. Transplacental passage; no evidence of fetal toxicity or subsequent immunodeficiency in non-transplant recipients. Termination unnecessary, drug better avoided or stopped if possible
	Lactation: inadequate data but better avoided on present evidence
Hydroxychloroquine	*Pregnancy:* adverse effects unlikely from limited data; termination not justified, drug can be continued
	Lactation: inadequate data; probably safe
D-penicillamine	*Pregnancy:* experimental fetal wastage. No convincing evidence of adverse effects in humans; better avoided but termination not mandatory
	Lactation: drug should be avoided on theoretical grounds but no compelling evidence for stopping in doses <600 mg/day
Gold	*Pregnancy:* no convincing evidence of adverse effects with IM or oral gold. Termination unnecessary but drug better discontinued
	Lactation: infant serum gold levels similar to maternal levels; no deleterious effects
Biologic therapies	*Pregnancy and lactation:* contra-indicated

Management summary for treating RA

- Fig. 5.1 summarizes the management of RA.
- There remains a need for the development of early predictors of long-term outcome in RA, allowing better patient selection for early intervention. Early functional impairment remains a crude but reliable indicator of poor prognosis. A high RF titre, ↑ ESR or CRP at diagnosis, ♂ gender, radiographic evidence of erosions, and rheumatoid nodules are features associated with aggressive disease. Further evaluation of early onset disease, combination therapies, and newly developing strategies in therapeutics will reduce a common and still severe disease to a milder if not minimally destructive condition. Of all patients with RA, 20% will have mild disease, 75% moderate disease with relapses and remissions, and 5% will have severe destructive disease.
- Patients are at risk of early cardiovascular disease. It is important to assess cardiovascular risk factors such as cholesterol, blood pressure, diabetes, corticosteroid use, smoking, etc. and modify them if possible.
- The multidisciplinary team are important in patient care and should be involved at an early stage.
- DMARD monitoring is needed to ensure patients do not suffer serious side-effects.

Patients should be involved directly in any decisions about their care.

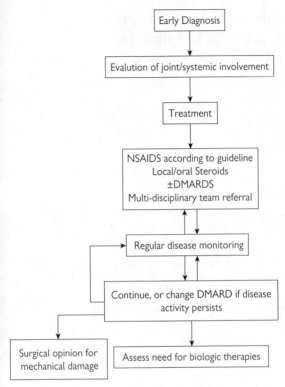

Figure 5.1 An algorithm for the management of adult rheumatoid arthritis

Rheumatoid factor positive polyarthritis in childhood

- This subset of juvenile idiopathic arthritis (see Chapter 7 for further details of classification) is clinically and genetically indistinguishable from adult RA. Approximately 25% of cases have a family history of seropositive RA.
- The disease usually presents as a polyarthritis (>five joints) of the small joints of the hands and feet. In presentation before the age of 10 years there is often associated early involvement of the wrists, knees, ankles, and hindfeet as well. All other features of adult RA may be seen in children.
- Fever is rare.
- The ILAR criteria suggests that three consecutive positive tests for serum IgM RF should be taken twice over the course of 3 months before the diagnosis is made. This is because transient positive titres are seen in infection. It is also important to bear in mind that a ↑ RF is also found in SLE (see Chapter 9), some vasculitides (see Chapter 14), hypergammaglobulinaemia, and sarcoidosis (see Chapter 18). The clinical features may also appear similar to juvenile psoriatic arthropathy (see Chapter 8).
- Radiological changes with periostitis and local osteoporosis tend to occur early in the disease. One-third of cases progress to severe functional limitation within 10–15 years.
- Differences from adult RA include the problem of growth retardation, a tendency to early fusion of the carpal bones, and erosions at the distal interphalangeal joints.
- A few cases of aortic regurgitation and pericarditis have been reported. Pulmonary manifestations of RA are, however, relatively uncommon.
- In the few cases that have been followed through pregnancy, there appears to be an almost universal post-pregnancy relapse of the RA.
- Treatment of RA in children is much the same as for adults. Early introduction of a DMARD is encouraged and most centres use as first-line therapy. MTX is well-tolerated in children. Oral therapy is first-line, but S/C administration is increasingly used, and has been shown to be effective in those with poor adherence or side-effects to oral treatment. A recent study using leflunomide found high rates of clinical improvement, but not as great as with MTX. If corticosteroid therapy is started, the preferred regimen is an alternate-day dosing.
- Cytotoxics tend to be spared for use in those with associated amyloidosis, vasculitis, pulmonary fibrosis, or aortic valve disease in the presence of active arthritis.
- NICE in the UK has reviewed the use of etanercept and recommended its use in active polyarticular disease when patients have been intolerant of, or not responded to, MTX.

Osteoarthritis (OA)

Introduction

Epidemiology and pathology

- Osteoarthritis (OA) is a chronic degenerative disorder characterized by cartilage loss and is the commonest condition to affect joints in humans. It is estimated that 15% of the population of the United Kingdom >55 years have symptomatic OA of the knee. In England and Wales, 1.3–1.7 million people have symptomatic OA.
- In elderly people in the West, OA is second to cardiovascular disease as a cause of disability.
- Although there are recognized associations between OA, age, and trauma, advances in cartilage biochemistry and the recognition of crystal-associated disease have renewed interest in OA as a dynamic condition of cartilage loss (chondropathy) with a periarticular bone reaction. At present, however, OA is assessed and managed clinically as a structural rather than physiological condition, with emphasis on late, rather than early, disease.
- OA is now viewed as a dynamic process with episodic progress. Chondrocyte dysfunction leads to metalloproteinase enzyme release causing collagen and proteoglycan degradation. Synovial inflammation is present, with production of cytokines such as Il-1 and TNFα that also induce metalloproteinase production.
- Macroscopic changes in OA include cystic bone degeneration, cartilage loss, and growth of irregular abnormal bone at joint margins (osteophytes). Microscopic changes include flaking and fibrillation of articular cartilage with variations in vascularity and cellularity of sub-chondral bone, leading to sclerosis and new bone formation.
- Most surveys of OA rely on radiographic features for definition and severity. These are problematic not least because correlation of radio-graphic change with clinical status, symptoms, and function, can be poor; it is best at the hip, then knee, and poor in the hand and spine. The correlation between pathology and radiology is shown in Table 6.1.
- There are various subgroups of OA and these are described below in the section on clinical features.

Risk factors

- Although no gender difference occurs in mild disease, there is a ♀ preponderance in severe disease and >50 years, There is also a polyarticular form of hand OA, 'nodal generalized OA', that has a predilection for peri-menopausal ♀.
- OA of the hip is more common in Europeans than Chinese and Afro-Caribbeans.
- The Framingham study found that 27% of those aged 63–70 years had radiographic evidence of knee OA, rising to 44% in those >80 years.

- Susceptibility factors include:
  - obesity (close association with knee OA, but not hip)
  - family history (particularly nodal generalized OA)
  - high bone density such as osteopetrosis (there is a negative correlation between OA onset and low bone density)
  - trauma
  - femoral dysplasia (for hip OA)
  - hypermobility (rigorous studies required, though one recent large study suggests hypermobility to be protective against hand OA).
- There is increased concordance for OA in monozygotic compared to dizygotic twins.
- Smoking appears to be protective (knee OA).
- Suggested risk factors for hip OA include previous hip disease (Perthes' etc.), acetabular dysplasia, avascular necrosis of the femoral head, severe trauma, generalized OA, and occupation (farming).
- There is little evidence to link OA with repetitive injury from occupation, except perhaps knee-bending in men.
- Dockers and miners have a higher incidence of knee OA.

Table 6.1 Radiographic–pathological correlates in OA

Pathological change	Radiographic abnormality
Cartilage fibrillation, erosion	Localized joint-space narrowing
Subchondral new bone	Sclerosis
Myxoid degeneration	Subchondral cysts
Trabecular compression	Bone collapse/attrition
Fragmentation of osteochondral surface	Osseous ('loose') bodies

Clinical features of OA

- The clinical features of pain and stiffness, functional impairment, and anatomical change, are interrelated but often discordant.
- There are several potential mechanisms for pain and none are completely understood. Pain may arise from inflammatory mediators or intra-articular hypertension, stimulating capsular, periosteal, and synovial nerve fibres. Pain may also arise from enthesopathy or bursitis that can accompany structural alteration, muscle weakness, and altered joint use.
- Although stiffness is a common complaint in OA, prolonged early morning stiffness should lead the clinician to consider the presence of an inflammatory arthropathy.
- Bony enlargement and deformity, crepitus, restricted movement, joint instability, and 'stress' pain also occur. Muscle weakness and wasting may be present.
- There are several subsets of OA that are worth noting. They are not absolute, and one set of characteristics may dominate the evolving disease at any one time. These subsets are:
  - primary OA:
    — Nodal generalized OA
    — Erosive ('inflammatory') OA
    — Large joint OA (knee and hip)
    — Spinal OA
  - secondary OA (see Table 6.2).

Nodal generalized OA

- This common condition is characterized by:
  - polyarticular finger involvement
  - Heberden's nodes (distal interphalangeal joint)
  - Bouchard's nodes (proximal interphalangeal joint)
  - predisposition to OA of knee, hip, and spine
  - good functional outcome in the hands
  - ♀ preponderance
  - peak onset around the menopause
  - strong family history.
- There is a tendency to greater distal joint disease. The first carpometacarpal (CMC), metacarpophalangeal (MCP), and interphalangeal joints (IPJ) of the thumb are also often involved, as are the index and middle MCP.
- The more proximal joints of the hand and wrist are otherwise relatively spared.

Erosive OA

- This uncommon condition is characterized by:
  - hand interphalangeal involvement
  - tendency to joint ankylosis
  - florid inflammation (episodic)
  - radiographic subchondral erosive change.
- Unlike nodal OA, proximal and distal IPJs are equally involved and, less frequently, the MCPs.

- IPJ instability is common. Given the additional risk of ankylosis, functional impairment is more likely than nodal OA.
- The principal hallmark of the condition is subchondral erosive change that can lead to remodelling.

Large joint OA

- The knee is commonly affected and most frequently in the patello-femoral and medial tibiofemoral compartments; severe bone and cartilage loss at the latter site causes instability and the classic varus (bow knee) deformity.
- Subdivision of hip disease is usually made on the basis of local radiographic patterns. There are two principal groups:
  i. Superior pole: common pattern, often unilateral, more common in ♂, and likely to progress.
  ii. Central (medial): less common, usually bilateral, more common in ♀, and less likely to progress.
- Indeterminate 'concentric' radiographic patterns also exist.

Secondary OA

Secondary OA is seen in association with a wide variety of disorders as illustrated in Table 6.2.

Natural history of OA

- Progression in the knee may take many years. Cohort studies have found that radiographic deterioration occurs in one-third.
- Progression of hip disease is variable. A Danish study found that 66% of hips worsened radiologically over 10 years, though symptomatic improvement was common.
- Hand disease is relapsing and remitting with episodic inflammatory phases associated with redness and swelling. Flares then reduce in frequency, and pain also improves.

Table 6.2 Secondary causes of OA

Trauma	Inflammatory arthritis
Metabolic/endocrine	**Crystal deposition disease**
Haemachromatosis	Calcium pyrophosphate
Acromegaly	Uric acid
Hyperparathyroidism	Hydroxyapatite
Ochronosis (alkaptonuria)	
Neuropathic disorders	**Anatomical abnormalities**
Diabetes mellitus	Bone dysplasia

The investigation of OA

- OA is a clinical and radiological diagnosis. There are no specific laboratory tests.
- Difficulty arises when one appreciates that radiological changes of OA appear in asymptomatic joints. In some cases, investigation may only play a small part in deciding if OA is the cause of a particular problem or not.
- Laboratory tests may be warranted if OA is considered secondary to an undiagnosed primary condition.
- Analysis of synovial fluid for crystals may be helpful.
- Plain radiographs classically show joint space narrowing, osteophytes, subchondral sclerosis, and bone cysts. They are cheap and available but are not an accurate record of disease progression due to the slow rate of joint-space narrowing that takes place in OA.
- MRI may delineate cartilage loss better, but fibrillation and preclinical disease cannot be evaluated. CT is no better than plain radiography, and isotope bone scans lack anatomical detail.
- There are potential markers of tissue destruction and inflammation that may be of use clinically in the future. A profile of several markers with genetic analysis may in the future provide an individual assessment for disease development and response to therapy. Examples of markers include:
  - cartilage oligomeric matrix protein (COMP)
  - pyridinoline and bone sialoprotein
  - metalloproteinases
  - hylauronan.

The management of OA

Successful management

Successful management centres on:
- A good history:
  - symptoms and impact on life
  - functional disability
  - functional requirements
  - patient expectation
  - psychological factors.
- A good examination:
  - extent of abnormality
  - origin of pain
  - degree of inflammation
  - instability of joint
  - muscle condition
  - other medical, soft-tissue, and neurological disease.
- A multi-disciplinary approach.

Modalities for management

- Exercise is an important intervention, to build muscle strength, encourage weight loss, improve endurance and joint proprioception. Advice alone is not as good as a specific programme with follow-up. Evidence-based guidelines for exercise in hip and knee OA have recently been published[1]. In more marked disease, support splints and walking aids may be necessary.
- Education has been shown in meta-analyses to have a significant effect on pain and function, but only 20% as effective as NSAID treatment.
- Analgesia is effective. It is recommended that initial therapy is with paracetamol 4 g daily, using paracetamol/opiate combinations if needed. NSAIDs are probably no more effective than paracetamol, but may be of use for short periods during disease flares. They are not recommended for long-term use, especially in the elderly. The selective Cox-2 inhibitors are as efficacious as standard NSAIDs, but there remains concern over cardiovascular safety and they should be used with caution and avoided in at risk groups.
- Intra-articular injections of corticosteroid are very useful in treating inflammatory disease flares, and may result in sustained symptom improvement, although response duration is variable. Many practitioners also add local anaesthetic, although there is no clear evidence that this improves the efficacy of the treatment. Most data is available for knee OA. For weight-bearing joints, strict non-weight-bearing for 24 hours post-injection improves the efficacy of the injection. Infection is rare (< 1 in 10 000 incidence), but care should be taken to clean overlying skin, and injection through in-fected/psoriatic skin should be avoided. Other side-effects to warn patients about are skin depigmentation and fat atrophy. It is advised that patients receive no more than 2 or 3 injections per year.
- Intra-articular injection of hyaluronic acid derivatives (visco-supplementation) reduce pain and swelling and may provide benefit for

6–12 months. In the short-term they may be as efficacious as intra-articular corticosteroid injections.

- Glucosamine and chondroitin sulphate are found in articular cartilage. Evidence suggests that when given as oral supplements these agents have an analgesic effect in mild-to-moderate OA of the knee. There is little evidence for use in OA at other sites. Some studies have suggested a disease modifying effect, but further research is needed. Evidence is difficult to interpret due to the heterogenicity of study methods, patient groups and glucosamine ± chrondroitin preparations used. Evidence for a disease-modifying effect is poor in humans.
- Acupuncture has been shown in randomized controlled trials to be better than placebo acupuncture in improving symptoms.
- There is some evidence that avocado/soybean unsaponifiable (ASU) supplementation, evening primrose oil, and omega-3 fish oils improve pain.
- The clinician should also seek ways to reduce the impact of disability. Options include:
  - occupational therapy: splints, tools, safe environment
  - treat depression, anxiety, fibromyalgia
  - coping strategies—behavioural therapy
  - patient education.
- Surgery may be required when medical therapy is unsuccessful. Procedures include:
  - arthroscopy
  - osteotomy
  - arthroplasty.

1 Roddy E, Zhang W, Dohetry M et al. Evidence-based recommendations for the role of exercise in the management of osteoarthritis of the hip or knee: the MOVE consensus. *Rheumatology* 2005; **44**: 67–73.

Juvenile idiopathic arthritis (JIA)

Introduction

- The classification of childhood onset arthritis has seen several changes over recent years. In this chapter we will discuss juvenile arthritis using headings and criteria from the International League of Associations for Rheumatology (ILAR). The terms 'juvenile rheumatoid arthritis' and 'juvenile chronic arthritis' were discarded in the ILAR classification. The term 'juvenile idiopathic arthritis' was adopted to indicate arthritis present for at least 6 weeks and currently of no known cause in a patient <16 years. It is a diagnosis of exclusion.
- JIA is one of the most common chronic disorders of childhood, with an estimated UK prevalence of 1 per 1000, and a UK incidence of 1 per 10 000.
- The categories of JIA are:
  - systemic arthritis
  - oligoarthritis (4 or fewer joints) ('persistent' or 'extended')
  - polyarthritis (rheumatoid factor positive and negative)
  - psoriatic arthritis
  - enthesitis related arthritis
  - undifferentiated arthritis.
- Where features of other rheumatic diseases are particular to child-hood, these are discussed at the end of the relevant chapter.
  - rheumatoid factor positive polyarthritis (see Chapter 5)
  - psoriatic arthritis and enthesis related arthritis (see Chapter 8)
  - SLE (see Chapter 9)
  - back pain (see Chapter 20).
- The classifications were derived for research purposes and are not primarily meant as diagnostic criteria. For a review of classification of JIA we recommend Hofer et al. (2002).[1] For an overview of the spectrum of paediatric and adolescent rheumatology we recommend Davies and Copeman (2006)[2].

General management principles in juvenile rheumatic diseases

- A multi-disciplinary approach is essential. Allied health professionals provide help with patient and family education, exercise, activities of daily living (home and school), maintenance of psychological well-being in patient and family, and advice on financial and disability support.
- Monitoring of height and weight is needed, and appropriate nutritional advice given if needed.
- Ophthalmic input is required if uveitis is present.
- The dose of corticosteroid should be kept to the lowest possible to reduce the development of growth retardation. That said, higher doses of steroid are often required than in adults to gain initial control of disease. Bone density scanning (DEXA) should be considered and calcium and vitamin D should be given. Bisphosphonates should only be given under specialist guidance.
- A close liaison with the child's school is needed. Fatigue is a common symptom and may require changes to the child's school timetable. It is important to continue education as much as possible during hospital admissions.

- Excellent communication skills are required to explain often complex treatments to patient and family. Coming to terms with a chronic disease is a difficult process and again will need a close working relationship between members of the multi-disciplinary team.
- The onset of adolescence brings new challenges. It is important to encourage the patient to be more active in decisions about disease management. Adolescence is a time of huge emotional and physical changes, and a chronic illness can make these changes more difficult. Discussion of personal issues such as sexuality, smoking, and alcohol require a good rapport with the patient. Parents should be encouraged to help develop the patient's independence in making treatment decisions, though this can be a long process. Adolescence is also the time to introduce the subject of transition from care by paediatric to adult health professionals. This is a gradual process and should be managed sensitively.

1. Hofer M, Southwood T. Classification of childhood arthritis. Best practice and research in Clinical Rheumatology 2002; **16**: 379–96.
2. Davies K, Copeman A. The spectrum of paediatric and adolescent Rheumatology. Best practice and research in Clinical Rheumatology 2006; **20**: 179–200.

Oligoarthritis (previously termed pauciarticular JCA/JRA)

- This is the most commonly encountered subset of the childhood chronic arthritides, accounting for 40–50% of all JIA.
- The condition is more common in ♀ than ♂ (4:1) and peaks between the ages of 1–3 years, though it can appear in the teenage years. Overall, the disease affects an estimated 30 per 100 000 children.
- ILAR classification criteria requires the presence of arthritis affecting 1–4 joints during the first 6 months of disease. The persistent subtype affects no further joints in the disease course. The extended subtype affects a total of >4 joints after the first 6 months of disease.
- Certain other distinct characteristics include:
  - tendency to involve large joints, excluding the hip and shoulder
  - chronic anterior uveitis (more common in girls)
  - presence of antinuclear antibodies
  - unique immunogenetics.
- The ILAR classification has the following exclusion criteria:
  - family history of psoriasis confirmed by a dermatologist in at least one first- or second-degree relative.
  - family history consistent with medically confirmed HLA B27 associated disease in at least one first- or second-degree relative.
  - a positive rheumatoid factor test.
  - HLA B27 positive male with onset of arthritis >8 years of age.
  - Presence of systemic arthritis (see next section).
- The aetiology of the condition is unknown. Several lines of evidence indicate that genetic factors (HLA associations) are involved in disease susceptibilty.

Clinical features

- JIA is always a clinical diagnosis of exclusion. There are no specific signs, symptoms, or laboratory tests. Nevertheless, the clinical picture is often quite recognizable (as above), and usually milder than conditions such as reactive or infective arthritis.
- Constitutional symptoms of fever, malaise, weight loss, and anorexia are not part of oligoarthritis. If present, this virtually excludes the diagnosis.

Joints

- Joint swelling, rather than pain, is the more common complaint. Stiffness may occur but rarely seems to limit function. Two-thirds of cases present with single joint disease, and a further 30% with 2 joints involved. There may be associated juxta-articular muscle atrophy. The child may simply present with a limping gait.
- The most common joints to be involved are the knee, ankle, and elbow. Disease in 1 or 2 small joints of the hand is uncommon but seen and need not predict progress to polyarticular disease. Shoulder and hip involvement are very rare; disease here should prompt a search for another condition. Occasionally patients may develop disease of the temporomandibular joint and cervical spine.

- A period of 2–5 years of active arthritis is a typical course for the condition. A patient who remains 'pauciarticular' for 5 years is unlikely to progress to polyarticular disease. A minority of cases will progress but the criteria for judging this likelihood remains unclear; that said, some 40% of patients with concomitant uveitis develop polyarticular disease and therefore risk factors for uveitis might be considered partly as criteria for risk of polyarticular disease.
- Leg length discrepancy can occur due to unequal limb growth. When disease begins before 3 years of age there is a risk of the affected limb being longer. Flexing the knee on the affected side compensates for the discrepancy and this in turn will exacerbate any flexion contractures.
- Disease onset after the age of 9 years may result in a shorter affected limb; this is a consequence of early epiphyseal closure.
- Synovial cysts occur and respond to intra-articular steroid injections (which may have to be given under general anaesthetic).
- They can rupture, presenting as acute intense limb pain and swelling.
- Over 80% of children suffer little or no musculoskeletal disability at 15 years follow-up.

Eyes

- ⚠ Uveitis is an important complication to be aware of. Up to 20% of cases develop a chronic, insidious, and potentially sight-threatening uveitis (most often anterior chamber).
- The risk of uveitis is associated with the mode of onset of arthritis and not the later extent of articular disease.
- Risk factors include:
  - ♀ gender (♀:♂ up to 7.5:1)
  - young onset disease (mean age 4 years)
  - oligoarthritis
  - positive antinuclear antibody.

- The uveitis is commonly asymptomatic, only 25% of patients complaining of redness in the eye, pain, or visual disturbance. Up to two-thirds of patients have bilateral disease though not necessarily at the same time. As such, regular ophthalmic examination is required (see Table 7.1).
- Uveitis and arthritis develop at different times. Uveitis may predate arthritis in up to 10% of cases. Otherwise, it is usually detected within 7 years (mean 2 years) of the onset of arthritis.
- The main determinants of poor outcome of uveitis are the extent of initial disease at presentation, and uveitis documented before the onset of arthritis. Early intervention is probably the single most important factor in determining outcome.
- Chronic asymptomatic uveitis persisting into adulthood is recognized.
- Treatment is with topical corticosteroids. Oral corticosteroids may be used for severe disease but concerns remain regarding growth retardation. Methotrexate is used.

Investigations in oligoarthritis

- There are no diagnostic tests.
- The acute-phase reactants are usually mildly raised.
- A persistent high ESR, with no other evidence of inflammation on other laboratory tests, might suggest the rare, congenital disorder hyperfibrinogenaemia. A high ESR should prompt a search for infection, occult inflammation, or malignancy, e.g. leukaemia.
- ANA are present in 40–75% of children. There is no evidence that ANA precede the development of the condition, or that titres correlate with disease activity.
- Rheumatoid factor is rare; positive in <5% of cases.
- Plain radiographs are valuable for assessing joint damage; however, the expertise of a paediatric radiologist familiar with normal variants of skeletal development should be sought.
- Clinical assessment and investigation should seek to exclude the common conditions of childhood rheumatic disease (see Table 7.2).

Table 7.1 Uveitis surveillance: recommended frequency of slit-lamp examination

Condition	Frequency
Systemic onset	Yearly
Oligoarthritis and rheumatoid factor negative	
Onset before age 7:	ANA positive: 2–3-monthly for 4 years then 6-monthly for 3 years. Then yearly
	ANA negative: 6-monthly for 7 years. Then yearly
Onset after age 7:	6-monthly for 4 years. Then yearly

Table 7.2 The differential diagnosis of oligoarthritis

Condition	Examples
Monoarticular disease	Septic arthritis
	TB
	Trauma/haemarthrosis
	Patellofemoral pain
	Pigmented villonodular synovitis (requires tissue biopsy)
	Foreign-body synovitis
	Thalassaemia/sickle cell/haemophilia
Short-lived inflammatory arthropathy	Lyme disease
	Viral arthritis
	Reactive arthritis
	Post-streptococcal arthritis
The spondylarthropathies	
Pain conditions	Hypermobility/regional pain syndromes
	Algodsytrophy
	Avulsion fractures
	Aseptic (avascular) necrosis
	Enthesitis
	Osteoid osteoma/bone pain

Treatment of oligoarthritis

- The main principles are the maintenance of normal joint function during active disease, and the early treatment of ocular inflammation. A team approach is required.
- Initially NSAIDs are given (ibuprofen or naproxyn most often).
- Intra-articular steroid injections may be useful in several situations:
  - the very young (unable to take oral medication)
  - marked persistent joint swelling
  - synovial cysts causing limitation of movement.
- Cases with prolonged disease or extension to polyarticular disease require more aggressive treatment. MTX is the preferred choice. Etanercept is increasingly used, in cases unresponsive to MTX. These agents should only be used under specialist paediatric supervision.
- Motor development and activity is very important. There should always be assessment of growth, development, and social interaction. Physical therapy makes an important contribution to the overall management of the condition.
- Joint surgery is rarely necessary.
- Uveitis can be more of a therapeutic challenge than the joint disease. Corticosteroid eye drops and mydriatics to prevent synechiae (fibrous bands that adhere the iris to the lens) are the typical initial regimen in mild disease. More severe disease requires oral prednisolone. MTX and etanercept may also help eye disease.
- There is limited experience with azathioprine and chlorambucil; ciclosporin A has been used in severe, refractory uveitis.
- Surgery may be necessary for cataracts, keratopathy, glaucoma, etc.

Systemic arthritis (previously systemic onset JCA/JRA)

- Systemic onset disease accounts for approximately 10–20% of juvenile arthritis.
- There is an equal sex incidence in systemic onset disease.
- The peak age of onset is 2–3 years.
- The non-articular features of the condition make a viral aetiology an attractive hypothesis, but there is little evidence for this.
- HLA studies demonstrate genetic heterogeneity with no clear associations.

Clinical features

- While arthritis is required to confirm the diagnosis, true joint
- inflammation may not be present at the onset of disease; some patients have developed inflammation as late as 9 years after the onset.
- The ILAR classification criteria require the presence of arthritis with, or preceded by, a daily fever of at least 2 weeks duration in association with one or more of the following: an erythematous evanescent rash, generalized lymphadenopathy, hepatomegaly and/or splenomegaly, and serositis (see Table 7.3).
- Most patients have arthritis at disease onset, and 50–60% will develop chronic persistent symptoms. In >75% of cases, the wrists, knees, and ankles are involved. Hip involvement occurs in about 50% of cases and is almost always bilateral, and associated with polyarticular disease. Hip and wrist joints are the most common sites of progressive destructive arthropathy, and one-third of patients with hip involvement will require hip arthroplasty. Tenosynovitis of the carpus and tarsus is common, and of the small joints, the hands are often affected more than the feet.
- Fever is the one extra-articular feature essential to making the diagnosis. The fever pattern is described as quotidian, often rising to 39°C before falling rapidly to normal, and typically in the late afternoon or early evening following a regular daily pattern. The patient often appears toxic during the fever, with chills and rigors, severe arthralgia and myalgia, and very often a rash. The fever should be present for at least 2 weeks and quotidian in character for at least 3 days to satisfy the diagnosis. Fever may persist for months even with treatment.
- The rash of systemic arthritis is a salmon-pink colour, most prominent over the chest, abdomen, back, and intertrigenous areas. The rash is usually macular, though occasional urticarial, with individual lesions 3–5 mm in diameter which may coalesce into larger ones. It has a tendency to come and go with the fever spike.

Table 7.3 Clinical features of systemic arthritis

Frequency	Feature
Very common	Spiking fever (with chills and sweats)
	Evanescent rash
	Myalgias
	Arthralgias—oligo/polyarthritis—usually after first 6 months from onset
	Growth abnormalities
Common	Generalized lymphadenopathy
	Hepatosplenomegaly
	Polyserositis
	Anorexia
	Weight loss
Rare	Myocarditis
	Coagulopathy
	Eye disease
	CNS involvement
	Haemophagocytic syndrome
	Primary pulmonary disease
	Renal disease
	Amyloidosis

- Hepatomegaly, splenomegaly, and lymphadenopathy are common findings and usually asymptomatic. Mild ↑ serum transaminases occurs frequently and is usually not significant clinically. This makes assessment of potentially hepatotoxic medications difficult. Chronic liver disease does not occur. It is, however, a feature of adult onset Still's disease. Very rarely an acute fulminant liver failure occurs with encephalopathy, disseminated intravascular coagulation, and bleeding.
- This syndrome is associated with considerable morbidity and mortality, treatment being supportive with corticosteroids and cyclosporin.
- Involvement of the serosal surfaces is one hallmark of systemic arthritis. Pericarditis, pleuritis, and sterile peritonitis are recognized manifestations of the disease; pericarditis is by far the more common of these. Most children will have echocardiographic evidence of pericarditis during systemic flares though <15% will be symptomatic. Rarely, the patient may have myocarditis, suggested clinically by persistent tachycardia, cardiomegaly, and congestive cardiac failure. There should always be a high index of suspicion in these cases as the mortality rate is high. Valvular disease is almost never seen. This may help to separate systemic arthritis from acute rheumatic fever with carditis.

- Abnormalities of growth are often as a consequence of hypercatabolism, poor nutrient intake, and concomitant use of corticosteroids. Suppression of disease activity and adequate nutrition are the most effective therapy. Growth hormone supplementation is reserved for patients whose growth is persistently below the third percentile on height charts and before epiphyseal fusion has occured.
- Amongst the rarer features, CNS manifestations are dominated by irritability and lethargy during fever spikes; renal involvement may occur as a complication of treatment or indicate the onset of amyloidosis; and ocular involvement is distinctly unusual relative to other forms of JIA, though asymptomatic uveitis does occur.
- Amyloidosis is a serious complication of all subtypes of JIA and is associated with significant morbidity and mortality. The most common cause of death with amyloidosis is renal failure (80% of cases in most series), followed by infection (10% of cases).

Differential diagnosis

- The differential diagnosis of systemic arthritis should always be kept in mind and looked for as many infectious and post-infectious disorders, other inflammatory diseases, and malignancy have similar clinical manifestations.
- Features that may raise suspicion of another diagnosis include:
  - leucopenia, thrombocytopenia
  - child looks ill even during afebrile episodes
  - bony tenderness
  - 'hard' hepatosplenomegaly/lymphadenopathy
  - recent antibiotic use
  - monoarthritis
  - persistent diarrhoea
  - marked weight loss.

Investigations in systemic arthritis

- There are no specific diagnostic tests.
- Characteristic haematological abnormalities include anaemia, thrombocytosis, and leucocytosis; the latter two abnormalities are hallmarks of the condition, so much so that normal counts raise suspicion about the diagnosis.
- Acute phase markers are usually ↑; the ESR, CRP, gammaglobulins, and serum complement (this may help to differentiate the disease from SLE). The ESR may be normal or ↓ in haemophagocytic syndrome complicating systemic arthritis.
- Hypoalbuminaemia may be multifactorial in aetiology (poor diet, reduced synthesis, intestinal leak), but should prompt the search for proteinuria, which, if 'heavy', would suggest amyloidosis and the need for renal or rectal biopsy, or scintigraphy using iodinated serum amyloid-P to detect deposits.
- Most children are seronegative for ANA and RF. No antinuclear antibody specificities have been consistently identified.

The following tests are suggested for all patients in the initial diagnostic investigation of systemic arthritis:
- Full blood count and blood film
- Renal and liver function tests
- Coagulation screen
- Serum immunoglobulins
- Serum albumin
- Antinuclear antibody titre
- Blood cultures
- Chest radiograph
- Plain radiographs of selected affected joints
- Abdominal and pelvic ultrasound
- Electrocardiograph
- Ocular slit lamp examination.

The following tests should also be considered:
- Muscle enzymes
- Rheumatoid factor
- Viral serology—parvovirus, adenovirus etc.
- Antistreptolysin antibody titres
- Serum IgD
- Urine homovanillic and vanillylmandelic acid
- Joint aspiration (for monoarthritis)
- Tissue biopsy (including bone marrow aspirate)
- Echocardiogram
- Upper gastrointestinal barium series
- Isotope bone and/or gallium scan.

The radiological abnormalities seen are listed in Table 7.4.

Table 7.4 Radiological abnormalities seen in systemic JIA

Feature	Percentage
Soft tissue swelling	80%
Joint space narrowing	50%
Growth abnormalities	50%
Erosions	40%
Subluxation	20%
Ankylosis	20%
Joint destruction	15%
Protrusio acetabulae	10%
Periosteal new bone	10%

The treatment of systemic arthritis

- The general approach to the management of the arthritis assumes the same principles as oligoarthritis. However, there is increased drug-related toxicity in systemic JIA. This is seen with salicylates, NSAIDs, and DMARDs, particularly gold and sulphasalazine.
- The most effective treatment consistently for systemic onset disease is corticosteroids. Likewise corticosteroids are the treatment of choice during an acute 'flare'. MTX may help in some cases. MTX is not as effective in this situation as in oligoarticular JIA.
- Chlorambucil is used in patients who have developed amyloidosis; however, it may not control systemic features and has been associated with an increased risk of leukaemia.
- Azathioprine is rarely used because of hepatotoxicity.
- Ciclosporin A appears to have a minimal effect on synovitis and systemic symptoms. The toxicity seems to outweigh the benefit. Perhaps more impressive has been the use of pulsed methylprednisolone and cyclophosphamide. However, this has only been tried on a small number of cases and given the difficulty of conducting randomized controlled trials in this condition, the long-term follow-up of these patients should be reported before this approach can be recommended.
- Initial control of fever, joint pain, and serositis should be with NSAIDs; ibuprofen, naproxen, or indometacin are commonly used. The dose should be decreased in the presence of severe hypoalbuminaemia as the drugs are protein-bound. NSAIDs should be tried for at least 1 week before being deemed to have failed. Indometacin is particularly useful for pericarditis; otherwise this may respond to pulsed methylprednisolone, as does myocarditis.
- When NSAIDs fail to control symptoms, regular or pulsed corticosteroid treatment is indicated. Steroids will control symptoms but they do not limit the duration or alter the prognosis of the disease and should be used judiciously. The daily dose should be at least 1 mg/kg in divided doses.
- Significant cardiac compromise from carditis may require pericardiocentesis.
- At present IV immunoglobulin remains experimental and reserved for those who fail to respond to steroids or who are hypogammaglobulinaemic.
- Anti-TNFα therapies may be effective in systemic JIA with persistent polyarthritis. High levels of TNF are found in the circulation. High levels of interleukin-6 (IL-6) and its soluble receptor are found, and studies (on-going) using IL-1 receptor antagonists or recombinant human anti-IL-6 antibody (MRA) have shown acute reduction in disease activity.

Rheumatoid factor negative polyarthritis in childhood (previously

termed polyarticular onset JCA)

General points

- There are two subtypes; rheumatoid factor (RF) negative (80%) and factor positive (20%).
- The RF should be checked on 2 occasions, 3 months apart. RF positive disease tends to occur most often in ♀ and follows a pattern similar to adult RA (see Chapter 5).
- The arthritis usually affects 5 or more joints within the first 6 months of disease. There must be no psoriasis in the patient or in any first-degree relative.
- Polyarticular onset occurs in about 30% of all patients with JIA.
- In the ILAR criteria, polyarthritis with positive RF is excluded.

Clinical manifestations of RF-negative polyarthritis

- Extra-articular manifestations may be present; however, in general features like fever are low grade and of short duration, if present at all. In the very young, there may be a transient rash lasting 1–2 days early in the disease. There is generally no lymphadenopathy, hepato-splenomegaly, or visceral involvement.
- Rapidly progressive joint disease dominates the clinical manifestations. Swelling may limit mobility, resulting in local bone demineralization and muscle wasting. Chronic hyperaemia may induce local accelerated growth and cartilage fusion.
- Carpal fusion and tendonopathies are common in the hands, leading to classical features such as boutonniere and swan-neck deformities. Flexion contracture is the first manifestation of elbow involvement, and the shoulders are commonly affected.
- In the lower limb, similar consequences are seen with tarsal fusion, tenosynovitis and bursitis, flexion deformities of the knee, and flexion deformities and aseptic necrosis at the hip.
- Cervical spine involvement is common with features akin to RA; apophyseal joint fusion, instability, and risk of cord compression. There is often fusion of the apophyseal joints of C3–C5 leaving rigid segments that sublux above and below. Atlantoaxial subluxation, seen in RF-positive arthritis and juvenile ankylosing spondylitis, is rare in RF-negative polyarthropathy.
- Temperomandibular joint involvement is common, leading to reduced growth and micrognathia. Dental malocclusion may require surgery when growth is completed.
- Some specific features have led to a proposed subclassification of this condition (see Table 7.5).

Table 7.5 Proposed subclassification of RF-negative polyarthritis

Subclassification	Percentage of cases	Characteristics
1. Positive for ANA—painful synovitis	About 40%	Female preponderance
		Most cases in very young (<3 years of age)
		Possible increased risk of eye disease
		Severe polyarthritis
2. With 'boggy' synovitis	15%	Mild pain
		Thick pannus
		Equal in sexes
		Functional impairment late
		Tenosynovitis common
3. 'Dry' polyarthritis	15%	Little joint swelling
		Progressive stiffness
		Chronic muscle wasting
		Often referred late in to onset
4. With spondylarthropathy	About 20%	Mid-childhood (8–10 years of age)
		Male preponderance
		At risk of spondylitis within 5–10 years

Laboratory investigations

The laboratory features are non-specific in RF-negative polyarthritis. The ESR, CRP, leucocyte count, and platelet count can be ↑ or normal. A low red cell count is unusual and should prompt a search for an alternative diagnosis.

Treatment

- The management of this condition involves a common approach as discussed in the first two sections of this chapter, with adaptations according to the different subtypes shown.
- Treatment should start with a trial of an NSAID for 4–8 weeks, moving to a second NSAID for the same period of time if the first fails. Ibuprofen, naproxyn, and diclofenac are commonly used.
- In non-responders to NSAIDs, intra-articular steroid injections may be necessary. Topical steroids should also be used from the onset with eye disease.
- DMARDs should also be introduced for at least 3 months.
- Methotrexate is the first-line drug of choice. Sulfasalazine may be used if there are features of spondyloarthropathy. Treatments should be continued for at least 6 months following remission; studies are ongoing to determine the benefit of continuing methotrexate for 6 and 12 months post remission. The biologic etanercept is used for patients intolerant of or unresponsive to, methotrexate.
- In all cases surgery and rehabilitation play an important role in management, and physiotherapy and occupational therapy advice should be employed early.

Chronic, infantile, neurological, cutaneous, and articular syndrome (CINCA)

- Closer scrutiny of paediatric inflammatory arthropathies has led to the description of syndromes that can be distinguished from systemic JIA. Among these syndromes is chronic, infantile, neurological, cutaneous, and articular syndrome (CINCA), different from JIA in its involvement of the central nervous system. The pathophysiology of this condition is unknown; no immune complex, autoantibody, or immunodeficiency has been found.
- The first symptoms are often present at birth, generally after an uneventful pregnancy. Three-quarters of neonates (the rest usually within 6 months of birth) have a non-pruritic urticarial rash that resembles that of Still's disease. Intermittent 'flares' of the condition are associated with fever, and enlargement of the lymph nodes and spleen.
- Central nervous system and sensory anomalies are important manifestations of CINCA. Chronic meningitis may result in recurrent headaches and seizures. There may also be transient episodes of hemiplegia.
- Sensory anomalies are progressive. These include perceptive deafness and optic atrophy. Other eye involvement includes uveitis, chorioretinitis, keratitis, and conjunctivitis.
- The skull tends to have an increased cranial volume and there is delay in closure of the anterior fontanelle, and sometimes calcification of the falx and dura.
- Joint involvement is variable but most often involves the knee. The main finding is an overgrowth of the epiphyseal plate, resulting in bony enlargement. Progressive contractures and loss of movement and function ensue. There is progressive growth retardation and, despite normal growth hormone profiles, a height below the third percentile is very frequent.
- Common morphological changes are also a feature. These include skull enlargement (often frontal bossing), a saddle-back nose, clubbing of the fingers and toes, and short and thick hands and feet.
- Treatment is symptomatic with NSAIDs and physiotherapy.
- Immunosuppressive drugs have little effect, and disease-modifying drugs are ineffective. Trials are underway with biologic therapies. Corticosteroids may help control fever and pain but have not been shown to have any effect on joint or skin disease.
- The reader is referred to Chapter 8 of this book for the section on enthesitis related and childhood spondylarthropathy.

Still's disease

- This condition has similar clinical and laboratory features to systemic JIA. 75% of cases range between the ages of 16–35 years at onset.
- The fever pattern is identical and 90% of cases develop the typical rash.
- One feature not seen in juvenile disease is the complaint of sore throat during fever spikes. Pulmonary and ocular disease seem to be more common in adult Still's, and carditis less so.
- Patients with a chronic articular course do not do well. Several factors predict a poor outcome in terms of progressive articular damage:
  - a polyarticular onset
  - axial arthritis
  - need for steroids within 2 years of onset of disease
  - history of childhood arthritis
  - rash.
- The treatment of 'adult-onset' Still's disease should follow the same lines as that for systemic JIA.

The spondylarthropathies

Introduction

- The seronegative spondylarthropathies are classically characterized by the following:
  - sacroiliac/pelviaxial disease
  - peripheral inflammatory arthropathy
  - enthesopathic syndrome
  - an extramuscular syndrome.
- The group is made up of several conditions that often overlap. These are:
  - ankylosing spondylitis
  - juvenile enthesitis related arthritis
  - psoriatic arthritis
  - reactive arthropathy
  - enteropathic arthritis
  - undifferentiated spondylitis.
- The undifferentiated conditions include subsets of cases where features such as dactylitis, uveitis, or sacroiliitis exist without the full criteria for a diagnosis.
- Some physicians also include pustulotic arthro-osteitis—SAPHO syndrome—(seen in Japan but rare in Europe and the United States) as part of the group.
- Doubt exists as to whether Whipple's disease and Behçet's disease should be considered part of the spectrum.
- Pathological changes are mainly at the insertion of tendons and ligaments into bone, and extra-articular changes may also develop in the eye, aortic valve, lung, and skin.

Diagnostic criteria and clinical subsets

- There is a general consensus that most criteria are too restricted given the wide spectrum of disease. For example, radiographic evidence of sacroiliitis in the absence of symptoms, or unilateral sacroiliitis with only dactylitis or uveitis, would be excluded from most criteria and yet could be part of the spondylarthropathy spectrum. Criteria with acceptable sensitivity and specificity are shown in Table 8.1.
- A variety of symptoms and signs are present and Table 8.2 highlights the differences between these conditions.
- The specific expression of disease is a product of inter-related genetic and environmental factors. The precise link between triggers such as infection and pathogenesis, and indeed the exact role of the HLA B27 molecule remains a mystery.
- The HLA B27 molecule has an association with the spondylarthropathies ranging between 50–95%. Interpretation of a positive result is complicated by the presence of this allele of the HLA B gene in up to 5–10% of the normal population. It may be of use in assessing symptomatic first-degree relatives of HLA B27+ probands with ankylosing spondylitis (AS); here the risk of developing the same disease is approximately 1 in 3. However, most physicians would not advocate the routine use of this marker generally.
- There are, however, a number of interesting observations in the study of HLA B27, which include the following:
    I. HLA B27 is inherited as an autosomal codominant characteristic, 50% of first-degree relatives of probands with HLA B27 possessing the antigen.
    II. 5–10% of HLA B27 positive individuals develop AS over time and 20% of individuals with B27 develop a reactive arthropathy after contact with agents such as chlamydia or salmonella.
    III. Only 50% with psoriatic or enteropathic spondylitis are positive.
    IV. The association between AS and B27 in non-Caucasians (50%) is much less than that of Caucasians (95%).
    V. Relatives of probands with both sacroiliitis and HLA B27 frequently remain disease free.
    VI. Concordance in identical twins is 70% vs 13% in non-identical twins.
    VII. Uveitis is a common accompaniment of AS. HLA B27 is found in up to 40% of cases of uveitis, even in the absence of underlying rheumatic disease.

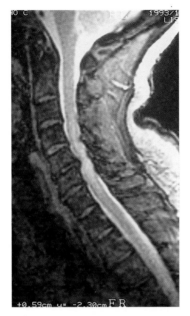

Plate 1 MR scan of the neck showing loss of height and signal affecting several discs with multisegmental spondylotic bars, compression of the cord from protrusion of the C5/6 disc and myelopathic changes (high signal) in the cord.

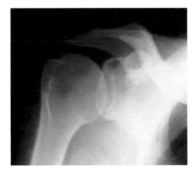

Plate 2 Patterns of radiographic abnormality in chronic SAI: sclerosis and cystic changes in the greater tuberosity.

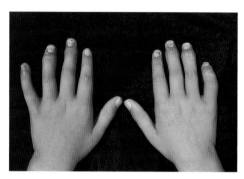

Plate 3 Dactylitis, nail changes, and DIPJ arthritis in psoriatic arthritis.

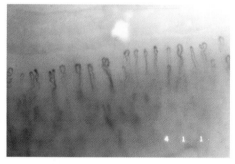

(a)

(b)

Plate 4 (a) Normal nailfold capillaries. (b) Nailfold capillaries in scleroderma showing avascular areas and dilated capillaries in an irregular orientation (original magnification ×65).

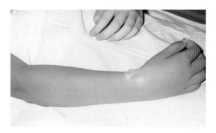

Plate 5 Diffuse arm and hand swelling in chronic regional pain syndrome (reflex sympathetic dystrophy) in a 13-year-old girl.

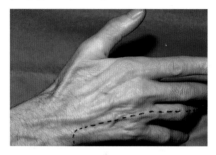

Plate 6 Slight flexion of fourth and fifth fingers as a result of an ulnar nerve lesion at the elbow. The area of sensory loss is indicated by the dotted line.

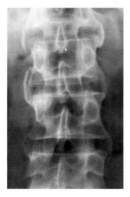

Plate 7 Psoriatic spondylitis: Non-marginal and 'floating' (non-attached) syndesmophytes.

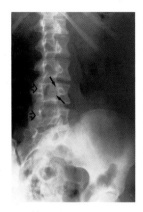

Plate 8 Spondylolysis. The defect in the pars interarticularis (black arrows) may only be noted on an oblique view. The patient has had a spinal fusion (open arrows).

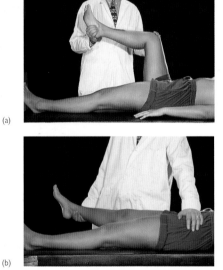

(a)

(b)

Plate 9 Testing passive hip flexion and rotational movements (a) and hip abduction (b). The pelvis should be fixed when testing abduction and adduction.

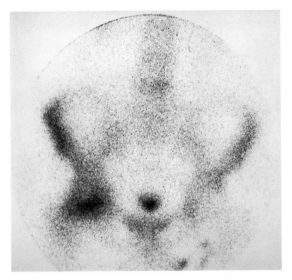

Plate 10 Bone scintigraphy showing osteonecrosis of the left femoral head (on the right-hand side as this an anterior view). Photopenia (an early sign) corresponds to ischaemia.

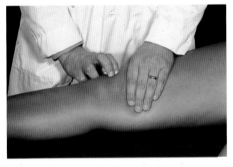

Plate 11 The 'patellar tap' test. Any fluid in the suprapatellar pouch is squeezed distally by the left hand. The patella is depressed by the right hand. It will normally tap the underlying femur immediately. Any delay in eliciting the tap or a feeling of damping as the patella is depressed suggests a joint effusion.

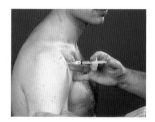

Plate 12 Injection of the glenohumeral joint via the anterior route.

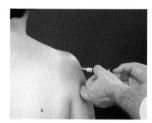

Plate 13 Injection of the subacromial space.

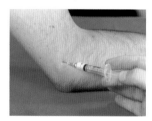

Plate 14 Injection of tennis elbow (lateral humeral epicondylitis/enthesitis).

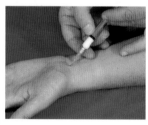

Plate 15 Injection of the carpal tunnel to the ulnar side of palmaris longus tendon.

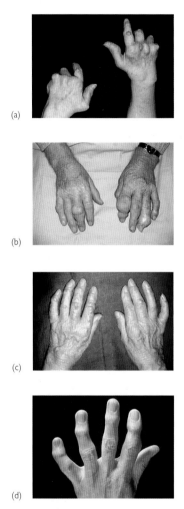

Plate 16 Nodules associated with joint diseases. (a) RA: typically over extensor surfaces and pressure areas. (b) Chronic tophaceous gout: tophi can be indistinguishable clinically from RA nodules though may appear as eccentric swellings around joints (Image provided courtesy of Dr R. A. Watts). (c) Multicentric reticulohistiocytosis: nodules are in the skin, are small, yellowish-brown, and are often around nails. (d) Nodal OA: swelling is bony, typically at PIPJs and DIPJs.

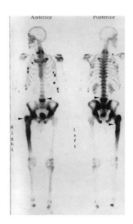

Plate 17 Bone scintigraphy (^{99m}Tc MDP) of a 65-year-old man with widespread bone pain and weakness suspected to have metastatic malignancy. Undecalcified transiliac bone biopsy confirmed severe osteomalacia. There was coincidental Paget's disease (arrowed lesions).

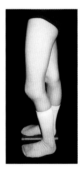

Plate 18 Increased growth of the left lower limb owing to chronic knee inflammation in (RF–) JIA.

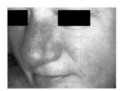

Plate 19 Lupus pernio presenting as a bluish-red or violaceous swelling of the nose extending onto the cheek.

Table 8.1 Criteria for diagnosing spondylarthropathies (Amor 1991)

Symptom(s)	Points
Clinical symptoms or past history of:	
1. Lumbar or dorsal pain at night or morning stiffness of the same areas	1
2. Asymmetrical oligoarthropathy	2
3. Alternating buttock pain	1
4. Dactylitis—sausage-like fingers or toes	2
5. Well-defined enthesopathic pain	2
6. Iritis	2
7. Non-gonococcal urethritis/cervicitis within 1 month of onset of arthritis	1
8. Acute diarrhoea within 1 month of onset of arthritis	1
9. Presence or history of psoriasis or inflammatory bowel disease	2
Radiological finding:	
10. Sacroiliitis	3
Genetic background:	
11. Presence of HLA B27 and/or family history of ankylosing spondylitis, reactive arthritis, uveitis, psoriasis, or chronic enterocolopathies	2
Response to treatment:	
12. Clear-cut improvement with NSAIDs	2

A patient is considered as having a spondylarthropathy if the sum of the points is > 6.

Reference: Amor B *et al. Annales de Medicine Interne*, 1991; **142**: 85–9.

Table 8.2 Comparison of the seronegative spondylarthropathies

Feature	AS	REA	PA	EA
Sex	More ♂	♂ = ♀	More ♀	♂ = ♀
Age onset (years)	20–30	Any age	Any age	Any age
Onset	Gradual	Sudden	Variable	Gradual
% HLA B27 +ve	95		20 (50 if sacroiliac disease is present)	
Sacroiliitis	Always	Often	Often	Often
Peripheral joint disease	Lower limb > upper	Usually lower limb	Usually lower limb	Usually lower limb
Enthesitis	Present	Present	Present	Present
Uveitis	Common	Not common	Not common	Not common
Conjunctivitis	Not seen	Not common	Not seen	Not seen
Urethritis	Not seen	Rare	Not seen	Not seen
Skin disease	Not seen	Rare	Very common	Rare
Mucosal disease	Not seen	Not seen	Not seen	Not common

AS, ankylosing spondylitis; REA, reactive arthritis; PA, psoriatic arthritis; EA, enteropathic arthropathy.

Ankylosing spondylitis

Epidemiology

- Few clinicians rely solely on the criteria; most would consider the diagnosis of ankylosing spondylitis (AS) in any case of symptomatic inflammatory back pain with radiographic evidence of sacroiliitis. The criteria for AS are shown in Table 8.3. The difficulty comes in recognizing early disease or subtle radiological change. There is often an insidious onset of back pain and morning stiffness that tends to improve with exercise. Occasionally sacroiliitis is a chance finding in the absence of pain. More sophisticated investigations than the plain pelvic radiograph, such as magnetic resonance imaging, may be inappropriate and unhelpful.
- Patients are typically <40 years of age with a ♂ to ♀ ratio of approximately 3:1.
- The condition occurs more frequently in Caucasian populations. In American Indians, where HLA B27 prevalence is high, AS is particularly frequent, whereas the condition is less common in Black Americans, and rarer still in Black Africans, as the prevalence of B27 gene ↓ respectively.
- Prevalence estimates in Caucasians range from 0.05–0.23% in adults. This may be an underestimate as people with mild symptoms may not seek medical advice.
- As previously stated, HLA B27 typing has led to greater understanding of the spondylarthropathies, but should not be considered a diagnostic test or necessary for the diagnosis of AS. Up to 5% of Caucasian patients with AS are negative for HLA B27.

Clinical features of AS

- The principal feature of the condition and allied diseases is the fibrosis and ossification of ligament, tendon, and capsule insertions into bone (the entheses), mainly in the region of the discs and sacroiliac joints.
- Synovitis also occurs, typically in the larger peripheral joints (hips and knees in particular). 20–40% of patients have some degree of peripheral joint disease at some stage during their illness, ♀ more so than ♂. Approximately 50% of patients with adult AS will develop hip arthritis and a proportion of these will need surgery.
- The standardized mortality ratio is increased at 1.5, mainly due to cardiac valve and respiratory disease, amyloidosis, and fractures.
- Like other forms of chronic disease, AS patients have a significant risk of having to alter or give up work.
- Though recognized as typical of AS, few patients progress to the classical late 'bamboo spine'. When the spine does fuse, with 'syndesmophytes' bridging the gap between vertebral bodies, microfractures can occur leading to acute episodes of severe pain and spondylodiscitis, a term given to collapse of the vertebral end-plate and destruction of the disc–bone border. This process is usually self-limiting, requiring rest and analgesia for up to 3 weeks. Most spinal disease is limited to chronic low-grade pain and stiffness with clinical evidence of a symmetrical reduction in spinal mobility.

Table 8.3 Diagnostic criteria: Modified New York Criteria

Clinical criteria:

Low back pain and stiffness for >6 months improving with exercise but not relieved by rest

Limitation of lumbar spine movements in saggital and frontal planes

Limitation of chest expansion relative to normal values for age and sex

Radiological criteria:

Greater than or equal to Grade II bilateral sacroiliitis

Grade III or IV unilateral sacroiliitis

Combined diagnostic criteria:

Definite AS if 1 radiological and 1 clinical criterion

Probable AS if 3 clinical criteria or a radiological criterion without signs or symptoms satisfying the clinical criteria

Van der Linden *et al.* Evaluation of diagnostic criteria for ankylosing spondylitis: a proposal for modification of the New York Criteria. *Arthritis Rheum*, 1984; **27**: 361–8.

- Patients may have insertional tendonitis at several other common sites including the Achilles tendon, intercostal muscles, plantar fascia, and dactylitis of the hands and feet.

Extra-articular disease in AS

- Constitutional features of fatigue, weight loss, low-grade fever, and anaemia are common. Fatigue as opposed to pain or stiffness can be the most troublesome symptom for a number of patients.
- Iritis occurs in up to 40% of cases but has little correlation with disease activity in the spine. There are no known triggers for this condition and although self-limiting, topical or systemic steroids may be required in severe cases. Iritis is usually unilateral.
- Upper lobe, bilateral pulmonary fibrosis is a recognized feature of the disease. Occasionally the fibrotic area is invaded by aspergillus with changes mimicking tuberculosis. Treatment of the fibrosis is of no avail. Pleuritis can occur as a consequence of insertional tendonitis of the costosternal and costovertebral muscles. Fusion of the thoracic wall leads to rigidity and reduction in chest expansion. Ventilation is maintained by the diaphragm; however, there is a three-fold increased risk of death from a respiratory cause compared with the normal population.
- Cardiac involvement includes aortic incompetence, cardiomegaly, and conduction defects. Of the 20% of patients with aortic valve disease, the majority are clinically undetectable.
- Neurological complaints per se are not a feature of AS, although nerve root entrapment or spinal cord/cauda equina compression can occur as a result of spinal fusion or fractures.
- Primary renal involvement is uncommon and if present may be due to coexistent medical conditions, NSAID use, or renal amyloidosis.

- Osteoporosis is an under-recognized finding. Estimates of prevalence range from 20–60%, ↑ with age and disease duration, and disease is largely confined to the axial skeleton. Bone density scanning may be inaccurate in the lumbar spine due to the presence of syndesmophytes late in disease. Studies would suggest that bone loss occurs early and during the acute inflammatory stage of the disease and that further bone loss, long-term, is rarely seen. Micro fractures may occur with trauma but the classical vertebral compression and wedge fractures of osteoporosis are rarely seen. Further work needs to be done to establish the need for, and efficacy of, current anti-catabolic and anabolic bone treatments.

Investigations in AS

- There is little correlation between any of the inflammatory markers and disease activity or clinical symptoms.
- It is not surprising that radiological evaluation is the most helpful form of investigation. Plain anteroposterior view radiographs are of the most value, but may not show early changes. A false positive result is common due to projection artifacts. Early changes include loss of the subchondral sclerotic line. Changes may initially be asymmetrical. Later findings include the more classical findings of subchondral sclerosis, erosions, and finally ankylosis. Radionuclide scanning may be sensitive but is non-specific and may be more confusing than helpful. CT provides excellent views of the SI joints. However the radiation dose is significant. MRI may demonstrate joint erosions, and also bone oedema and fatty change in marrow which are not detected by CT or plain radiographs.
- The main radiological features of 'primary' AS and that associated with inflammatory bowel disease are:
  - symmetrical sacroiliac changes
  - ascending spread of disease
  - facet joint involvement
  - squaring of vertebrae
  - syndesmophytes
  - ossification
  - osteitis pubis.
- It is said that AS associated reactive arthritis or psoriatic arthropathy (PsA), i.e. secondary AS, tends to differ in being far less severe radiologically, with often asymmetrical sacroiliac disease and random spinal involvement.
- It is important to differentiate syndesmophytes from osteophytes; the former most often moving vertically, the latter horizontally and in association with disc-space narrowing.
- AS should also be distinguished from diffuse idiopathic skeletal hyperostosis (DISH). The two conditions are compared in Table 8.4.

Table 8.4 Differentiating diffuse idiopathic skeletal hyperostosis (DISH) and ankylosing spondylitis (AS)

Feature	DISH	AS
Age of onset (years)	Usually > 50	Usually < 40
Kyphosis	No	Yes
Reduced mobility	Occasionally	Very often
Pain	Common	Very common
Reduced chest expansion	No	Common
Radiological findings:		
Hyperostosis	Yes	Yes
Sacroiliac joint erosions	No	Yes
ALL ossification	Yes—common	No
PLL ossification	Yes—occasionally	No
Syndesmophytes	No	Very common
Erosive enthesitis	No	Very common
Non-erosive enthesitis	Very common	Common

ALL, anterior longitudinal ligament; PLL, posterior longitudinal ligament.

Disease status and prognostic indicators in AS

- There are validated self-administered instruments defining disease status in AS. Since one lacks the advantage of valuable laboratory tests, it is helpful that there is a good correlation between the self-reporting of symptoms and observed clinical status of patients with AS.
- Instruments for assessing disease status include indices produced by the Royal National Hospital for Rheumatic Diseases, Bath, UK, namely The Bath Ankylosing Spondylitis Functional Index (BASFI), Disease Activity Index (BASDAI), Metrology Index (BASMI), and Radiology Index (BASRI). Several of these disease status scores are used in the UK for determining the introduction of anti-TNFα therapy.
- It is difficult to define outcome for individual patients when considering prognosis. The main predictive factors in AS appear to be:
  - early hip involvement
  - an ESR > 30
  - poor initial response to NSAIDs
  - early loss of lumbar spine mobility
  - presence of dactylitis
  - oligoarticular disease
  - onset < 16 years
  - low social–educational background
  - sporadic disease rather than familial.

The treatment of ankylosing spondylitis

- General principles include the following:
  - patient education
  - exercise

- physiotherapy and hydrotherapy
- avoid smoking
- NSAIDs for spinal disease
- self-help groups.

- Emphasis is placed on the need to maintain posture and physical activity. Extension exercises are important as the natural history of the disease is towards flexion and loss of height. Physiotherapy and rehabilitation provide benefit in the short-term but it remains unclear as to the benefits in the long-term. Spa treatment has been shown to improve function for up to 9 months, with subsequent reduction in health resource use. Spa therapy is expensive and not widely available.

- Fatigue may be a major concern, hampering exercise. In some cases, low-dose amitriptyline at night may ameliorate this problem.

- For the majority of patients, NSAIDs remain the treatment of choice. Some patients will still be taking the older NSAID phenylbutazone, that requires regular monitoring of the FBC (CBC) due to risk of marrow suppression. The majority will be taking regular NSAIDs such as diclofenac or naproxen. Indometacin was widely used but less so now because of its GI side effects. COX-2 selective drugs have less GI side effects and equal efficacy but care must be taken in patients with cardiovascular disease or the elderly.

- Sulfasalazine has been shown in meta-analysis to be efficacious when compared with placebo for peripheral joint disease only. However, improvement in symptoms and quality of life is often not dramatic and sulfasalazine has a small role to play, perhaps mainly in peripheral inflammatory disease.

- Mixed results have been found with MTX, but all trials have been non-randomized and small case series. Again, benefit that has been shown has been in peripheral and not axial disease.

- Joint inflammation can be managed in acute, severe cases with intra-articular corticosteroids, as can dactylitis and tendonitis by local steroid infiltration. Care should be taken injecting around tendons, as rupture can occur. Injection around the Achilles tendon is not recommended. Systemic steroids are rarely used, though there is evidence that low dose IV therapy can produce a short-lived improvement in symptoms.

- Infliximab and etanercept in combination with NSAIDs have been used in spinal and peripheral disease with good results in clinical outcome measures, but with limited effect on spinal mobility. There is no evidence for their benefit in peripheral disease or evidence that concurrent use of methotrexate is beneficial.

- The British Society for Rheumatology (BSR) has drawn up guidelines for use of anti-TNFα therapies in AS in the UK. The National Institute for Clinical Excellence (NICE) is also due to report on their use in 2006. Patients must satisfy the modified New York Criteria for AS, have a BASDAI (see Table 8.5) of at least 4 and a spinal pain visual analogue score of at least 4 cm on 2 occasions at least 4 weeks apart without any treatment change. Patients must also have failed 2 or more NSAIDs taken sequentially at maximum tolerated/recommended dose.

Table 8.5 Bath Ankylosing Spondylitis Disease Activity Index (BASDAI)

The assessment comprises 6 questions with an analogue score answer of 0 ('none') to 10 ('very severe') for each on a 10 cm scale.

The questions are:

1. How would you describe the overall level of fatigue/tiredness you have experienced?

2. How would you describe the overall level of AS neck, back or hip pain you have had?

3. How would you describe the overall level of pain/swelling in joints other than neck, back, or hips you have had?

4. How would you describe the overall level of discomfort you have had from any areas tender to touch or pressure?

5. How would you describe the overall level of discomfort you have had from the time you wake up?

6. How long does your morning stiffness last from the time you wake up? (for this score the 10 cm scale is divided evenly so that 30 mins lies at 2.5 cm, 1 hr at 5 cm, 1 and a half hours at 7.5 cm, and 2 or more hours at 10 cm).

The score is calculated by adding each of the measures for question 1 to 4 to the mean of the sum of questions 5 and 6, and then dividing the whole by 5. The maximum score therefore is 10.

- Inevitably some patients require joint replacement, most commonly at the hip. Response to such surgery is usually excellent provided there are not major periarticular contractures secondary to ankylosis. Surgery for spinal deformity is possible but carries considerable anaesthetic and surgical risk and should be carried out in specialist centers.
- Topical steroid eye drops should be used to treat uveitis. If the symptoms persist for > 3 days an ophthalmological opinion should be sought. Infliximab and etanercept have been used to treat resistant iritis.
- Any associated psoriasis, inflammatory bowel disease, or concern over reactive inflammation secondary to an infection should be treated accordingly.
- There is no treatment for pulmonary fibrosis associated with AS. Given the added potential concern of reduced chest expansion, patients should be advised not to smoke in an attempt to avoid further lung disease.
- Nevertheless, it is important to remember that the majority of patients have minimal functional impairment despite their disease, and lead full, active lives.

Psoriatic arthritis

Epidemiology and clinical features

- The association between psoriasis and an inflammatory arthropathy is well-recognized. It may affect any peripheral joint as well as the axial skeleton and sacroiliac joints. Epidemiological studies support the notion of a distinct disease as opposed to the random finding of coexisting common conditions such as psoriasis and RA. Psoriasis affects 1–2% of the population, and 10% of these develop arthritis.
- The condition affects ♀ and ♂ equally, usually between the ages of 20–40.
- RF can be present in up to 10% of patients with psoriasis, 90% remaining seronegative, and most patients with psoriatic arthritis run a benign course. In about 20% of cases there is a chronic, progressive, and deforming arthropathy with an often asymmetrical pattern, including distal interphalangeal joint involvement, and specific radiological features that can distinguish it from RA.
- Nail lesions may be the only clinical feature that can identify patients with psoriasis destined to develop arthritis. These lesions occur in 90% of patients with psoriatic arthritis (PsA) and in 40% of patients with psoriasis alone. A comparison between PsA and RA (see Chapter 5) is made in Table 8.6. The joint symptoms most commonly occur after the diagnosis of psoriasis, but may predate or occur simultaneously in a minority.
- The clinical patterns of psoriatic arthritis are:
  - distal, involving the distal interphalangeal joints (DIPJ)
  - asymmetric oligoarthritis
  - symmetrical polyarthritis, indistinguishable from RA
  - arthritis mutilans
  - spondylarthropathy.

- The radiological features associated with PsA which help to differentiate it from RA include:
  - absence of juxta-articular osteoporosis
  - DIJP disease
  - 'whittling' (lysis) of terminal phalanges
  - asymmetry
  - 'pencil-in-cup' deformities
  - ankylosis
  - periostitis
  - spondylitis.
- The patterns of arthritis may change over time in > 60% of patients.
- It is not clear though if the patterns of disease have any prognostic significance and the changes and prognosis are variable.
- The frequency of spinal involvement can vary between 2% in isolated back disease, to 40%, when associated with peripheral arthritis.

Table 8.6 Comparison of psoriatic arthritis and rheumatoid arthritis

Feature	Psoriatic arthritis	Rheumatoid arthritis
Sex ratio	♂ = ♀	♀ > ♂
Symmetry of joint disease	Less common	Very common
DIP(J) involvement	Common	Uncommon
Spine involvement	Common	Uncommon
Skin/nail changes	Common	Uncommon
Enthesopathy	Common	Uncommon
Ankylosis	Common	Uncommon
Osteopenia	Uncommon	Common

- Dactylitis, swelling of the whole finger, occurs in over one-third of patients. Tenosynovitis and enthesitis are also common, particularly at the plantar fascia insertion and Achilles tendon.
- Hyperuricaemia, probably related to high skin cell turnover, is not uncommon. The possibility of gout, particularly in young females, should be borne in mind.

Treatment of PsA

- This should include the treatment of the skin as well as the joints and many patients are also under the care of a dermatologist.
- Patient education, physiotherapy, occupational therapy, and surgery all have a role to play akin to that already described above for RA and AS.
- Initial treatment in mild cases is with NSAIDs, adding a DMARD if inflammation and joint damage persist. The reader is referred to the section on 'Treatment of RA' in Chapter 5 for further details on specific agents. Azathioprine, sulfasalazine, penicillamine, gold, and leflunomide may all be used with some effect; there are anecdotal reports of 'flares' of skin psoriasis with hydroxychloroquine. The most commonly used agent is MTX; it also can have a dramatically improving effect on the skin disease. Sulfasalazine may be more efficacious in those with both spinal and peripheral joint involvement.
- Oral and IM steroids should be avoided, but intra-articular steroids may be used, avoiding joints surrounded by psoriatic plaques for fear of introducing infection. Steroids have the potential for causing a flare of psoriatic plaques.
- Patients with severe and unresponsive disease can be offered ciclosporin A and retinoids.
- Etanercept and adalimumab are licensed for the treatment of PsA and have positive effects on skin as well as joint disease. In the UK the BSR have produced guidelines for use of anti-TNFα therapies in PsA and NICE is currently undertaking an appraisal. Treatment of patients with purely axial disease should follow the AS guidelines mentioned earlier. Inclusion criteria for patients with peripheral disease are the failure of 2 standard DMARDs alone or in combination, and active joint disease with 3 or more tender and swollen joints.

Reactive arthropathy

Clinical presentation

- Reactive arthritis is an aseptic inflammatory arthritis triggered by an infectious agent outside the joint.
- Spondylarthropathies can be defined as 'reactive' if urethritis/cervicitis (sexually transmitted reactive arthritis or SARA) or diarrhoea (gut associated reactive arthritis or GARA) are present. The features of the spondylarthropathies can vary in the 'reactive' subgroup from one patient to another, and in the same patient at any given time in the course of the disease.
- The onset of reactive arthritis may be acute, with fever, weight loss, and diffuse polyarticular involvement. More often, however, there is limited joint synovitis and a low-grade, or absent, fever.
- Mucocutaneous features include painless balanitis circinata of the glans penis, and pustular psoriasis of the palms or feet (keratoderma blennorhagica), often associated with a more severe outcome.
- Conjunctivitis is observed early. Uveitis is less frequent early in disease, often occurring in recurrent disease and between episodes of arthritis.
- Acute diarrhoea may precede the musculoskeletal symptoms by up to 1 month. The GI symptoms may be so mild as to be ignored by the patient and often the provoking agent has cleared from the gut before the joint symptoms arise. Several triggering agents have been isolated from stools and these include, *Shigella*, *Salmonella*, *Clostridium*, and *Yersinia*. Chronic diarrhoea does not appear to be associated with reactive arthritis. However, the demarcations can be blurred and some patients may have inflammatory bowel-associated arthropathies, or silent inflammatory lesions that appear to manifest as 'reactive-like' and are best described as undifferentiated spondylarthropathy.
- Urethritis, prostatitis or cervicitis may be present at prompt suspicion of infection. Rigorous investigation is required to ensure pathogenic mycoplasmas and ureaplasmas are identified and eradicated. The commonest non-gonococcal, sexually acquired urethritis is due to Chlamydia.
- Recurrent or repeated infections do not always lead to a recurrence of arthritis and may occur in the absence of further sexual intercourse. There are some important differential diagnoses outside the spondylarthropathies that include HIV-associated arthritis, Lyme disease, parvovirus arthropathies, and Behçet's disease (see p.512).

Investigation and treatment of reactive arthritis

- The inflammatory nature of the condition can be confirmed by the presence of a ↑ ESR and CRP. For therapeutic decisions in some cases, but mainly for epidemiological purposes, many tests can be done looking for a causative agent. Most screens are negative and in this sense there is merit in just taking a close history and limited investigation rather than a full diagnostic work-up. If required, the clinician should request stool, urine, and blood cultures, urethral and vaginal swabs, and aspirate a swollen joint looking for cells, crystals, and infection. It may be helpful to enlist the expertise of colleagues in infectious diseases for the assessment of sexually acquired infections.

- The use of monoclonal antibodies, or DNA and RNA hybridization, in the search for products of triggering agents, is limited to research purposes. Likewise, tests for detecting antibodies to bacteria have no specific place in current clinical practice and do not have a predictive value on outcome.

- In the early stages of disease there are no radiological signs except in a very small number of cases where changes in the sacroiliac joints may be seen and probably pre-date presentation.

- There is no specific cure. NSAIDs and local corticosteroid injections are the mainstay of therapeutic intervention. If symptoms persist > 6 months and there is clinical evidence of ongoing synovitis and joint destruction then a disease-modifying agent such as sulfasalazine, MTX, or azathioprine should be considered. There is no proven role for systemic steroids in this situation.

- Taking account of all symptoms, the bulk of patients are in complete remission at the end of 2 years, the majority within 6 months. The metatarsophalangeal joints and the heel often remain sites of persistent pain, and balanitis and keratoderma may persist, acting as markers of potential poorer prognosis. Other factors that may be predictive of poor outcome include oligoarthritis of the hip, persistently ↑ ESR, poor response to NSAIDs, dactylitis, and involvement of the lumbosacral spine.

- Aseptic urethritis and early conjunctivitis resolve quickly and spontaneously. Antibiotic therapy will clear underlying infections but this may not have any affect on the duration of disease.

- Uveitis should be treated in the usual way with topical steroid drops and a referral to an ophthalmologist if there has been no response within 3 days.

- Patient education, particularly in the context of food hygiene and of prevention of exposure to sexually acquired infection, is important. Contact tracing is vital in cases of sexually transmitted infection.

Enteric arthropathy

Clinical presentation

- The arthropathies of ulcerative colitis and Crohn's disease have many similarities and the combination of peripheral and axial skeletal disease, enthesopathies, mucocutaneous, and ocular disease fits neatly into the diagnostic realm of the spondylarthropathies.
- The exact pathology is unknown, but is thought to be due to impairment of the gut-mediated immunity and increased bowel permeability, allowing bacteria to pass through the bowel wall into the circulation.
- Mono- or asymmetrical oligoarthritis can be coincident with the onset of bowel disease or arise during the course of the disease. There is a close association between exacerbation of bowel and peripheral joint disorders, and enteropathic arthritis (EA) tends to remit after removal of diseased bowel tissue. The knees and ankles are most commonly involved.
- In contrast to peripheral arthritis, sacroiliitis is not clearly associated with either the onset or exacerbation of the bowel disease and may be present for years prior to the onset of colitis or ileitis.
- Other non-articular features to look for include:
  - uveitis (in about 10%),
  - erythema nodosum
  - pyoderma gangrenosum
  - aphthous stomatitis.
- Arthropathy associated with inflammatory bowel disease often improves with treatment of the bowel symptoms. Intra-articular steroids, sulfasalazine, and MTX can be used in resistant cases. NSAIDs should be used with caution as they can cause a flare of Crohn's disease. Anti-TNFα therapies used in treatment of Crohn's disease may also improve joint symptoms.

Spondyloarthropathies in childhood

Epidemiology and clinical presentation

- This umbrella term covers a heterogenous group of diseases associated with HLA B27 that affect children under the age of 16 and produce a spectrum of symptoms in adulthood.
- The disease group includes:
  - enthesitis and arthritis syndrome
  - juvenile ankylosing spondylitis
  - juvenile reactive arthritis
  - juvenile psoriatic arthritis(JPsA)
  - arthritis associated with inflammatory bowel disease
  - anterior uveitis.
- Using the ILAR classification, the spectrum of diseases is called enthesitis-related arthritis (ERA).
- Incidence is estimated at 1.44 per 100 000 children. Prevalence has increased over the last 30 years.
- IgM RF and antinuclear antibodies are not found. 90% patients will be HLA B27 positive.
- The diagnosis is often more difficult in childhood as symptoms of back pain and radiological changes are uncommon. The diagnosis rests more often on the presence of lower limb large joint arthritis associated with enthesopathy, acute uveitis, psoriasis, or bowel pathology, and may be difficult to separate from JIA. The reader is referred to Chapter 7 for a description of the classification criteria for childhood arthropathies.
- Apart from an increased incidence of peripheral disease and rare axial symptoms, juvenile onset spondyloarthropathies resemble the adult forms. This lack of early axial disease may lead to initial misdiagnosis as oligoarticular JIA.
- The Rome and New York criteria for the diagnosis of adult AS have not been validated in children; nevertheless, a small proportion of children fit these critieria and are considered to have juvenile AS. Approx 5–8% of children attending rheumatology clinics have AS. This compares with 75% having JIA. Juvenile AS commonly presents with lower limb large joint arthritis (often knees and ankles) with the early course often episodic. It also appears to differ from adult AS in the precocious destruction of the hip joint. The condition is reported more often in ♂ than ♀ and 50% of cases go on to develop AS in adult life.
- Enthesitis and arthritis syndrome usually affects the feet and can be disabling. The disease is usually episodic, but some cases are chronic, resulting in bony erosions and joint ankylosis. Over 70% patients with enthesitis syndrome will fulfill diagnostic criteria for AS after 5–10 years from onset.
- Childhood reactive arthritis and enteropathic arthropathy are essentially similar to adult disease.

JPsA

- JPsA is defined in the ILAR criteria as either arthritis in the presence of psoriasis, or arthritis and at least 2 of:
  - dactylitis
  - nail abnormalities (pitting or onycholysis)
  - family history of psoriasis confirmed by a dermatologist in at least one first-degree relative.
- The incidence of JPsA is estimated at 3 per 100 000, with a prevalence of 15 per 100 000.
- Oligo or polyarthritis may occur and can affect large or small joints, the spine, and sacroiliac joints. Anterior uveitis is seen in 10–20%.
- JPsA, traditionally grouped with the spondylarthropathies, has greater clinical and laboratory similarity to JIA; important dissimilarities with the spondylarthropathies include a lack of association with HLA B27, and AS as an outcome.
- JPsA is also more common in ♀ than ♂.
- Childhood reactive arthritis and enteropathic arthropathy are essentially similar to adult disease.

Treatment of JPsA

- The principles of treatment include education, physiotherapy, splints, orthotics, NSAIDs, and intra-articular corticosteroids for peripheral arthritis. Oral corticosteroids may be used for severe arthritis or enthesitis.
- In the presence of significant axial disease, polyarthritis, or persistent oligoarthropathy, sulfasalazine may be started (initially at 12.5 mg/kg/day, increasing weekly over 1 month to 50 mg/kg/day in 2–3 divided doses). However SZP may be no better than placebo, as seen in recent trials.
- MTX has shown little effect in spondyloarthropathy patients without JPsA. MTX and ciclosporin have been used successfully in the treatment of JPSA alone or in combination.
- Infliximab and etanercept have been used and appear to be as effective as in adult spondyloarthropathy treatment. They have also been used to treat uveitis.

Prognosis in juvenile spondyloarthropathy

Remission rates vary widely in studies, with estimates of 10–20% in remission at 10 years. A large proportion of children will therefore have persisting disease in adult life, with associated disability.

Systemic lupus erythematosus (SLE)

Introduction

- Systemic lupus erythematosus (SLE) is a complex clinical syndrome characterized by inflammation of multifactorial aetiology in most of the body's organs or systems. The diversity of clinical symptoms is matched by that of the autoantibodies detected in the condition.
- Patients will present to a variety of specialists, with variable clinical and serological expression of lupus. This may bias the reporting of cases given the wide spectrum of pathology. It is important to remember that there are also variations in the incidence of clinical features between ethnic groups. With this in mind, the physician needs a keen sense of awareness of a variety of multisystem pathologies and to appreciate that SLE has taken on the mantle of syphilis as the great mimic of other conditions.
- The American Rheumatism Association (ARA), now the American College of Rheumatology, published its revised criteria for the classification of SLE in 1982 (see Table 9.1). As stated in other sections of this book, criteria are for the classification of the disease for epidemiological and research purposes mostly, and not as a diagnostic tool. In practice, however, these criteria naturally tend to form the corner stone for clinical diagnosis.

Table 9.1 Revised criteria of the ARA for the classification of SLE

1	Malar rash	
2	Discoid rash	
3	Photosensitivity	
4	Oral ulcers	
5	Arthritis	
6	Serositis:	Pleuritis or pericarditis
7	Renal disorder:	Persistent proteinuria of >0.5 g/24 h or cellular casts
8	Neurological disorder (having excluded other causes):	Seizures or psychosis
9	Haematological disorders:	Haemolytic anaemia or
		Leucopenia <4.0 × 10^9/litre on 2 or more occasions
		Lymphopenia <1.5 × 10^9/litre on 2 or more occasions
		Thrombocytopenia <100 × 10^9/litre
10	Immunological disorders:	Raised antinative DNA antibody binding
		Anti-Sm antibody
		Positive antiphospholipid antibodies
11	Antinuclear antibody in raised titre	

SLE may be diagnosed if 4 or more of the 11 criteria are present either serially or simultaneously.

The clinical features of SLE

Lupus is 10–20 times more common in ♀ than ♂, and most likely to develop between the ages of 15–40 years. There are several non-specific features that are in common with many other chronic diseases. Of these, lethargy and fatigue are often the most disabling. Weight loss, nausea, and persistent lymphadenopathy are also features.

Musculoskeletal

- Polyarticular, frequently symmetric and episodic arthralgia occurs in 90% of cases. About 50% will also have morning stiffness. In most cases symptoms outweigh objective clinical signs, and overt joint damage from synovitis is confined to < 10% of patients. Intense tendonitis is more common than synovitis and can lead to deforming reversible subluxation of joints without erosive disease (Jaccoud's arthropathy).
- Avascular necrosis occurs in 5–10% of patients; most cases being associated with previous steroid use.
- Myalgia has been reported in up to 60%, but true myositis in < 5%, and myopathy may be a consequence of steroid and chloroquine treatment.

Skin

Although the 'butterfly' rash of the nasal bridge and malar bones is classically described, it is found in only about one-third of patients. The cutaneous manifestations of SLE are listed in Table 9.2.

Cardiovascular disease

- Pericardial disease is the most common component of heart involvement in lupus. Most cases are clinically silent and a mild pericarditis with a rub is more common than a significant accumulation of pericardial fluid, and pericardial thickening is a more likely feature than an effusion on echocardiography.
- ⚠ When a pericardial effusion does evolve it can be rapid, constrictive, and life-threatening.
- Up to 15% of patients with lupus can develop clinical myocarditis, defined by combinations of tachycardia, dysrhythmias, a prolonged PR interval on electrocardiography, cardiomegaly, and congestive cardiac failure. Histological studies suggest that a mild non-specific perivascular inflammatory infiltrate is a common feature. Corticosteroid therapy, although indicated for inflammatory cardiac disease, is itself an added risk factor for atherosclerosis given its propensity to induce hypertension, hypercholesterolaemia, and obesity.
- Systolic murmurs, probably due to a hyperdynamic circulation secondary to anaemia, are common. The classic endocarditis described by Libman and Sachs can be identified in up to 50% of cases at autopsy but rarely causes clinically significant lesions. As most lesions of Libman–Sachs endocarditis are too small to be assessed accurately by echocardiography, any valve vegetations identified in a patient who is febrile should raise the possibility of bacterial endocarditis.
- Women with SLE have a 5–6% ↑risk of coronary heart disease compared to general population. This risk is increased 50% in women 35–44.

Table 9.2 Cutaneous manifestations of SLE

Frequency of occurrence	Feature
Common (20–50%)	Butterfly rash
	Photosensitivity
	Chronic discoid lesions
	Non-scarring alopecia
	Purpura/petechiae
	Vasculitis of the digits
Less common (5–20%)	Mucosal ulcers
	Urticaria
	Hyperpigmentation
	Limb ulcers
	Subcutaneous nodules
Occasional (5%)	Periorbital oedema
	Jaundice
	Severe scarring alopecia
	Pruritis
	Bullae
	Panniculitis
	Psoriaform lesions

Pulmonary disease

- Because of the tendency for disease to be subclinical, chest radiographs and pulmonary function tests invariably indicate a greater degree of involvement than is evident clinically, and patients present quite late in the disease process following a history of slow onset non-productive cough and increasing shortness of breath on exertion. Pulmonary function tests typically show both diminished total lung capacity and peak flow rates.
- Pleuritic pain/pleuritis is present in up to 60% of cases.
- Pleural effusions are a feature in one-third of patients but they are usually small and clinically insignificant.
- Interstitial fibrosis, pulmonary vasculitis, and pneumonitis are found in up to one-fifth of lupus patients. This said, it is difficult to separate 'true' pulmonary disease such as pneumonitis from that occurring as a consequence of concurrent infection, congestive cardiac failure, and renal failure. Pulmonary haemorrhage is rare in lupus.
- ⚠ Pulmonary hypertension is unusual and has been linked to the presence of antiphospholipid antibodies. There is great interest in antiphospholipid antibodies and thrombotic events in lupus. Patients presenting with compromising pleuritic pain and/or pulmonary hypertension should be investigated for the presence of pulmonary emboli and antiphospholipid syndrome.

Renal involvement

- Assessment of blood pressure for hypertension, urine for protein, blood, and casts, and the serum creatinine and urea is an essential part of regular monitoring. Symptoms suggesting renal failure rarely become obvious until substantial damage has occurred. If early disease is suspected, the physician should consider 24-h urinalysis for proteinuria and creatinine clearance. The glomerular filtration rate and renal function may also be assessed by nuclear medicine techniques.
- The World Health Organization has subdivided renal lupus into five categories according to biopsy findings. The classification has some drawbacks. Tubulointerstitial disease is not considered and allowance is not made for the varying degree of severity within each category.
- There remain differences of opinion as to when and whether a renal biopsy is undertaken. Nephritis can transform from one type to another and the same biopsy may have more than one histological appearance. There are differing reports on the value of biopsy as an indicator of poor prognosis. Doubt has also been thrown on the ability to reproduce activity and chronicity scores accurately. Few studies on the relationship between renal histology and outcome have addressed the question as to what information renal biopsy adds to the clinical data. However, glomerulosclerosis is a poor prognostic feature. It must also be remembered that a renal biopsy has complications in itself.
- Although not uniformly agreed, it can be recommended that lupus patients with microscopic haematuria and/or proteinuria with a ↓ glomerular filtration rate should be considered for renal biopsy. However, the information provided about prognosis should not be overestimated and it is advised that the biopsy material be assessed in centres with a high degree of experience.

Haemopoietic involvement

- A high ESR is a common finding.
- A normochromic, normocytic 'anaemia of chronic disease' presents in up to 70% of patients with lupus. Renal failure, NSAID-induced gastric bleeding, Coombs' positive and microangiopathic haemolysis, and red cell aplasia, are factors that may contribute to the anaemia.
- Leucopenia and lymphopenia are common abnormalities of the white cell count in 50% and 80% of patients respectively. A leucocytosis is rare, suggesting infection or steroid therapy.
- There are several forms of clinical thrombocytopenia. Chronic, indolent, and uncomplicated thrombocytopenia ($<100 \times 10^9$/litre) is present in up to 20% of patients. ⚠ A rarer acute and life-threatening severe thrombocytopenia is also recognized. This requires aggressive therapy initially with high-dose systemic steroids, and patients may require splenectomy. Some patients may also present with what initially appears to be an idiopathic thrombocytopenia (ITP), later followed by other manifestations of lupus.

Table 9.3 Other clinical features of SLE

Vascular	Raynaud's phenomenon
	Cutaneous vasculitis
	Digital ulcers and gangrene
Gastrointestinal	Hepatomegaly (25%)
	Abdominal pain (10–20%)
	Splenomegaly (10%)
	Aseptic peritonitis (rare)
	Mesenteric vasculitis (rare)
	Pancreatitis (rare)
Biochemical	Hypergammaglobulinaemia (60%)
	Hypoalbuminaemia (50%)
	Normal CRP*

* The CRP may be raised in some lupus patients but generally a raised CRP would suggest either infection, erosive arthritis, or possibly serositis.

Nervous system disorders

- Features of neurological disease range from the common migraine headache (in up to 40% of patients) to psychoses and seizures (in 5–10% of patients over the course of their disease). Thromboembolic disease associated with antiphospholipid antibodies can cause major cerebrovascular damage (see Chapter 10).
- Approximately 10% of patients will develop a sensory (or less often sensorimotor) peripheral neuropathy. Cranial nerve involvement is less common and is usually associated with active systemic disease.
- Up to 70% prevalence of psychiatric illness has been quoted in the literature. However, this includes anxiety and depression, rarely separated in studies from the non-specific stresses associated with debilitating and often painful disease, as opposed to the disease *per se*. This said, it does emphasize the degree of the problem and that depression must be assessed and managed seriously in lupus.
- Detailed psychometric testing can identify subtle impairment, in up to 20% of lupus patients. Emotional lability, personality change, and impaired judgement and cognition suggest organic involvement.
- Whilst it is accepted that corticosteroids can induce psychiatric symptoms, in general it is felt the drugs given in lupus are not responsible for most of the psychiatric manifestations observed.

- Examination of the cerebrospinal fluid in neuropsychiatric disease is not considered useful and not routinely done. It may be of value in ruling out infection in the immunosuppressed or in demonstrating oligoclonal bands and high protein levels in cerebral lupus.
- Electroencephalography is often non-specific and is not recommended. CT is of most help in distinguishing cerebral infarction from haemorrhage, or a mass lesion. MR imaging and positron emission CT (SPECT and PET) are neither specific for, nor well-correlated with, central nervous system involvement. For example, it is difficult to distinguish between small vessel vasculitis and multiple thrombi.

Other clinical features

Other clinical features are listed in Table 9.3.

Antiphospholipid (antibody) syndrome and SLE

- There are recognized associations between anticardiolipin antibodies and the lupus anticoagulant in systemic lupus erythematosus. Anticardiolipin antibodies form part of a spectrum of antiphospholipid antibodies of which the lupus anticoagulant is part.
- A statistically significant association has been shown between the presence of these antibodies in lupus patients, and the following clinical conditions:
  - venous and arterial thrombosis
  - thrombocytopenia
  - cerebral disease
  - recurrent fetal loss
  - pulmonary hypertension
  - livedo reticularis.
- A small cohort of patients with anticardiolipin antibodies develop renal impairment due to multiple small thrombi.
- Neither the lupus anticoagulant nor anticardiolipin antibodies appear to correlate with age, duration of disease, or a variety of established lupus clinical features, including polyarthritis, vasculitis, or serositis.

Further details, including management, may be found in Chapter 10.

Pregnancy and SLE

- There is a disparity in the literature as to whether pregnancy is associated with an ↑ risk of lupus 'flare'. However, pregnancy does not appear to worsen the long-term outcome of SLE, nor do flares of disease activity necessarily affect the outcome of pregnancy. A major complication, however, is pre-eclampsia. Preexisting renal disease may be an important risk factor.
- ⚠ SLE is associated with an ↑ rate of fetal death late in pregnancy and overall approximately 25% of lupus pregnancies result in fetal loss.
- Anti-Ro antibodies are associated with fetal heart block.
- The antiphospholipid antibody syndrome and its associated complications during pregnancy is discussed in Chapter 10.
- Drugs commonly used in SLE are similar to those used in RA and are discussed in Chapter 5. This includes an outline of drug safety in pregnancy.

Diagnosis and investigation of SLE

- The majority of investigations are aimed specifically at end-organ disease. Investigation in the form of radiographs, FBC, coagulation screen, ESR, CRP, and renal and liver biochemistry, urinalysis, and blood pressure may lead to other tests, e.g. of haemolysis or pleuritic pain. For clinical patterns and markers of SLE activity, the physician is directed to autoantibody and complement tests (see Table 9.4).

- There are a variety of circulating autoantibodies to a range of nuclear, cytoplasmic, and plasma membrane antigens. Most patients (98% or more) will have antinuclear antibodies. Approximately 60% have ↑ levels of dsDNA antibodies (detected as the immuno-fluorescent Crithidia test or by specific ELISA or radioimmunoassay). Some patients have varying combinations of antibody profile that may change over the course of the disease. The antibodies, their prevalence and clinical association are shown in Table 9.4.

- Lupus is associated with deficiencies of the early classical pathway of complement (e.g. C1q, C1r, C1s, C2). The overall consequence is ↓ clearance and ↑ deposition of complexes. Reduced levels of complement C3 and C4 are common in SLE.

- Disease activity may be assessed using dsDNA antibody and serum complement levels as surrogate markers. Antibodies to DNA tend to ↑, and serum complement levels ↓, during active disease. However, these markers are not 100% sensitive to changes in disease activity and should be interpreted in the context of clinical findings. A subset of patients will be 'serologically active but clinically quiescecent', meaning they will have low complement levels and raised dsDNA titres but no signs of active disease. Patients should always be treated on the basis of symptoms rather than blood tests alone.

- Some individuals may have high levels of RF and features of an erosive RA type disease. This 'overlap' syndrome is termed 'rhupus'. The mix of clinical features and autoantibodies is not peculiar to SLE and all the autoimmune rheumatic diseases are subject to the phenomenon of 'overlap' or 'undifferentiated' disease. In this situation a number of clinical features and antibodies common to several diseases are present without the absolute criteria for any one specific disease; treatment is determined by the end-organ disease that is present. The concept of 'mixed connective tissue disease' as a specific diagnosis, rather than 'undifferentiated' disease remains controversial.

- The assessment of disease activity is central to patient management. Several global activity indices have been produced that correlate well and are reliable. Awareness of changes in lupus activity, whether improvement of disease or not, is an essential part of decision-making and drug treatment. Global scoring systems such as the Systemic Lupus Erythematosus Disease Activity Index (SLEDAI) are of some value, both in the context of clinical trials and long-term follow-up of patients. A better overview of disease activity is provided by the British Isles Lupus Assessment Group (BILAG) activity index that records activity in eight organs/systems.

Table 9.4 Autoantibodies of systemic lupus erythematosus used in clinical practice

Autoantibody		Prevalence (%)	Associations
Intracellular:	DNA	40–90	Renal disease
	Histone	30–80	Drug-induced lupus
	Sm	30 (Africans, Caribbeans), 10 (Caucasians)	
	U1 RNP	20–30	Renal disease
	rRNP	5–15	? Neuropsychiatric lupus
	Ro/SS-A	25–40	Sjögren's syndrome, cutaneous lupus, congenital heart block
	La/SS-B	10–15	As Ro/SS-A
Cell membrane:	Cardiolipin	20–40	Recurrent abortion, thrombosis
	Red cell	< 10	Haemolytic anaemia
	Platelets	< 10	Immune thrombocytopenia
Extracellular:	RF	25	Cross reacts with histones and Ro
	Complement C1q	50	A rise can precede nephritis

- Equally constructive is the concept of an index of damage as distinct from disease activity. For example, a patient with shortness of breath may have an active but reversible vasculitis or an irreversible fibrosis; the distinction between the types of damage is important since the treatments are different. A SLICC (systemic lupus international collaborating clinics) damage index has been developed and is currently being assessed and modified. The reader is referred to two articles by Gladman et al.[1,2] as the background for current scoring systems.

1. Gladman DD et al. Senitivity to change of 3 systemic lupus eythematosus disease activity indices: international validation. *Journal of Rheumatology*, 1994; **21**: 1468–71

2. Gladman DD et al. The development and initial validation of the Systemic Lupus International Collaborating Clinics/American College of Rheumatology damage index for systemic lupus erythematosus. *Arthritis and Rheumatism*, 1996; **39**: 363–9

Drug-induced lupus (DIL)

- Many drugs have been implicated in causing DIL. Those definitely and most commonly associated with DIL are:
  - minocycline
  - hydralazine
  - procainamide
  - isoniazid
  - quinidine
  - methyldopa
  - chlorpromazine
  - salazopyrine (sulfasalazine).
- Hydralazine-associated DIL is considered to be dose dependent, and procainamide, time dependent.
- Up to 90% of cases taking procainamide develop a positive antinuclear antibody (ANA) and 30% of these develop DIL.
- Renal, central nervous system, and skin features of SLE are rare in DIL. Other features of SLE such as articular, pulmonary, and serosal disease are common.
- In the majority of cases the condition subsides on withdrawing the drug. There is no contraindication to using these drugs in idiopathic SLE.

The treatment of SLE

- Several general measures are important:
  - rest as appropriate; try to avoid stress.
  - avoid overexposure to heat and sunlight using sun creams of factor 15+.
  - try to adhere to a low-fat diet and add fish oil derivatives.
  - control cardiovascular risk factors.
- Advice should include intake of calcium and vitamin D for healthy bones. Patients on steroids >5 mg should be offered a bisphosphonate (assuming not contra-indicated e.g. premenopausal women) as prophylaxis against steroid-induced osteoporosis.
- Vaccinations, apart from 'live' vaccine (e.g. yellow fever, live polio) in patients on immunosuppressives, are not contraindicated though the degree of response differs from the healthy individual.
- Medium-to-high oestrogen contraceptive pills should be avoided. Progesterone only, the lowest oestrogen pill, or other methods of contraception are advised. Many patients tolerate hormone replacement therapy (HRT) but use in the menopause is controversial; one in seven patients may experience a 'flare' of their disease with HRT.

Reduction of cardiovascular disease risk factors

- Management of traditional risk factors (smoking, hypertension, diabetes)
- Status treatment for hypercholesterolaemia
- ± Aspirin
- Tighter control of SLE disease activity.

Table 9.5 outlines the common therapies used to treat the various clinical manifestations of SLE.

The management of SLE as an acute rheumatological emergency is discussed in Chapter 21.

New therapies in SLE

Rituximab

Encouraging results have been seen using this anti-CD20 monoclonal antibody in patients with active systemic disease that have failed, or only had partial response to, conventional treatments. Further studies are needed to determine optimum dose and long-term tolerability.

Mycophenolate mofetil (MMF)

MMF ↓ disease activity and mortality in mouse models of lupus. It has been studied in the management of lupus nephritis, where similar rates of remission, relapse, and infection were seen in comparison to the standard treatment of cyclophosphamide induction followed by azathioprine maintenance therapy. MMF was not associated with marrow suppression or amenorrhoea. MMF has also been seen to be effective in maintaining remission in lupus nephritis in comparison to long-term intravenous cyclophosphamide.

Autologous haemopoietic stem cell transplantation (HSCT)

HSCT is used to treat haematological diseases, but has been used in patients with severe refractory SLE. The procedure is effective in inducing remission but is curative in <50%. Mortality is high and long-term effects are unknown. New autoimmune conditions have been reported after HSCT. It is currently used only in those with life-threatening SLE.

Table 9.5 Recommendations for drug use in SLE

Symptom	Drug	Regimen
Arthralgia/fever	NSAIDs (caution with renal disease)	No special recommendation
Arthralgia/myalgia/lethargy	Hydroxychloroquine	400 mg daily for 3 months then reduce dose to 200 mg if responding. Initial ophthalmic check-up recommended—patient then to report if visual disturbances
Malar/discoid rash	Prednisolone, hydroxychloroquine, thalidomide	
Arthritis/serositis/myositis	Prednisolone	20–40 mg daily for 2–4 weeks, then reducing dose 5 mg steps each week. Require bone prophylaxis against osteoporosis if dose remains at 7.5 mg or above for more than 3 months.
Autoimmune anaemia or thrombocytopenia (ITP)	Prednisolone, azathioprine	60–80 mg prednisolone daily for 2 weeks, reducing in 10 mg steps per week after depending on response. 2.5 mg/kg azathioprine. ITP might also require immunoglobulin or splenectomy
Renal	Prednisolone and azathioprine. Cyclophosphamide	Severe disease may require monthly IV steroid and cyclophosphamide for 6 months then 2–3 monthly for 2 years
Central nervous system	Prednisolone, ?anticonvulsant	Up to 80 mg daily
Raynaud's disease	See Chapter 12	

Other agents

The efficacy of anti-TNFα therapy in SLE is at present not clear. 16% of RA patients on these therapies develop double-stranded DNA antibodies, and 0.2% a transient lupus-like syndrome. A small, open label study has shown benefit in lupus nephritis but further work needs to be done.

IL-1 receptor antagonist (anakinra) has been shown to be well-tolerated in early studies for arthritic symptoms.

LJP-394 is a B cell toleragen that leads to serological improvement but not a reduction in number of renal flares.

Pooled immunoglobulin (IVIG) may be of use in severly ill patients not responding to other therapies, and perhaps more so in situations where sepsis is the trigger and life-threatening. It may have a role in drug-resistant membranous and membranoproliferative nephritis, cutaneous lupus, and has been used in severe autoimmune thrombocytopenia with effect.

Prognosis and survival in SLE

- Many studies of the duration of disease and survival rates are confounded by inadequate attention paid to the ethnic group, age of onset, and socioeconomic status of individual patients. The number of patients lost to follow-up is also high. With the division of patients into those with or without overt nephritis, it is reasonable to state a 5-year survival in lupus of 90%. At 15 years, only 60% of those with nephritis will be alive compared with 85% of those patients without renal disease.

- A bimodal mortality curve is considered to exist. Patients who die within 5 years usually have very active disease, requiring high doses of immunosuppressives. Those patients dying later tend to do so from cardiovascular disease, renal disease, and possibly infection.

- The combined effect of the disease and its treatment is to render the immune system prone to infection. It is often difficult to apportion responsibility to one or other. The possibility of infection must always be kept in mind and treated aggressively as outcome from sepsis can be very poor.

- Controlling risk factors for cardiovascular disease is important.

- Studies to date do not show any major link to the use of immunosuppressive agents and malignancy in SLE.

Childhood SLE

- This is a rare disease with an estimated incidence of 0.4 per 100 000. There are several features of childhood SLE that differ from the adult disease, though essentially the main features and treatment are in common. General management strategies (i.e. not including pharmacological agents) for child welfare are the same as those employed in the management of all paediatric arthritides—see Chapter 7.
- The overall prepubertal ♀:♂ ratio is 3:1, suggesting a higher male frequency in childhood SLE as compared to that seen in adults; the ratio reverts to the more classic adult ratio of 9:1 post-puberty.
- The disease is more common and severe in those of Afro-Caribbean and Asian origin.
- The main features at presentation are arthritis, myalgia, fever, and rash (all features with a frequency of approximately 60–80% of cases at diagnosis). Malar rash is present in 30% of cases at diagnosis, and renal disease at onset of disease is high (up to 60%). True myositis with proximal weakness occurs in <10% of cases. Neuropsychiatric disease is present in up to 40% cases.
- Avascular necrosis is more common in children than adults with SLE (10–15% of cases), and is more common in SLE than other paediatric autoimmune rheumatic diseases where prolonged high-dose steroids are used. Unlike in adults with SLE, paediatric Raynaud's phenomenon and vasculitis are not associated with greater risk of avascular necrosis.
- True discoid lupus lesions are rare below the age of 18. Alopecia is present in up to 50% of paediatric cases, and scarring is unusual.
- Raynaud's phenomenon is less common in childhood lupus and occurs in 10–20% of patients.
- As in adult disease, hydroxychloroquine and NSAIDs can be used for mild skin and joint disease.
- Oral or IV corticosteroids are given for disease not responding to the above measures, or in moderate-to-severe multisystem disease. Growth retardation secondary to corticosteroids is a major concern, and the lowest possible dose of steroid should be used. Bone protection with calcium and vitamin D should also be given.
- Cyclophosphamide, azathioprine, methotrexate and mycophenolate mofetil are used as in adult disease. Case reports of successful autologous stem cell transplantation have been described.
- The 10-year survival for SLE in childhood is currently estimated at 85%.

Neonatal SLE ⚠

- This is a rare condition found in the newborn and characterized by discoid skin lesions, haemolytic anaemia, hepatitis, thrombocytopenia, and congenital heart block (CHB).
- It is associated with placental transmission of maternal Ro and La antibodies.
- The non-cardiac manifestations resolve within 1 year. Cardiac involvement often requires early pacemaker insertion, and mortality in the first 3 years of life is up to 30%.
- In women with anti-Ro/La antibodies there is a 5% chance of their first child being born with CHB; this rises to 15% with subsequent pregnancies.
- Fetal monitoring with echocardiography in the antenatal period is essential.

The antiphospholipid (antibody) syndrome (APS)

Introduction

The antiphospholipid syndrome (APS) was first described in the 1980s and comprises arterial and venous thrombosis with or without pregnancy morbidity in the presence of anticardiolipin (ACL) antibodies or the lupus anticoagulant (LAC). It can be 1° or 2° in association with other autoimmune diseases, most commonly systemic lupus erythematosus (see Chapter 9).

APS can affect almost any body system or organ, and presents to many medical specialties, including rheumatology, dermatology, neurology, and cardiology.

Classification criteria were produced in 1999 (see Table 10.1).

Table 10.1 Classification criteria for the antiphospholipid syndrome

Clinical Criteria	
Vascular thrombosis	1 or more episodes of arterial, venous or small vessel thrombosis in any tissue or organ confirmed with imaging or histopathology, with the exception of superficial venous thrombosis. Histopathology should show thrombosis without significant inflammation in the vessel wall.
Pregnancy morbidity	1 or more unexplained death of a morphologically normal fetus at or beyond 10 weeks gestation
	OR
	1 or more premature births of a morphologically normal neonate at or before 34 weeks gestation due to severe pre-eclampsia, eclampsia or severe placental insufficiency
	OR
	3 or more unexplained, consecutive, spontaneous abortions before 10 weeks gestation and excluding maternal anatomical or hormonal abnormalities, and excluding maternal and paternal chromosomal causes.
Laboratory criteria	Medium/high titre of IgG and/or IgM isotype anticardiolipin antibody in blood on 2 or more occasions at least 6 weeks apart using standard assays.
	Lupus anticoagulant present in plasma on 2 or more occasions at least 6 weeks apart.

Adapted from Wilson *et al.* International consensus statement on preliminary classification criteria for definite antiphospholipid syndrome: report of an international workshop *Arthritis Rheum* 1999; **42**: 1309–11

Epidemiology and pathology

- Antiphospholipid (APL) is the overall term used with ACL and LAC being subgroups.
- Antibodies are directed at protein–phospholipid complexes. Recently antibodies to β_2-glycoprotein I (β_2GPI) have been found to be the main target antigen involved in the binding of anticardiolipin antibodies to anionic phospholipids.
- Case control studies estimate the prevalence of ACL in the normal population to be 1–4%. Prevalence in those >65 years increases to 12–50% depending on the study. Prevalence of ACL and LAC in SLE patients is estimated at 20–40% and 10–20% respectively. These differences arise due to the lack of uniformity of assay methods. New standardization criteria have been developed that will help resolve these issues.
- The LAC and ACL antibody tests are the most useful antibodies for identifying patients with the syndrome. The LAC test cannot be performed reliably if a patient is receiving heparin or oral anticoagulant. The ACL antibody assay is the most sensitive test available. The two tests can be discordant in up to 40% of cases and their unrelated behaviour in the course of disease and in the individual patient means that both assays are required to identify cases of APS.
- Apart from a clinical suspicion leading to a request for antiphospholipid antibody assays, a clue to their presence lies in finding a prolonged clotting time in assays for the 'internal pathway'-clotting cascade.
- The specificity of antiphospholipid antibodies probably differs in various disorders. Studies suggest that LAC and high titres of IgG ACL antibodies are associated with greater risk of thrombosis; the risk is much lower in patients with infection-related or drug-induced antibodies, that tend to be of the IgM isotype. The role of anti-β_2GPI antibodies in disease diagnosis is still debated. 10% of patients with APS only have antibodies to β_2GPI. There is evidence that β_2GPI titre and simultaneous presence of ACL or LAC are associated with disease severity. Currently it is not recommended for routine testing.
- The differential diagnosis of unexplained thrombosis includes deficiencies of protein C and S, and antithrombin III; however, these are usually associated with recurrent venous thrombosis. Most striking about APS is the feature of thrombosis in the setting of thrombocytopenia. The main differential diagnosis is thrombotic thrombocytopenic purpura. This is mainly a microvascular disorder most often associated with neurological features of confusion, seizures, and changes in conscious level rather than the larger vessel thromboses seen in APS.
- Only a third of all patients with APL/ACL ever experience thrombosis. 75% of those with an initial venous event will have another; 93% of those with an initial arterial event will have another.

Clinical features of APS

Table 10.2 summarizes the main clinical features of APS and some of the less common findings.

Thrombosis

- Apart from cases of severe thrombocytopenia, antiphospholipid antibodies are paradoxically associated with thrombosis rather than haemorrhage.
- Vessels of all sizes, venous or arterial, may be affected without evidence of an inflammatory infiltrate, i.e. vasculitis. This distinction is important not only in trying to understand the pathogenesis of the disorder but also in the choice of treatment. Unlike other known clotting disorders, arterial thrombosis is a major feature of APS. The antibodies should be sought particularly in the younger stroke patient where they may account for up to 20% of cases.
- Widespread thrombosis is the feature of life-threatening 'catastrophic antiphospholipid syndrome'. In this situation the patient may present with acute medical collapse, severe thrombocytopenia, multi-organ failure (notably cerebral and renal), and adult respiratory distress syndrome.

Thrombocytopenia

This is common though usually not severe enough to cause bleeding. ACL antibodies have been found in up to 30% of cases of presumed immune thrombocytopenic purpura (ITP). Some patients also develop a concomitant Coomb's positive haemolytic anaemia (Evan's syndrome).

Fetal loss

Recurrent spontaneous pregnancy loss is a common complication of APS. This is most frequent in the second trimester, differing from the first trimester pattern of loss in the general population. Screening for the antibodies in the general population is not of value. Previous pregnancy history is of importance in determining the significance of a positive antibody titre. For example, estimates suggest a 30% risk of fetal loss in the first pregnancy in lupus patients with APS, rising to 70% in a pregnancy if there is a history of at least two previous spontaneous abortions.

Other features of APS

- Transient and recurrent neurological symptoms resembling multiple sclerosis or epilepsy are features of APS. Though rare, it is important to be aware of these conditions as anticoagulation therapy may be effective in such cases.
- Transverse myelopathy, though rare, has a strong association with the presence of antiphospholipid antibodies.

- Cardiac manifestation are seen in up to 40% of patients. However only a small proportion (5%) have significant morbidity. In a European cohort, myocardial infarction was the presenting feature of APS in 3% of patients, and was seen during follow-up in 5.5%. The prevalence of ACL in patients with myocardial infarction is estimated at 5–15%, however screening is not indicated, except in younger patients, those with other symptoms and signs of APS, and those with a family history of autoimmune disease. Mitral and aortic valve thickening and dysfunction is commonly seen on echocardiography, but significant morbidity is uncommon.

Table 10.2 Clinical features of the antiphospholipid syndrome

Feature	Subgroup	Frequency
Major features:		
Thrombosis	Overall	
	Venous:	85%
	All	55%
	Lower limb	66%
	Pulmonary	25%
	Arterial:	45%
	All	45%
	Stroke	50%
	Transient ischaemia	33%
Recurrent fetal loss	Overall	33%
	First trimester	33%
	Second trimester	50%
	Third trimester	20%
Thrombocytopenia		25%
Associated features:	Leg ulcers, livedo reticularis, thrombophlebitis	
	Heart valve lesions and myocardial infarction	
	Transverse myelitis, chorea, and epilepsy	
	Haemolytic anaemia, Evan's syndrome	
	Pulmonary hypertension	
Less common findings:	Splinter haemorrhages, digital gangrene, leg ulcers	
	Migraine, Guillain–Barré, pseudomultiple sclerosis	
	Amaurosis fugax, retinal artery and vein occlusion	
	Labile hypertension and accelerated atherosclerosis	
	Renal artery stenosis/thrombosis	
	Ischaemic bone necrosis	
	Addison's disease	

Treatment of APS

Treatment of APS is summarized in Table 10.3.

- Studies suggest that lifelong and oral anticoagulation is an effective therapeutic option in the 2° prevention of thrombosis. Care should be taken to balance the intensity of anticoagulation with the associated bleeding risk.
- Levels of ACL antibody do not necessarily correlate with risk of thrombosis. This finding supports the recommendation that prophylaxis in the asymptomatic individual is not warranted.
- Mild thrombocytopenia need not be treated. Severe cases (<50 x 10^9/litre) should be treated with oral corticosteroids in the first instance. In those failing to respond, gamma-globulin, danazol, and splenectomy have been used with varying success.
- The presence of antiphospholipid antibodies in pregnancy, in the absence of a history of thrombosis or fetal loss, is not an indication for treatment.
- Prophylactic heparin at surgery is recommended.
- ⚠ Women with APS on warfarin should be converted to standard heparin or low-molecular-weight heparins preferably prior to conception, although the reader should be aware that the latter may not be licensed for this purpose. Aspirin should also be introduced.
- Other advances have been the realization that high-dose immuno-supression is unwarranted and that combined care between rheumatology, obstetrics, and haematology, with judicious monitoring and timely intervention, has a significant impact on outcome in pregnancy.

Table 10.3 The treatment of APS

Clinical situation		Treatment
Asymptomatic		Observation and/or low-dose aspirin
Thrombosis	Deep venous—1st event	Lifelong warfarin (INR 2–3)
	1st stroke	Lifelong warfarin (INR 2–3) and/or low-dose aspirin
	Transient ischaemia	Low-dose aspirin
	1st non-cerebral arterial event	Warfarin (INR 2–3) and aspirin
	Recurrent arterial/venous event	? warfarin (INR 3–4) or LMWH
	Catastrophic APS	Warfarin
		Corticosteroids
		Immunoglobulin
		Plasmapheresis
		Cyclophosphamide
Pregnancy	No previous history	Observation and/or low-dose aspirin
	First trimester abortion Second/third trimester fetal loss	Low-dose aspirin and LMWH
	Repeat fetal loss despit Heparin	?gammaglobulin
Thrombocytopenia	Mild (100–150 count)	Observe
	Moderate (50–100)	Observe
	Severe (<50)	Corticosteroids (as ITP), ?role of splenectomy

LMWH = low molecular weight heparin

Catastrophic APS (CAPS) ⚠

Introduction

- This rare variant of APS affects small vessels and visceral organs and was first described in 1992. It is an important and serious condition that can present to many medical specialties.
- It can present in previously asymptomatic patients.
- The trigger is an infection in 20% cases. Other precipitating factors include trauma/surgery, malignancy, warfarin withdrawal in a patient with APS, and pregnancy.
- CAPS is associated with other autoimmune conditions such as SLE (see Chapter 9), RA (see Chapter 5) and SScl (see Chapter 12).
- Despite these risk factors it is estimated that 45% cases have no known trigger.
- Mortality is high at 50% and most patients require the Intensive Care Unit.

Clinical features

- Diffuse peripheral and central thrombosis occurs leading to:
  - limb arterial and venous occlusion
  - intra-abdominal organ infarction including renal failure
  - pulmonary emboli and adult respiratory distress syndrome
  - small vessel cerebrovascular disease
  - aortic and mitral valve defects and myocardial infarction
  - other thrombotic complications such as ovarian, testicular, and retinal vessel occlusion.
- Livedo reticularis, gangrene, and purpura are visible markers of the disorder on the skin.
- Bone marrow infarction has also been reported.
- Classification criteria have recently been produced[1].

Laboratory features

These include:

- Moderate-to-severe thrombocytopenia
- Haemolysis
- Disseminated intravascular coagulation
- High levels of IgG ACL antibodies.

The differential diagnosis

The clinician should consider the following conditions

- Thrombotic thrombocytopenic purpura (red cell fragments more numerous than in CAPS)
- HELLP syndrome (haemolysis, elevated liver enzymes and low platelets)
- Haemolytic–uraemic syndrome
- Cryoglobulinaemia
- Vasculitis.

---

1 Cervera R, Font J, Gomez-Puerta JA *et al.* Validation of the preliminary criteria for the classification of the catastrophic antiphospholipid sydrome. *Ann Rheum Dis*, 2005; **64**: 1205–1209.

Treatment and prognosis
- Apart from techniques and therapies used in the intensive support of multiple organ failure, IV heparin, corticosteroids, and immunoglobulin (for 4–5 days at a dose of 0.4 g/kg/day) is warranted.
- Plasma exchange may help but cyclophosphamide is not considered to be effective.
- Case reports exist in single patients describing the use of prostacyclin, defibrotide, fibrinolytics, and rituximab.
- Mortality remains >50% and 25% of survivors will develop further APS -related events.
- Recurrence of CAPS is very rare.

Sjögren's syndrome (SS)

Epidemiology and pathology

- Sjögren's syndrome (SS) is a chronic autoimmune disease of unknown aetiology, characterized by lymphocyte infiltration of exocrine glands resulting in xerostomia and keratoconjunctivitis sicca.
- The condition may be 1°, associated with specific extraglandular (systemic) disease, or 2° in association with a number of other autoimmune rheumatic diseases, including RA (see Chapter 5) and SLE (see Chapter 9).
- ⚠ It is also a disorder in which a benign autoimmune process can terminate in a lymphoid malignancy.
- The syndrome affects ♀ more than ♂ in a ratio of 9:1, and tends to occur at 40–50 years of age. It can, however, occur in any age group.
- Population prevalence is estimated at 1%, similar to that of RA.
- The triggering of autoimmunity and the development and continuation of an autoimmune response remain a great source of interest as much in SS as in other areas of autoimmune rheumatic disease. The links between environmental stimulus and immunogenetics, and the studies of humoral and lymphocyte activity may help to untangle the mechanisms whereby immunological dysregulation can lead to malignant transformation of B cells involved in the immune process.
- Epstein–Barr and retroviruses have been implicated in pathogenesis.
- HLA DR–3 is strongly associated.
- Antibodies to nuclear components Ro and La are found and are thought to be formed when these antigens are exposed on the surface of apoptotic cells.
- RF and antinuclear antibodies are also common and patients may be erroneously diagnosed with RA.
- Recently discovered autoantigens in SS include fodrin and muscarinic acetylcholine receptor M3.

The Classification criteria for SS requires the presence of at least 4 of 6 of the following:

- **Occular symptoms** e.g. daily persistent troublesome dry eyes for >3 months, recurrent sensation of sand/gravel in eyes, or use of tear substitutes >3 times per day
- **Oral symptoms** e.g. daily feeling of dry mouth for >3 months, recurrent or persistently swollen salivary glands, or frequent use of liquid to aid swallowing of dry food
- **Positive Schirmer's test** (see text)
- **Abnormal lower lip biopsy**
- **Low unstimulated whole salivary flow** <1.5 ml per minute
- **Antibodies to Ro and/or La**

Exclusions include head and neck irradiation, hepatitis C, AIDS, pre existing lymphoma, sarcoidosis, graft versus host disease, antichloinergic drug use.

For further information the reader is referred to Vitali C, Bombardieri S, Moutsopoulos HM. Calssification criteria for Sjögren's syndrome; a revised version of the European criteria proposed by the American-European consensus group. *Ann Rheum Dis,* 2002; **61**: 554–8.

Clinical manifestations of SS

Glandular disease

- The initial manifestations can be non-specific and 8–10 years can elapse before the symptoms of the full-blown syndrome develop.
- Typical initial features of 'sicca' syndrome include subjective dry eyes (xerophthalmia) in >50% at presentation, dry mouth (xerostomia) in 40%, and parotid/salivary gland enlargement in 25%. The prevalence of these manifestations ↑ with the duration of disease. There may be concurrent corneal and conjunctival damage (keratoconjunctivitis sicca), and dental caries from poor tear and salivary flow respectively.
- A number of other conditions can lead to a dry mouth or parotid/salivary gland swelling, and these should be borne in mind during assessment.
- Some causes of xerostomia/ophthalmia include:
  - age (frequent in the elderly)
  - drugs—psychotropic, parasympathetic, antihypertensive, diuretics
  - dehydration
  - psychogenic
  - irradiation
  - congenital gland malformation or absence.
- Some causes of parotid gland enlargement include:
  - neoplasia
  - bacterial and viral (mumps, influenza, EBV)
  - CMV, HIV, coxsackie A infection
  - recurrent parotitis/chronic sialadenitis
  - sarcoidosis
  - endocrine—diabetes mellitus, acromegaly.

Extraglandular (systemic) disease

Extraglandular disease is seen in one-third of patients with primary SS. The main symptoms are fatigue, low-grade fever, myalgia, and arthralgia (see Table 11.1).

Joints

Joint pain is common; radiographs rarely reveal pathological changes. Non-erosive arthritis is more frequent in patients with Raynaud's phenomenon, and the latter can pre-date SS by many years. In contrast to SScl (see Chapter 12), Raynaud's in SS is not associated with digital ulceration and infarcts.

Table 11.1 The incidence of extraglandular manifestations of primary Sjögren's syndrome

Condition	Frequency (%)
Arthralgia/arthritis	60
Raynaud's phenomenon	40
Lymphadenopathy	14
Pulmonary disease	14
Renal disease	9
Liver disease	5
Lymphoma	5
Vasculitis	5
Splenomegaly	3
Peripheral neuropathy	2
Myositis	1

Skin

- The skin may be involved with itchy annular erythema, alopecia, and hyper/hypopigmentation. A hypersensitivity vasculitis may also develop.
- Vascular involvement in SS affects small and medium-sized vessels. The most common manifestations are purpura, urticaria, and skin ulceration. Skin vasculitis in SS is more benign and treatment with corticosteroids is not always needed.

Pulmonary disease

Pulmonary function abnormalities are seen in 25% patients, though they are not usually clinically significant. Lymphocytic infiltration occurs around bronchioles, leading to a picture of cryptogenic organizing pneumonia. This responds well to corticosteroids.

Renal disease

- Overt renal disease is found in 10% of patients with primary SS. An abnormal, subclinical, urine acidification test is found in up to 40% of cases but some patients develop distal tubular acidosis and concurrent renal stones. Fanconi syndrome is less common.
- Glomerulonephritis is rare and seen mainly in those with SS/SLE overlap. In many cases a consistent finding is cryoglobulinaemia and hypocomplementaemia.

Gastrointestinal and hepatobiliary disease

- Dysphagia due to dryness of the pharynx and oesophagus is common. Chronic atrophic gastritis may occur due to lymphocytic infiltration similar to that seen in the salivary glands.
- Subclinical hyperamylasaemia is a common finding in up to 25% of cases and there may be a close link between 'autoimmune cholangitis' of SS and primary biliary cirrhosis (PBC). Sicca syndrome is found in approximately 50% of cases of PBC.
- Transaminase ↑ may be due to hepatitis C. Hepatitis C can cause a Sjögren's-like disease often in association with a 'mixed' cryoglobulinaemia.

Neuromuscular disease

- Mononeuritis multiplex as a consequence of vasculitis is well recognized as is the isolated involvement of cranial nerves, particularly the trigeminal and optic nerve. A peripheral sensory neuropathy is also seen. Specific involvement of the central nervous system remains a controversy. Multiple sclerosis-like syndromes may be seen.
- Myalgia is common, myositis rare and responds to cyclophosphamide (see Chapter 13, Polymyositis).

Lymphoproliferative disease ⚠

- Patients with SS have approximately a 40-fold higher relative risk of developing a lymphoma, compared with age, sex, and race-matched normal controls. The lymphomas are primarily B cell in origin, usually expressing the monoclonal IgMk, and of two major types, either highly undifferentiated, or well-differentiated immunocytomas.
- The clinical picture is diverse. The approach to therapy should be determined by the stage and histological grade of the disease.
- The salivary glands are the main site of lymphomatous change. The presence of lymphadenopathy, organomegaly, or persistent, painful, and continuously enlarged salivary glands, in the absence of infection, should raise suspicion and warrants biopsy. Other organs and systems may be affected including the reticuloendothelial system, lungs, kidneys, and GI tract.
- Risk factors include monoclonal gammopathy, cryoglobulins, hypocomplementaemia and major salivary gland swelling.

Cardiovascular system ⚠

Anti-Ro and La antibodies cross the placenta and can cause fetal congenital heart block. Mothers with these antibodies have a 1 in 20 risk. Fetal heart rate monitoring in specialist centres is needed. Oral dexamethasone given to mothers early following detection of heart block may reverse the condition. Neonatal lupus is also seen, its most common manifestation being a florid rash.

Other pathology in SS

- Over 50% of patients have antithyroid antibodies and altered thyroid biochemistry without necessarily overt clinical symptoms.
- Non-bacterial interstitial cystitis due to an intense inflammation of the mucosa can cause frequency, nocturia, and perineal pain.
- Mild normochromic, normocytic anaemia is common; leucopenia and thrombocytopenia rare. The ESR is often raised and the CRP usually normal.

Other autoimmune diseases

In a recent retrospective case review of 114 patients with primary SS, 33% had an additional autoimmune disease, 6% two diseases, and 2% three diseases. Hypothyroidism was most common condition seen.

Investigation of SS

- Common laboratory findings in primary SS are detailed in Table 11.2.
- To evaluate the glandular component of the disease, various tests are used. Setting a cut-off point between the normal and abnormal individual is difficult.
- Salivary flow rates (sialometry) can be measured for whole saliva or separate secretions from different salivary glands, with or without stimulation. Patients with overt SS have ↓ flow rates. This technique is simple and effective.
- Anatomical changes in the ductal system can be assessed by radio contrast sialography. This can, however, be painful and there is some controversy as to its sensitivity and specificity.
- Scintigraphy, with uptake of ^{99}Tc, may provide a functional evaluation of all the salivary glands by observing the rate and density of uptake and the time for it to appear in the mouth after IV administration. Scanning has a high sensitivity but low specificity. Neither sialography or scintigraphy are suggested as routine investigations.
- Schirmer's test is used for the evaluation of tear secretion. Strips of filter paper 30 mm in length are slipped beneath the inferior eye-lid by a fold at one end of the strip. After 5 min the length of paper that has been made wet by the tears is measured; wetting of <5 mm is a strong indication of diminished tear secretion.
- A lower lip salivary gland biopsy may show lymphocytic infiltration and glandular atrophy. Although often performed, the procedure is invasive with a risk of sensory nerve damage.

Table 11.2 Common laboratory findings in primary SS

Finding		Frequency (%)
General	Anaemia	20
	Thrombocytopenia	2
	Leucopenia	6
	Raised ESR	60
	Raised CRP	6
Cryoglobulinaemia		Up to 30
Serology	ANA	90
	Rheumatoid factor	60
	Ro/SS-A	60
	La/SS-B	40
	Antimitochondrial	6
	Sm	2
Hepatitis C		?True frequency

Treatment of SS

Table 11.3 summarizes the treatment options for Sjögren's syndrome.

Table 11.3 The treatment of Sjögren's syndrome

Condition	Treatment
Dry eyes	Regular bathing with artificial tears. Avoid smoky rooms or dry air-conditioning. Glasses may help protect against wind on the face. Contact lenses may protect the cornea but need regular wetting. Mucolytics such as acetylcysteine. Avoid certain drugs. Occasionally individuals may benefit from a tarsorraphy or procedure to dilate the lacrimal ducts or obstruct tear clearance via the nasolacrimal duct
Dry mouth	Good oral hygiene. Regular fluids avoiding sugary drinks. Sugar-free flavoured lozenges (may contain pilocarpine). Artificial salivas and fitted saliva sumps in denture caps. Oral bromhexine 48 mg/day may help
Sicca manifestations	May improve with the cholinergic agent pilocarpine (side-effects include flushing/sweating) or cemiveline (less side-effects)
Vaginal dryness	Patients may respond to propionic acid gels. Rigorous treatment of infection. Advice on lubricants etc. if there is pain with intercourse
Salivary gland	Infection—tetracycline (500 mg 4 times/day) and NSAIDs. Persistent pain and swelling—Biopsy
Arthralgia	Hydroxychloroquine 200–400 mg/day (see Drugs in RA, for monitoring)
Systemic vasculitis	Necrotizing vasculitis and glomerulonephritis—prednisolone and/or cyclophosphamide. Leucocytoclastic vasculitis—no specific therapy
Liver disease	Cholestasis may respond to ursodeoxycholic acid 10–15 mg/kg/day
Interstitial lung disease	Prednisolone

Other treatments

- There is no evidence that azathioprine, low dose steroids, ciclosporin or methotrexate are useful. Hydroxychloroquine ↓ ESR and immunoglobulin levels, but has no effect on salivary flow rates. Many clinicians use it to treat fatigue, myalgia, and arthralgia.
- Infliximab has been used successfully in primary SS. Rituximab, in limited studies to date may improve symptoms in an SS patient treated for lymphoma.
- Oral interferon alpha improves salivary flow but long-term use may be limited.

Systemic sclerosis and related disorders

Epidemiology and diagnostic criteria

- Scleroderma is a spectrum of rare disorders ranging from limited to generalized, non-systemic to systemic, and environmental to autoimmune rheumatic disease. Generalized scleroderma, systemic sclerosis, predominantly affects ♀ and is associated with ↑production of connective tissue, notably collagen, widespread microvascular damage, and inflammation.
- The spectrum of scleroderma and scleroderma-like syndromes includes:
  - raynaud's phenomenon—primary, secondary
  - scleroderma (localized)—morphoea, linear, *en coup-de-sabre*
  - scleroderma (systemic)—limited cutaneous, diffuse cutaneous, scleroderma sine scleroderma
  - chemical induced—environmental, occupational, drugs
  - scleroderma-like disease (see Table 12.1)—metabolic, immunological, localized sclerosis, and visceral disease.
- There is no single diagnostic test for systemic sclerosis (SScl) although there are specific autoantibodies. For the purpose of separating it from other autoimmune rheumatic diseases and identifying case profiles, preliminary criteria were developed in 1980 by the American Rheumatism Association. These criteria have a 97% sensitivity and specificity for definite SScl, but are less sensitive for the largest subset of patients with limited cutaneous disease, failing to identify 10% of such cases.
- Currently the most widely used classification of SScl (see Table 12.2) defines 2 subsets divided into limited cutaneous (lcSScl) and diffuse cutaneous (dcSScl). Over 60% of cases are in the 'limited' subset, where visceral involvement is late, some 10–30 years after onset of Raynaud's. The term 'limited cutaneous' is now preferred to CREST (calcinosis, Raynaud's, eosophageal dysphagia, sclerodactyly, telangiectasia).
- ⚠ DcSScl is more serious, of rapid onset, and associated with organ failure often within the first 5 years of presentation.
- Clearly these models will continue to change and develop as knowledge of pathogenesis advances and immunological findings are matched to clinical subsets.

Table 12.1 Scleroderma-like syndromes

Metabolic/inherited	Insulin-dependent diabetes mellitus (digital infarcts)
	Carcinoid syndrome
	Acromegaly
	Phenylketonuria
	Amyloidosis
	Lichen sclerosis et atrophicus (acrodermatitis)
	Inherited premature ageing syndromes
Immunological/inflammatory	Chronic graft versus host disease
	Eosinophilic fasciitis
	Overlap/undifferentiated autoimmune rheumatic disease
	Lymphoedema
Local visceral disease	Idiopathic pulmonary fibrosis
	Infiltrating carcinoma/infiltrating cardiomyopathy
	Sarcoidosis
	Amyloidosis

- There are 3 main abnormalities in scleroderma. A vasculopathy is found that manifests clinically as Raynaud's phenomenon, and pathologically as endothelial cell injury. Vascular injury may be the primary event either by vasomotor instability or microvascular intimal proliferation and vessel obliteration. Intravascular pathology in the form of ↑ platelet activity, red cell rigidity, and thrombosis may also be a factor. Inflammation is also seen, but the morbidity and mortality associated with these diseases is due to the third process-fibrosis. Fibrosis is the hallmark of several diseases and in SScl it is widespread and non-organ-specific. Excess deposition of collagen and extracellular matrix protein is found in the skin and internal organs of patients with SScl. Current research is focusing on the role of several proteins including endothelin-1 and transforming growth factor beta.
- Several chemical agents have been implicated in the development of scleroderma, including:
  - silica
  - organic chemicals: aliphatic hydrocarbons—vinyl chloride, naphtha; aromatic hydrocarbons—benzene, toluene, epoxy resin, toxic oil, paraffins
  - drugs: hydroxytryptophan, carbidopa, fenfluramine, bleomycin, cocaine.

Table 12.2 The classification of systemic sclerosis

1. 'Prescleroderma'	Raynaud's phenomenon, nail capillary changes, digital ischaemia
	Disease-specific antinuclear antibodies: antitopoisomerase-1 (Scl-70) anticentromere (ACA) nucleolar
2. Diffuse cutaneous SScl	Skin changes within 1 year of Raynaud's. Truncal and acral (face, arms, hands, feet) skin involvement
	Tendon friction rubs
	Early, significant organ disease: interstitial lung disease oliguric renal failure myocardial disease gastrointestinal disease
	Nailfold capillary dilatation and 'drop out'
	Scl-70 antibodies in up to 60% of patients
3. Limited cutaneous SScl	Raynaud's phenomenon for many years
	Acral skin involvement
	Late incidence of pulmonary hypertension with or without interstitial lung disease
	Skin calcification and telangiectasia
	Nailfold capillary dilatation without 'drop out'
	ACA antibodies in 70–80% of patients
4. Scleroderma sine scleroderma	Raynaud's ±
	No skin involvement
	Presentation with lung fibrosis, renal crisis, cardiac or gastrointestinal disease
	Antinuclear antibodies may be present

Cutaneous features of scleroderma and their treatment

Scleroderma—'localized' skin changes

- This is distinct from SScl in its absence of vasospasm, vascular, and organ damage, and the distribution of skin lesions.
- Morphoea may be 'circumscribed' with just 1 or 2 lesions or 'generalized'. The rash is often itchy, violaceous or erythematous, and progresses to firm 'hide-bound' skin with hypo- or hyperpigmentation and subsequent atrophy. The 'circumscribed' condition tends to resolve within 3 to 5 years and treatment is often unnecessary. The acral parts are spared, the trunk and legs being most often involved. The 'generalized' form can be disfiguring, leading to contractures, ulceration, and occasionally malignancy. Generalized morphoea may respond to oral corticosteroids, D-penicillamine, methotrexate, intralesional interferon, ciclosporin, or IV immunoglobulin.
- Guttate morphoea is a variant with small 10 mm diameter papules and minimal sclerosis, resembling lichen sclerosus et atrophicus. The lesions usually localize to the neck, shoulders, and anterior chest wall.
- Linear scleroderma describes a band-like pattern of sclerosis, often in a dermatomal distribution. The sclerotic areas often cross over joints and are associated with soft tissue and bone atrophy, and growth defects. Treatment is similar to generalized morphoea as above. Physiotherapy and appropriate exercises may help to minimize growth defects in the childhood form.
- *En coup-de-sabre* is linear sclerosis involving the face or scalp and associated with hemiatrophy of the face on the same side. The lesion assumes an ivory and depressed appearance reminiscent of a scar from a sabre.

Scleroderma—'diffuse' skin changes

- The changes in the skin usually proceed through three phases of early, classic, and late. In the early stage there may be non-pitting oedema of the hands and feet, most marked in the mornings and often associated with Raynaud's. The skin then becomes taut, the epidermis thins, hair growth ceases, and skin creases disappear and the 'classic' changes of scleroderma become more pronounced. When limited to the fingers alone the term sclerodactyly is applied. The classic changes remain static for many years.
- Taut hypo- or hyperpigmented skin involvement proximal to the elbow, knee, or clavicle qualifies a patient as having dcSScl. In this group there is a preponderance of visceral involvement in the first 5 years of symptoms ⚠.
- The late phase may evolve at any time. Truncal and limb skin softens such that it can be difficult to know that a person ever had sclerosis. However, the hand changes rarely resolve and continue to show the ravages of fibrosis and contractures. During this phase of the disease digital pitting scars, loss of finger pad tissue, ulcers, telangiectasia, and calcinosis can occur.
- A practical scheme for assessing dcSScl and lcSScl by dividing the disease into early and late stages is shown in Table 12.3.

Table 12.3 Characterisitc findings in early and late systemic sclerosis

Diffuse cutaneous features	Early onset (<3 years from onset of disease)	Late onset (>3 years from onset of disease)
Constitutional	Fatigue, weight loss	Minimal
Vascular	Raynaud's (often mild)	Severe Raynaud's. Telangiectasia
Cutaneous	Rapid progression involving arms, face, and trunk	Stable or some regression
Musculoskeletal	Arthralgia, myalgia, stiffness	Flexion contractures
Gastrointestinal	Dysphagia and 'heart burn'	More severe dysphagia. Midgut and anorectal disease
Cardiorespiratory	Myocarditis, pericarditis, lung fibrosis	Progression of established disease/ Pulm. Hypertension
Renal	Maximum risk of scleroderma renal crisis	Crisis uncommon after 5 years

Limited cutaneous features	Early onset (<10 years from onset of disease)	Late onset (>10 years from onset of disease)
Constitutional	None	Digital ulceration or gangrene
Vascular	Severe Raynaud's. Telangiectasia	Stable, calcinosis
Cutaneous	Mild sclerosis on trunk and face	Flexion contractures
Musculoskeletal	Occasional joint stiffness	More severe symptoms common. Midgut and anorectal disease
Gastrointestinal	Dysphagia and 'heart burn'	Slow progressive lung fibrosis. Pulmonary hypertension.
Cardiorespiratory	Rarely involved	Right-sided heart failure
Renal	No direct involvement	Rarely involved

Raynaud's phenomenon (Table 12.4)

- The overall prevalence of this phenomenon is between 3–10% of the population worldwide, variation depending on climate, skin colour, and racial background in particular. In SScl Raynauds is present in approximately 95% of cases.
- The classical features are episodic pallor of the digits (due to ischaemia), followed by cyanosis (due to deoxygenation), and then redness and suffusion with pain and tingling. The last stage of redness is a reactive hyperaemia following the return of blood. Continuous blueness/cyanosis with pain is not Raynaud's.
- Symptoms that might suggest secondary Raynaud's include an onset in the young or >45 years, symptoms all year round, digital ulceration, and asymmetry.
- The antinuclear antibodies discussed earlier should be sought and in some centres nailfold capillaroscopy can be performed. Pathological changes seen on capillaroscopy include nailfold capillary dilatation, haemorrhage, and dropout. Both have a high predictive power for detecting those patients likely to develop SScl.

Table 12.4 The treatment of Raynaud's phenomenon

Treatment	Examples	Comments
Non-pharmacological	Hand warmers. Protective clothing	Universally helpful
	Evening primrose oil	Effective in clinical trials
	Fish-oil capsules	
Oral vasodilators	Nifedipine	Often idiosyncratic response and best tried in rotation
	Diltiazem	
	Amlodipine	
	Losartan	
Topical vasodilators	Fluoxetine/ketanserin	Named patient basis in the UK
	Glyceral trinitrate patch	
	1% hexylnicotinate	
Parenteral vasodilator	Prostacyclin	For severe attacks, digital gangrene, and prior to hand surgery
	Calcitonin gene-related peptide (CGRP)	
Surgery	Chemical or operative lumbar or digital sympathectomy. Debridement. Amputation	

Systemic features of the disease, investigation, and treatment

The gastrointestinal tract (Table 12.5)

- The GI tract is probably the most commonly involved system in SScl. Over 90% of all patients with lcSScl and dcSScl develop oesophageal hypomotility, with >50% of patients with lcSScl having serious disease. In the earliest stages of neural dysfunction most patients are asymptomatic. Prokinetic drugs such as metoclopramide may help. With progression from poor contractility to fibrosis and atrophy, these agents become less helpful; eventually restoration of function is not possible.
- Many patients develop reflux oesophagitis. Simple advice such as raising the head of the bed, taking frequent small meals, and avoiding late night snacks, may help. Patients should avoid NSAIDs and nifedipine, and often require an H_2-blocker or proton-pump inhibitor.
- Small bowel disease with hypomobility can lead to weight loss and malabsorption; 2° bacterial overgrowth may exacerbate the situation requiring rotational courses of antibiotics and the use of prokinetic drugs. Ultimately the small bowel may fail, necessitating total parenteral nutrition.
- Pancreatic insufficiency and biliary cirrhosis may require supplementation.
- Atony and hypomotility of the rectum and sigmoid colon may cause constipation and incontinence, best managed with bulking agents, although severe cases may need limited surgery or the use of implantable sacral stimulators.
- Anaemia due to vascular lesions in the GI mucosa is now widely recognized. The classic appearance in the stomach is now called gastric antrum venous ectasia (watermelon stomach), and these lesions may be treated by argon laser therapy if blood loss is significant.

Pulmonary disease (Table 12.6) ⚠

- Pulmonary disease ranks second to oesophageal in frequency of visceral disease. With the improvements in management of renal disease, pulmonary disease is now the major cause of death in SScl.
- The major clinical manifestations are parenchymal lung disease (interstitial lung disease, organizing pneumonia, and traction bronchiectasis) and pulmonary vascular disease (isolated pulmonary hypertension, pulmonary hypertension associated with interstitial lung disease, and pulmonary oedema). Parenchymal lung disease is found in two-thirds of cases, and pulmonary hypertension in 50%. Far less common conditions include plqeurisy, aspiration pneumonia, drug-induced pneumonitis, and spontaneous pneumothorax.

Table 12.5 Common gastrointestinal disorders in systemic sclerosis

Site	Disorder	Investigation	Treatment
Mouth	Caries. Sicca syndrome	Dental radiographs	Oral hygiene. Artificial saliva
Oesophagus	Hypomotility	Barium swallow	Metoclopromide
	Reflux		Avoid NSAIDS. Raise head of bed. Antacids
	Strictures	Endoscopy	Dilatation
Stomach	Gastroparesis		Metoclopromide
	Gastric ulcer	Barium swallow. Endoscopy	Proton-pump inhibitor
Small bowel	Hypomotility	Barium follow-through	Metoclopromide
	Malabsorption	Hydrogen breath test	Pancreatic supplements. Low-dose octreotide. Nutritional support, antibiotics
		Jejunal aspiration/biopsy	
		Stool cultures	
Large bowel	Hypomotility	Barium enema	Stool bulking agents
Anus	Incontinence	Rectal manometry	Surgery. Neurostimulator

Table 12.6 Cardiopulmonary disorders in systemic sclerosis

Disease	Frequency	Investigation	Treatment
Lung disease:			
Pulmonary fibrosis	Most common in dcSScl	Chest radiograph, lung function tests, high-resolution chest CT scan	Trials at time of writing. Combination of corticosteroid and cyclophosphamide
Pleurisy	Uncommon	Chest radiograph	NSAIDs. Low-dose oral prednisolone
Bronchiectasis	Rare	Chest CT scan	Antibiotics. Physiotherapy
Pneumothorax	Rare	Chest radiograph	Intercostal drain. Pleurodesis
Pulmonary hypertension	10–15% overall	Doppler echocardiogram. Catheter studies	Endothelial 1 receptor antagonists (Bosentan). Prostacyclin Sildenafil. Anticoagulation. Long-term oxygen therapy
Cardiac disease:			
Dysrhythmias and conduction defects	Rare	ECG. 24-h ambulatory cardiac monitor	Dependent on rhythm—drugs. pacemaker
Pericarditis	10–15% overall	Echocardiogram	As pleurisy, above
Myocarditis	Rare	'MUGA' scan	Prednisolone, Cyclophosphamide. Diuretics
Myocardial fibrosis	30–50% of dcSScl		Diuretics. ACE inhibitors

- Interstitial lung disease often develops insidiously and established fibrosis is currently untreatable. Early diagnosis is therefore vital. Most centres would now treat active disease with oral corticosteroids and either oral or IV cyclophosphamide. Trials are continuing at present using oral and IV regimes.
- The plain chest radiograph is not a sensitive test for early fibrosis. Lung function tests can be discriminatory. The single-breath diffusion test
- (DLCO) is abnormal in >70% of early cases and lung volumes are often ↓. In the case of a low DLCO and normal lung volumes, the clinician should think of pulmonary hypertension, which has a dismal overall prognosis responding poorly to intervention.
- High-resolution CT scanning now plays a major part in detecting and following interstitial lung disease and should be performed whenever possible.
- Fibrosis tends to be associated with dcSScl and Scl-70 antibodies, and PAH with lcSScl and anti-centromere antibodies.
- Recent studies suggest a prevalence of PAH of 10% in SSc. Right heart catheterization is the gold standard method of diagnosis, but screening using this method is not practical. Annual echocardiography by experienced practitioners, and lung function tests and clinical assessment are essential to help detect subclinical disease. Treatment of PAH associated with SSc has developed rapidly over the last 5–10 years. Continuous parenteral prostacyclin improves symptoms and pulmonary artery pressures, but not mortality. Studies are in progress using subcutaneous and nebulized prostacyclin. Bosentan, an oral endothelin receptor antagonist, improves function and is now an accepted treatment. Sildenafil inhibits phosphodiesterase type 5, and enhances relocution of Vascular Smooth Muscle as well as inhibiting their growth. A recent double-blind placebo-controlled study of patients with idiopathic or connective tissue disease associated pulmonary hypertension found that Sildenafil significantly ↑ 6-minute walk times and mean pulmonary artery pressure.

Cardiac disease

- There are many cardiac manifestations including pericardial effusion, arrhythmias, heart block and myocardial fibrosis. Many cases are subclinical and careful monitoring is needed. More epidemiological research is needed in this area.

Renal disease ⚠

- Renal disease has been superceded by lung disease as the main cause of death in SScl due to the impact of ACE inhibitors in the treatment of hypertensive renal crisis. It remains however a major, life-threatening complication of SScl.
- Both epithelial and endothelial damage occur before becoming clinically detectable.
- The most characteristic pattern of involvement is the renal hypertensive crisis, generally occurring with dcSScl within the first 5 years of disease onset. In high-risk patients the incidence may be as high as 20%, and associated with microangiopathic haemolytic anaemia, encephalopathy, and convulsions. Mortality may reach 10%.

- A more insidious pattern of renal involvement is also reported in which there is a slow ↓ in glomerular filtration rate accompanied by proteinuria. This probably reflects a more benign vascular and fibrotic process.
- Hypertension should be treated with angiotensin-converting enzyme inhibitors (ACE-I) and calcium-channel blockers. IV prostacyclin may help the microvascular lesions.
- Dialysis may become necessary. It is important to know that considerable recovery of renal function can be made after an acute crisis and that decisions involving renal transplantation should be withheld for up to 2 years.
- Corticosteroids are known to ↑ the risk of renal crisis in dcSScl. Doses >20 mg daily should be avoided.
- Other associated risks for hypertensive renal crisis include rapidly progressive skin disease and diffuse cutaneous disease.

The management of scleroderma renal crisis as an acute rheumatological emergency is discussed in Chapter 21.

Other organ involvement

Table 12.7 summarizes the involvement of other organs in SScl.

Malignancy

It is suggested that there is an ↑ in incidence of all malignancies in SSc patients. Potential causes include immunosuppressive drug use, ↑ incidence of cancers in scar tissue and oncogene over expression. However as these patients are closely monitored, there may be ascertainment bias. Further work is needed in this area.

Table 12.7 Other organ involvement in systemic sclerosis

Organ	Effect	Frequency
Thyroid gland	Spectrum of autoimmune disease. Hypothyroidism common	20–40%
Liver	Primary biliary cirrhosis	3% of lcSScl*
	Obstructive jaundice, calcification, nodules	Very rare
Nervous system	Trigeminal neuralgia	Common
	Carpal tunnel syndrome	3%
	Sensorimotor neuropathy	
	Autonomic neuropathy	
	Subacute cord degeneration	Rare
Genital	Cavernosal artery fibrosis causing impotence	Up to 50%

* Antimitochondrial antibodies found in up to 25% of patients with SScl and anticentromere antibodies found in 10–20% of patients with 1° biliary cirrhosis.

Antifibrotic and immunosuppressive therapies for systemic sclerosis

- Apart from the specific therapies alluded to in the sections on skin and systemic disease above, a number of general systemic therapies are under investigation though none have demonstrated marked benefit.
- Currently no treatment can induce complete remission of the disease. Some therapies can offer partial relief and control of end-organ damage. The evaluation of treatments is extremely difficult given the complexity, heterogeneity, and episodic nature of the disease, as well as the paucity of patients.
- D-penicillamine was been widely used in the past but a single randomized controlled trial has shown no benefit.
- Novel potential antifibrotic therapies may develop through understanding more about anti cytokine antibodies that block fibroblast activation (e.g. anti-TGF-β), or by antagonists/gene translocations that influence pre- and post-translational modification of collagen.
- Both antimetabolite and alkylating immunomodulatory agents have been used, particularly in early dcSScl. The majority of these therapies are currently being evaluated in controlled trials (see Table 12.8).
- Halofuginone, a type I collagen synthesis inhibitor has shown beneficial effects in treating scarring and has been used to mixed effect in bleomycin-induced scleroderma. Further work is needed to assess its use in SScl.
- A recent open label study of minocycline suggests this agent does not work.
- Studies are currently underway looking at the effect of anti-TNFα agents in early skin disease that is mainly inflammatory in nature.
- Autologous stem cell transplant has been performed in severe disease, but has a high mortality rate. Its place in treatment strategies needs further research.
- Acetic acid iontopheresis and ultrasound are being studied in the treatment of SScl related calcinosis.
- Other studies are looking at plasmapharesis and thalidomide.

Table 12.8 Antimetabolite and alkylating immunomodulatory agents being evalualted for use in treatment of SScl

Agent	Comment
Ciclosporin	Beneficial on skin sclerosis
	Watch for renal crisis
	Reduce dose if on calcium-channel blockers
Photophoresis	Benefit reported but needs good clinical trial
Plasmaphoresis	Equivocal and anecdotal
Pooled gammaglobulin	No formal evaluation
Antithymocyte globulin	Possible benefit in diffuse disease, high morbidity
Methotrexate	Control trial in progress for evaluation in dcSScl
Cyclophosphamide	Efficacy from trial data on lung fibrosis. Often given with steroids
Chlorambucil	Anecdotal and control trial failed to show superiority over placebo
Mycophenolate	Improvement in skin disease

Summary—the approach to systemic sclerosis

Diffuse cutaneous systemic sclerosis

History and physical examination generally establishes the diagnosis and autoantibody profiles may identify poor prognosis. The extent of visceral disease should be assessed by baseline investigations as follows:

- Urea and electrolytes
- Creatinine clearance and urinary protein (repeat annually)
- Barium swallow/GI endoscopy depending on symptoms
- Chest radiograph at baseline
- Lung function tests (annually)
- Electrocardiogram (annually)
- Doppler echocardiography (with estimate of pulmonary artery pressure) (repeat annually)
- High-resolution CT lung scan if lung function abnormal.
- Given the paucity of patients, it is important to be aware of local or national centres of expertise and patient suitability for clinical trials.

Limited cutaneous systemic sclerosis

By the time of presentation physical signs are usually diagnostic. Investigations are as above and treatment is mostly symptomatic, concentrating on vascular (Raynaud's and pulmonary hypertension) and GI disease, with annual review.

Prognosis

- SScl has the highest case-specific mortality of any autoimmune rheumatic disease. Estimates of 5 years mortality in scleroderma range from 34–73%. Standardized mortality ratios have been estimated at 3–4 times expected. Logistic regression modelling suggests 3 factors—proteinuria, ↑ ESR, and low carbon monoxide diffusion capacity—are >80% accurate at predicting mortality >5 years.
- Patients with renal crisis have been estimated to have a 50% mortality, although the use of ACE inhibitors and renal replacement therapies may have reduced this.
- Anti-topoisomerase and anti-RNA polymerase antibodies have also been associated with SScl-related mortality.
- Advances in the understanding of mechanisms leading to pulmonary hypertension has led to new therapies that, with time, may show significant impact in slowing disease progression.

Eosinophilia–myalgia syndrome

- This condition was first defined in 1989, as an epidemic in association
- with the ingestion of L-tryptophan. The clinical features resemble Spanish toxic oil syndrome, a condition described in 1981 and associated with a toxin in rapeseed oil. L-tryptophan was widely used, particularly in the United States, for insomnia, premenstrual syndrome, and depression.
- Both conditions share the features of eosinophilia and fasciitis with the disease of the same name, eosinophilic fasciitis. However, no toxin has been associated with eosinophilic fasciitis (see text below).
- The clinical features of the condition are shown in Table 12.9.
- Laboratory and imaging findings include:
  - leucocytosis
  - eosinophilia (>500 mm^3)
  - ↑ ESR
  - ↑ aldolase
  - ↑ creatine kinase
  - abnormal liver function tests
  - abnormal chest radiograph.
- Histologically there is an activation of eosinophils and fibroblasts that contribute to tissue injury and fibrosis.
- The treatment for this condition is essentially supportive and with steroids for pulmonary disease.

Table 12.9 Clinical features of eosinophilia–myalgia syndrome

Flu-like symptoms	Fatigue
	Arthralgia
	Myalgia
	Weakness
Pulmonary	Pneumonitis
	Pulmonary hypertension (in 5%)
Skin	Diffuse, truncal, erythematous macules
	Oedema followed by scleroderma-like changes
	Alopecia
Gastrointestinal	Dysphagia
	Odynophagia—pain on swallowing
	Diarrhoea
	Hepatomegaly
Nervous system	Cognitive impairment
	Neuropathy

Eosinophilic fasciitis

- This is an uncommon idiopathic condition that shares the haematological and skin features of eosinophilia–myalgia syndrome (see previous section). Organ disease is, however, uncommon.
- Cutaneous disease is the most common finding, evolving from oedema
- to fibrosis (especially in children) and induration. The arms and legs are most often involved and there may be localized morphoea, synovitis, and myositis.
- The condition may resolve spontaneously. Otherwise, 50% of cases respond to corticosteroids, though only 15% gain complete remission.
- The condition may be a paraneoplastic phenomenon. It is over represented in women and in the haematological malignancies in this respect. The paraneoplastic condition often fails to respond to steroids and resolves on successful treatment of the underlying malignancy.
- Several treatments have been shown to be of benefit including corticosteroids and ciclosporin.

Inflammatory myopathies— polymyositis (PM) and dermatomyositis (DM)

Epidemiology and diagnosis

- Polymyositis (PM) and dermatomyositis (DM) are the most common forms of 'idiopathic inflammatory myopathy', the latter distinguished by the presence of a characteristic rash. Overlap syndromes with other autoimmune rheumatic diseases occur in 15–20% of cases.
- These conditions are rare. PM has an estimated incidence of 2–8 per million. Incidence increases with age and is highest between the ages of 40–65 years. The ♀ to ♂ ratio is 2:1, but is lower in myositis associated with malignancy, and higher during the childbearing years (5:1). A small amount of evidence suggests that the incidence in Afro-Caribbean ♂ and ♀ compared to white Caucasians is 3–4:1.
- The uncertainty about aetiology makes classification of these conditions difficult. However, a modification of Bohan and Peter's classification (1975) shown in Table 13.1 serves this purpose at present.
- There are a number of 2° causes of myositis and myopathies. These will be discussed later in this chapter.
- The criteria for the diagnosis of PM and DM are shown in Table 13.2.

Table 13.1 Modification of Bohan and Peter's classification of PM and DM

1	Primary idiopathic polymyositis
2	Primary idiopathic dermatomyositis
3	1 or 2 above, with malignancy
4	Juvenile poly(dermato)myositis
5	Overlap syndromes with other autoimmune rheumatic diseases
6	Inclusion-body myositis

7	Rarer myositis:
	  granulomatous
	  eosinophilic
	  focal
	  orbital

8	Drug-induced

Table 13.2 Criteria for the diagnosis of poly/dermatomyositis

1	Compatible weakness. Symmetrical proximal muscle weakness developing over weeks or months
2	Elevated serum muscle enzymes, creatine kinase and aldolase
3	Typical electromyographic findings: myopathic potentials (low amplitude, short duration, polyphasic) fibrillation, positive sharp waves, increased insertional activity, complex repetitive discharges
4	Typical muscle biopsy findings

5	Dermatological features of DM:
	
	  Gottron's papules, involving fingers, elbows, knees, and medial malleoli
	
	  Heliotrope sign around the eyes
	
	  Erythematous and/or poikilodermatous rash

Clinical features of PM and DM

Myositis

- Muscle weakness is the main clinical feature in both conditions and is almost universal, tending to develop insidiously over months but occasionally developing with great speed.
- The weakness is usually symmetrical and diffuse, involving the proximal muscles of the neck, shoulders, trunk, hips, and thighs, the lower limb muscles tending to be clinically symptomatic first.
- Weakness of the distal muscles is rare but can occur late in the disease. The face and ocular muscles may also be involved.
- ⚠ Shortness of breath may be a consequence of diaphragmatic and intercostal muscle weakness (as well as other causes that will be discussed later), and should be looked for.
- Myalgia occurs in about 50% of cases; it is usually mild and sometimes difficult to distinguish from polymyalgia rheumatica.
- There may be atrophy in chronic disease, more so in PM than DM, and contractures may occur in disease of long duration.
- Often the distinction between autoimmune rheumatic disease overlapping with PM/DM versus an autoimmune rheumatic disease with myositis as a manifestation can be very difficult. The relative severity of clinical symptoms and the serological picture may be of help.

Cutaneous disease

- The rash of DM commonly precedes the weakness by weeks to months. The rash may parallel the weakness or remain independent, persisting after the myositis resolves. Erythematous or violaceous papules or plaques (Gottron's papules) or macular patches (Gottron's sign) may occur over the metacarpophalangeal and proximal (occasionally distal) interphalangeal joints. Occasionally these lesions may be found on the extensor surfaces of the knees, wrists, elbows, or medial malleoli. The rash is present in up to 80% of cases.
- A macular eruption may involve the upper chest, neck, shoulders, extremities, face, and scalp. This may develop into poikiloderma, hyper- or hypopigmentation with atrophy and telangiectasia. Typical features include the 'V' sign at the base of the neck anteriorly, and the 'shawl' sign at the back of the neck and across the shoulders.
- The heliotrope rash, found in 30–60% of cases, is a purple/lilac coloured suffusion around the eyes, often associated with periorbital oedema. It is characteristic but not pathognomic.

- Some patients have typical cutaneous DM but do not develop overt myositis. The term 'amyopathic DM' is applied. The same risk of malignancy and systemic complications remains.
- Calcinosis, cutaneous vasculitis, and ulceration, rare in adults, are more common in juvenile DM.

Malignancy

- Studies suggest a modest ↑ in malignancies within 1–2 years of onset in DM. The malignancy may pre-date, peri-date, or post-date the onset of myositis. In the majority of cases, cancer and myositis have an independent course.
- The largest population studies suggest the presence of malignancy to occur in 15% of cases of DM (relative risk in ♂ 2.4, in ♀ 3.4) and 9% of cases of PM (relative risk in ♂ 1.8, and ♀ 1.7). Cancer deaths in studies suggest an increase in DM but not PM, supporting a true association with DM, rather than a study bias due to intensive searching. The highest risk appears to be in ♂ >45years with DM who lack myositis autoantibodies or overlap autoimmune rheumatic disease.
- Tumours frequent in the general population are frequent in PM and DM. There does, however, appear to be an ↑ in ovarian, breast, lung, stomach, colon, and bladder cancers out of proportion to that of other tumours.
- The extent of investigation is controversial. Thorough physical assessment should always include rectal, pelvic, and breast examination. Specific investigations should include a chest radiograph, urinalysis, prostate-specific antigen in men, faecal occult blood testing, mammography, and cervical smear, and probably pelvic ultrasound and CA 125 levels in women. Further bowel investigations are open to debate and determined by individual patient symptoms. Remember that a ↑ ALT may be from muscle and need not indicate liver pathology.
- ⚠ Malignancy manifesting as paraneoplastic myopathy and its investigation is discussed in Chapter 4.

Systemic manifestations

Table 13.3 shows the systemic manifestations of PM and DM.

Assessment of disease activity and damage
- There is a need to be able to accurately assess disease activity and damage using valid and reliable instruments, as has been developed in systemic lupus erythematosus.
- A disease activity measure might contain the following information:
  - muscle strength measure
  - patient and physician global disease activity visual analogue scale
  - laboratory tests results
  - physical function measures (Health Assessment Questionnaire)
  - patient quality of life measures (e.g. Short Form-36).
- A damage score should contain information on damage to different organs.
- Several activity and damage measures are currently being validated e.g. MYOACT and MYODAM.

Table 13.3 Systemic manifestations of PM and DM

Organ/system	Features
General	Fatigue, malaise, weight loss
	Fevers—in 40% overall
	Raynaud's phenomenon
Pulmonary	Due to muscle weakness: aspiration pneumonia, ventilatory failure ($\downarrow$ TLC, VC, $\uparrow$ RV)*
	Due to local disease: interstitial fibrosis (20%), pulmonary vasculitis (rare), pulmonary hypertension (rare)
	Due to treatment: hypersensitivity pneumonitis, opportunistic infection
Gastrointestinal	Oesophageal dysphagia—in 30%
	Striated muscle dysfunction
	Cricopharyngeal dysfunction
	Low oesophageal dysfunction
	Stomach and bowel dysmotility[†]
Cardiac	Cardiomyopathy—<5%
	Pericardial effusion—up to 20%
	Heart block—rare
	Dysrhythmias—uncommon
Skeletal	Arthropathy
	Deformity, mild erosive arthritis
Renal	Very rare. Possible myoglobinuria

* TLC = total lung capacity; VC = vital capacity; RV = residual volume.
[†] Intestinal vasculitis, perforation, and pneumatosis cystoides intestinalis, features of juvenile DM, are very rare in the adult.

Investigation of PM and DM

The investigation of potential malignancy in DM has been discussed earlier in this chapter. Specific investigations for PM/DM include the following:

Muscle enzyme levels

- Serum levels of enzymes released from damaged muscle may be helpful both in diagnosis and monitoring of the disease; creatine kinase (CK) is most widely used.
- There are a number of causes of a ↑ CK level (see Table 13.4), and levels, particularly in DM, may not be ↑ despite active myositis and may be influenced partly by muscle bulk, i.e. relative chronic muscle atrophy. The latter is difficult to assess since measures of muscle mass do not necessarily correlate well with degree of inflammation. Tests that measure muscle mass are not currently practical for clinical use.

Table 13.4 The causes of a raised creatine kinase

Cause	Examples
Strenuous prolonged exercise	
Muscle trauma	
Diseases affecting muscle	Myositis
	Metabolic
	Dystrophy
	Myocardial infarction .
	Rhabdomyolysis
Drugs	Toxic myopathy
	Induction of myositis
	Inhibition of CK excretion (barbiturates, morphine, diazepam)
Metabolic abnormalities	Hypothyroidism
	Hypokalaemia
	Ketoacidosis
	Renal failure
Normal variants	Ethnic group (often higher normal values in the Black population)
	Increased muscle mass
	Technical artefact

Autoantibodies in myositis

- A high antinuclear antibody (ANA) and myositis-specific autoantibodies (MSA) favour PM/DM over other myopathies. The various associations with autoantibodies are shown in Table 13.5.
- A general correlation with anti-Jo-1 antibodies is observed but the usefulness of titres as an index of disease activity is not established.
- Antisynthetase antibodies may alert the physician to an ↑ risk of interstitial lung disease, or identify PM/DM in patients who present with prominent extramuscular disease.

Electromyography

- Electromyography (EMG) and nerve conduction studies cannot establish the diagnosis of PM/DM with certainty, but can demonstrate a myopathic process and help to exclude many other neuropathies and certain myopathies (Table 13.6 gives the differential diagnoses of myopathy and Table 13.7 lists drug-induced myopathies in more detail).
- 90% of patients will have abnormal EMG studies.
- Early findings include low-amplitude, short-duration, polyphasic potentials, with early recruitment and full interference patterns (more fibres are required to achieve a given force). The latter features are in contrast to neuropathies where there is ↓ recruitment and interference. With time, reinnervation of denervated fibres leads to high-amplitude, long-duration, polyphasic potentials. Other features include spontaneous activity in up to 75% of cases, fibrillations, and repetitive discharges akin to myotonia but of constant amplitude and starting and stopping abruptly.

Table 13.5 Antibodies in PM/DM

Antibody class	Antibody subclass	Percentage of PM/DM	Myositis subgroup
Myositis-specific:		In total 30–40	
Anticytoplasmic	Anti-Jo-1	20	Antisynthetase syndrome
	Anti-PL-7/PL-12/OJ/EJ	<3 each	
	Anti-SRP	4	PM
Antinuclear	Anti-Mi-2	8	DM
	Anti-56 kDa	90	All
Myositis-associated:	Anti-PM-Scl	8	PM/DM–scleroderma overlap
	Anti-U1-RNP	12	PM/DM overlap syndromes
	Anti-U2/U5-RNP	<2	PM
	Anti-Ro and Anti-La	5–10	Systemic lupus, Sjögren's syndrome

Table 13.6 The differential diagnosis of myopathy

Agent	Examples
Infectious diseases:	
Viral	Retroviruses
	Picornaviruses (entero.)
	Adenoviruses
	Influenza
	Hepatitis B and C
Bacterial	Pyomyositis
	Lyme myositis
	Tuberculosis
Protozoa	Toxoplasmosis
	Trypanosomiasis
Parasites	Trichinosis
	Cysticercosis
Fungal	Candida
Idiopathic:	
Inclusion body myositis	
Autoimmune rheumatic disease	
Other disorders	Granulomatous myositis
	Eosinophilic myositis
	Focal/orbital myositis
Other myopathies:	Dystrophies and congenital myopathies
	Enzyme deficiencies and lipid storage disorders
	Carcinomatosis
	Rhabdomyolysis
	Neurological: motor neuron disease, myasthenia gravis, Guillain–Barré syndrome
	Endocrine: hypo/hyperthyroidism, Cortisol Excess
	Metabolic: hypocalcaemia, hypokalaemia
	Malnutrition
	Drugs

Table 13.7 Drug-induced myopathy

Clinical picture	Examples
Drugs implicated in autoimmune myopathy	D-penicillamine
	Cimetidine
	L-tryptophan
	Zidovudine
Myopathy with weakness, myalgia, and high CK	Colchicine
	Hydroxychloroquine
	Lipid-lowering agents
	Cyclosporin
	Vincristine
	Carbimazole, propylthiouracil
	Alcohol
	NSAIDs—rare in aspirin, phenylbutazone
Rhabdomyolysis picture	Alcohol
	Illicit drugs—cocaine, heroin
	Amphetamines
	Barbiturates
	Statins (rare)
	Anaesthetics—malignant hyperthermia
	Psychotropics—neuroleptic-malignant syndrome

Imaging

- MR scan, with high sensitivity, sequentially identify areas of muscle inflammation, atrophy, or fatty infiltration. It is useful in helping to decide if weakness is due to disease activity or previous damage.
- Magnetic resonance spectroscopy, ultrasound, and ^{99}Tc and thallium have been used to assess the distribution of disease. None are advocated as part of current routine clinical investigation.

Muscle biopsy

- Most patients should have a biopsy; some feel all patients should have one. There is an argument for not doing so in, for example, the patient with proximal weakness, ↑ enzymes, typical EMG changes, a rash of DM, confirmed myositis-specific autoantibodies, or an overlap autoimmune rheumatic disease and myositis-associated autoantibodies.
- An open biopsy gives the best picture of muscle architecture and is required for certain functional enzyme studies. However, needle punch-biopsy causes less morbidity, is often quicker, may be easier to arrange, and is adequate in the majority of cases.
- Optimal processing and evaluation, minimizing risk of artefact, requires coordination with the pathologist prior to the biopsy taking place.
- Patients with a clinical diagnosis of PM/DM who do not respond to treatment as expected may benefit from a biopsy in order to confirm a diagnosis.

Other tests

- The ESR is ↑ in 50% of cases but correlates poorly with disease activity and response to therapy. The CRP is not specific; high levels would suggest a concurrent infection.
- Gammaglobulins may be ↑; if ↓, this may suggest the presence of a viral infection.
- Complement levels in PM/DM are usually normal.
- Proteinuria is often the result of myoglobinuria.
- Serial spirometry for respiratory muscle weakness may be required.

Treatment of PM and DM

- Treatment should be started promptly pending completion of investigations, particularly in acute onset weakness, dysphagia, respiratory insufficiency, and systemic complications.
- Most cases would be treated with oral corticosteroids alone, though initial therapy with a combination of steroid and immunosuppressive has its supporters. While not demonstrated by prospective randomized controlled trials, the effectiveness of steroids in initially improving muscle strength is generally accepted.
- There is a lack of randomized placebo-controlled trials in treatment of PM and DM.
- An exercise programme helps improve fatigue and muscle strength. Exercise should be used with caution during periods of disease activity, but there is no evidence that it causes prolonged ↑ in muscle enzyme levels or inflammation.

Corticosteroids

- Oral prednisolone at 60–80 mg/day is continued until a ↓ in CK and/or a substantial improvement in muscle strength is seen. Severe cases (or extraskeletal involvement) may be treated with IV methyl-prednisolone 1 g/day for 3 days before starting oral prednisolone. High doses may be required for months and a bisphosphonate should be considered early as prophylaxis against steroid-induced osteoporosis. Adequate calcium and vitamin D intake should always be maintained.
- Most patients will respond to treatment, but this can be slow and partial. The CK is often seen to change faster than any apparent ↑ in strength. Failure to respond may be due to one of several reasons:
  - incorrect diagnosis
  - hereditary myopathy or 'inclusion-body'
  - steroid myopathy
  - permanent loss of strength
  - unresponsive to steroid therapy.
- When the initial goals have been reached, the dose of steroid should be ↓ gradually over a 6-month period to maintenance dosage in the order of 5–10 mg prednisolone/day. This treatment may be required for 1–2 years.

Immunosuppressive agents

- These are required in up to 25% of cases. The trend is towards earlier introduction because of improved response and an aim to keep steroid therapy to a minimum. There is no consensus on the most appropriate regimen. Choice will depend on disease severity, drug safety profile, clinical experience and patient preference.
- Methotrexate (MTX) and azathioprine (AZA) have demonstrable efficacy in retrospective analysis and, in the case of AZA, a controlled study. MTX may have greater efficacy than AZA, particularly in antisyn-thetase antibody-positive, and ♂ patients. The risk of pulmonary fibrosis limits its use in myositis associated lung disease. AZA is less toxic but may take longer to show effectiveness. Studies have shown

a synergistic effect of MTX and AZA where a single drug has failed. The reader is referred to Chapter 5 for discussion on the monitoring of disease-modifying drugs.

- Ciclosporin is a useful therapy in patients where MTX and AZA have been ineffective or not tolerated. It has been used in combination with MTX or IV gammaglobulin.
- Cyclophosphamide has had variable results and is used in resistant cases or in those cases where there is severe extraskeletal involvement such as vasculitis or lung disease.
- Tacrolimus has been used in refractory patients with synthetase syndromes, with improvement in muscle strength, lung function, and cutaneous manifestations. It can be given as an ointment.
- Mycophenolate mofetil (MMF) and chlorambucil are also used.
- There are several reports of improvements in clinical and laboratory measures in patients with refractory PM/DM after receiving infliximab or etanercept. Further work needs to be done in this area.
- In open label studies, rituximab has been used in refractory DM with clinical improvement.
- Monoclonal antibodies against complement component C5 are also being used in the treatment of DM.

Intravenous gammaglobulin (IVIg)

IVIg is obtained from healthy donor serum and contains a large antibody pool. There is increasing evidence of the efficacy of this treatment in both PM and DM. High-dose regimens in the form of 2 g/kg/day for 2–5 days each month have been advocated. However, the effectiveness of each treatment is of limited duration (4–6 weeks), tapering and main-tenance regimens are empirical and tachyphylaxis may occur. It can be used safely in immunocompromised patients and there are no reports of transmission of infectious diseases. Further studies are needed to refine the place and optimum treatment dose.

Treatment of extramuscular disease in PM/DM

- The rash of DM may respond to the treatment of the myositis. If lesions persist, hydroxychloroquine at 200–400 mg/day may be of benefit, though it does not help the myositis. Photosensitivity can respond to sunscreens. Topical steroids are often not successful.
- The treatment of amyopathic DM is controversial. Sunscreens and hydroxychloroquine can be used and in some severe cases steroids or immunosuppressives are justified for the cutaneous disease. If treat-ment is withheld due to an absence of myositis, the patient should be followed closely, especially in the first 2 years after onset, to avoid delay in treatment should myositis develop.
- Calcinosis, principally a problem in juvenile disease, is difficult to treat. Treatment of the disease may help to prevent calcinosis, but it does not affect established calcinosis. Inflammation may respond to colchicine and surgical resection may help for accessible deposits.
- Physiotherapy and passive exercises help prevent contractures, though active exercise is discouraged in the acute period of muscle inflammation.

- Interstitial lung disease is managed as in other autoimmune rheumatic disease, with oral steroids and oral or IV cyclophosphamide.
- Distal oesophageal dismotility does not generally respond to immunosuppression, but measures similar to treatment of reflux may help.

Drug-induced myopathy

- Table 13.7 lists the drugs that commonly cause a myopathy.
- Recently most attention has been given to HMG-CoA reductase inhibitors (statins) used in lipid reduction therapy. These drugs are widely prescribed and are available 'over-the-counter'. In large-scale trials, myalgia has been noted in 11% of patients and significant myositis with ↑ CK levels in 0.5%. Myalgia and cramp are the most common symptoms reported, and may be exacerbated by the use of other drugs (ciclosporin and fibrates) or other diseases (hypothyroidism). Patients presenting with muscular symptoms should have their muscle enzyme levels checked and the drug stopped or reduced in dose.

Prognosis in PM and DM

- PM and DM are diseases with a high mortality and morbidity. One retrospective study estimated a mortality rate of 22%, mostly due to malignancy and pulmonary disease.
- The use of prolonged immuno-suppressive therapy increases the risk of infection, which may be with unusual organisms. Case reports have described atypical mycobacterial infections in patients with long-standing PM/DM.
- A worse prognosis is associated with increasing age, bulbar muscle, and cardiopulmonary involvement.

Inclusion-body myositis

- This is a distinct disorder that comprises 20–30% of idiopathic myositis. It usually begins after the age of 50 years and is 3 times more common in ♂. The difficulty in distinguishing it from PM and its insidious onset can lead to considerable delay in diagnosis.
- Distal weakness and wasting can be as common as proximal, often involving the lower limbs before the upper, and sparing the face.
- Dysphagia is a feature in 40% of cases and myalgia in 20%.
- The diagnosis is confirmed on muscle biopsy; however, lesions are often multiple and focal and serial biopsies may be required.
- Patients do not respond to treatment as well as do those with PM and as a consequence some cases may receive extensive treatment inappropriately if this is not recognized. Treatment usually begins with high-dose corticosteroid for 3 months, adding in MTX or AZA if there is clinical improvement; otherwise, some would advocate discontinuing treatment.
- Weakness will progress in most patients but this is often very slow. Patients may need assistance with daily activities within 10 years and some may be wheelchair bound within 15 years of onset of symptoms.
- Interferon beta may be efficacious in the treatment of inclusion-body myositis.

PM and DM in children

- The 1° clinical feature of both juvenile DM (JDM) and PM (JPM) is chronic, progressive, proximal muscle weakness. Fulfilment of the criteria of Bohan and Peter is needed to establish the diagnosis (see Table 13.8). In addition to the rash, 3 of the other 4 criteria need to be met for DM. These criteria need to be revised in children because biopsies and electromyography are now rarely done as they are invasive painful procedures. MR is increasingly used to define inflammatory changes and to guide biopsies if done.
- Incidence values for JDM and JPM range form 2.5–5 per million.
- The childhood peak for the disease is 5–9 years of age and JDM is 10–20 times more common than JPM.
- Children of African or Asian origin may be at increased risk of chronic myositis. In the United States, Caucasian children with DM are reported more frequently, with a ♀ to ♂ ratio of 2:1. In the United Kingdom, Ireland, and China the ratio is in the order of 5:1.
- JDM is a systemic disease, most commonly affecting the gut, lungs, and nervous system. This is thought to be due to vasculitis that is more marked than in adult disease.
- Antinuclear antibodies are seen in 20–70% of cases of JDM/JPM. Mysositis-associated antibodies seen in adult disease (Jo-1) are rarely seen in childhood disease.
- The ↑ frequency of malignancy seen in adults with DM within 2 years of onset of disease is not seen in childhood DM or PM.
- Several agents have been associated with the onset of juvenile DM, which may also explain some temporal, seasonal, and regional differences in disease onset. The most prominent agents to date have been RNA picornaviruses, group A β-haemolytic streptococci, and *Toxoplasma gondii*. The true pathogenesis of juvenile DM in relation to infectious agents remains unclear.
- HLA associations include B8 and DRB1.
- TNFα promoter polymorphisms have also been implicated in pathogenesis.
- In general the clinical features of juvenile DM/PM are similar to adult disease. Fever, abdominal pain, dysphagia, dyspnoea and peripheral arthritis are seen. Skin ulceration is seen in 20% of patients and can be severe and disabling. Lipodystrophy is a recognized skin finding. Calcinosis, is more common in childhood (10–30% of patients) and the outcome of this ranges from spontaneous resolution to chronic deposition and flexion contractures. Calcinosis is difficult to treat and causes long-term morbidity.

Table 13.8 Bohan and Peter's criteria for the diagnosis of juvenile DM/PM

Feature	DM	PM
Characteristic rash	Yes	No
Symmetrical proximal muscle weakness in the absence of other rheumatic/endocrine disease	Yes	Yes
Elevated muscle enzymes	Yes	Yes
Muscle histopathology	Yes	Yes
Electromyographic changes of inflammation	Yes	Yes

- Rapid disease control is important to help prevent damage. IV or oral corticosteroids are first line, followed by MTX.
- Other treatments that have been used include IV immunoglobulin and ciclosporin A. Cyclophosphamide is used for severe multisystem disease.
- Infliximab and IV bisphosphonates have shown some effect on muscle disease and calcinosis. Rituximab and autologous stem cell transplantation have been used in a small number of cases.
- Early physiotherapy and muscle strengthening is vital, and evidence suggests that this does not affect the inflammatory process.
- Disease activity and damage measures are now being used and validated, as in adult disease.

Primary vasculitides

Introduction

- The vasculitides are a heterogeneous group of relatively uncommon diseases that can arise as 1° conditions or as a 2° feature of an established disease such as RA (see Chapter 5) or SLE (see Chapter 9).
- Vascular inflammation leads to vessel wall destruction and necrosis. Focal large-vessel disease may cause haemorrhage or infarction of organs, small-vessel involvement tending to spare the internal organs and affecting the skin principally. However, more widespread small-vessel disease commonly affects the kidneys.
- There is considerable overlap between the vasculitides and the causes of vasculitis are largely unknown. During the 1980s a classification system developed based on vessel size with the inclusion of a division between 1° (unknown aetiology) and 2° vasculitis (see Table 14.1). In 1993 the Chapel Hill Consensus Conference (CHCC) developed definitions based on clinical and laboratory features. This classification does not address the pathogenic mechanisms, and in particular the relationship with autoantibodies.
- A modification of the CHCC definitions by Scott and Watts (1994) reflects not only vessel size but also the link with antineutrophil cytoplasmic antibodies (ANCA), immune-complex deposition, and response to immunosuppression (see Table 14.2).

The reader may wish to refer to Jeanette et al. (1994)[1] This paper details the CHCC classification. We present the classification from Scott and Watts (1994)[2] because it is both clear and practical.

Antineutrophil cytoplasmic antibody (ANCA)

- ANCA was first described in 1985. Two major staining patterns are seen: cytoplasmic (c-ANCA) directed against proteinase 3 and found chiefly in Wegener's granulomatosis (80% sensitive and 97% specific), and perinuclear (p-ANCA) directed against myeloperoxidase and typically found in microscopic polyangiitis.
- Proteinase 3 and myeloperoxidase are present in the azurophilic granules of neutrophils and monocyte lysozomes. Proteinase 3 is also found on the plasma membrane of resting neutrophils.
- ANCA can be detected using immunofluoressence and enzyme immunoassay. Atypical ANCA staining is seen in inflammatory bowel disease, infection such as agents leading to atypical pneumonia, and against antigens such as lactoferrin and elastase. Subtle differences in staining patterns are best resolved by using enzyme immunoassay.
- There is now evidence that ANCA is directly pathogenic by inciting a respiratory burst and degranulation of leucocytes, leading to endothelial injury.

1 Jeanette JC et al. Nomenclature of systemic vasculitides. Proposal of an international consensus conference. *Arthritis and Rheumatism*, 1994; **37**: 187–92.

2 Scott DGI and Watts RA. Classification and epidemiology of systemic vasculitis. *British Journal of Rheumatology*, 1994; **33**: 897–900.

Table 14.1 A classification of systemic vasculitis

Dominant vessel	1° disorders	2° disorders
Large arteries	Giant cell arteritis. Takayasu's. Isolated central nervous system angiitis	Aortitis in rheumatoid arthritis. Infection, e.g. syphilis
Medium arteries	Classical polyarteritis nodosa. Kawasaki disease	Infection, e.g. hepatitis B. Hairy cell leukaemia
Medium arteries/small vessel	Wegener's granulomatosis. Churg–Strauss syndrome. Microscopic polyangiitis	Vasculitis secondary to autoimmune disease. Malignancy. Drugs. Infection, e.g. HIV
Small vessels (leucocytoclastic)	Henoch–Schönlein purpura. Essential mixed cryoglobulinaemia. Cutaneous leucocytoclastic angitis	Drugs. Malignancy. Infection, e.g. hepatitis B/C

- Neither 'c' or 'p'-ANCA positivity has a 100% specificity. For example, the c-ANCA can be found in some cases of microscopic polyangiitis (15%) and Churg–Strauss syndrome (25%). However, it is rarely found in classical polyarteritis nodosa (2%) and it is very rare to find a false-positive result occurring in a non-vasculitic illness. The p-ANCA is seen in a wide spectrum of conditions including autoimmune rheumatic disorders and inflammatory bowel disease.

Disease and damage assessment

Several indices have been developed that are valid and reliable. The Vasculitis Damage Index (VDI) and Birmingham Vasculitis Activity Score (BVAS) are the indices most commonly used.

The following sections will deal with each of these conditions in turn, outlining specific criteria, clinical features, investigation, and management in each case.

Systemic vasculitis as an acute rheumatological emergency is discussed in Chapter 21.

Table 14.2 The relationship between vessel size and response to treatment

Vessel	Steroids	Cyclophosphamide + steroids	Other*
Large	+++	–	+
Medium	+	++	++
Medium/small	+	+++	–

* Includes plasmapheresis, antiviral therapies, and IV immunoglobulin.

Large-vessel vasculitis

- Large vessels include the aorta and its largest branches to the major body regions—subclavian, carotid, and femoral arteries. The 1° large-vessel vasculitides are those in which there is no known precipitating cause. These, and the 2° large-vessel diseases, are shown in Table 14.3.
- Occasionally medium-sized vessels may be involved but almost never small vessels. Similarly medium- and small-vessel vasculitides, such as Wegener's granulomatosis, rarely involve large vessels. In contrast, 2° vasculitides such as RA (see Chapter 5) can involve the whole spectrum of vessel size.
- The clinical features of large-vessel arteritis are protean. Arch aortitis presents with diminished or absent peripheral pulses, claudication, bruits, hypertension, and heart failure, often in the presence of systemic illness. Occlusion or stenosis of any of the major arteries can lead to transient or permanent ischaemic damage. Infective arteritis, in contrast, usually leads to aneurysm formation rather than stenosis.
- Assessment should include a screen for disease activity, organ damage, and aetiology. With respect to the latter this should include blood cultures, syphilis VDRL test, temporal artery biopsy, rheumatoid factor, ANA, ANCA, and antiphospholipid antibodies (see Chapter 10).

Table 14.3 The causes of large-vessel vasculitis

Primary	Takayasu's arteritis
	Giant cell arteritis*
	Behçet's disease
	Wegener's granulomatosis
	Cogan's syndrome
	Isolated CNS angiitis
Secondary[†]	Infection: bacterial, fungal, mycobacterial, spirochaetal
	Rheumatoid arthritis
	Seronegative spondylarthropathy
	Systemic lupus erythematosus
	Sarcoidosis
	Relapsing polychondritis
	Juvenile chronic arthritis

* Giant cell arteritis is discussed in this chapter in the section on polymyalgia rheumatica.
[†] The secondary causes of large-vessel vasculitis are discussed in their respective sections.

Takayasu's arteritis

- Takayasu's arteritis (TA) is a chronic granulomatous panarteritis affecting the aorta and large arteries, and, less frequently, the pulmonary arteries.
- It is very rare in the United States and the United Kingdom. It is commonest in Japan, Southeast Asia, India, and Mexico. Annual incidence is estimated at 2.6 per million in the United States.
- TA tends to affect ♀ (90% of cases) with adolescents and young adults between 20–40 years at most risk. Classification criteria distinguish TA from giant cell arteritis (GCA) by age at onset (TA <40 years, GCA >50 years).
- The hallmark of the disease is vascular ischaemic symptoms with bruits, claudication, or diminished pulses. Panarteritic inflammatory infiltrates cause luminal narrowing/occlusion. The most common abnormality (90%) is a bruit, most often occurring in the carotid arteries (70%).
- Lightheadedness, visual disturbance, and strokes can occur. Hypertension develops (30–70%) as a consequence of renal artery stenosis.
- Approximately 50% of patients develop musculoskeletal symptoms, mostly as arthralgia. Synovitis and myalgia are less common. Cardiac lesions occur in 40% with aortic incompetence, congestive cardiac failure, and systemic hypertension accounting for the majority of fatal outcomes. Coronary vessels may be involved and up to 50% of cases have disease of the pulmonary arteries with pulmonary hypertension. The diagnosis of TA has depended on arteriography to demonstrate characteristic changes of arterial dilatation, thrombosis, and aneurysm formation. High-resolution ultrasonography is sensitive in detecting carotid lesions. Magnetic resonance angiography (MRA) will likely become the technique of choice, replacing conventional angiography.
- PET scanning is useful in showing disease activity in cases where it is difficult to ascertain whether symptoms are due to disease activity or damage, especially if blood tests are unhelpful.

Treatment

- Initial medical treatment is with corticosteroids (prednisolone 60–80 mg/day). However, 40% of cases will require further immuno-suppression with MTX or AZA in the first instance, or cyclo-phosphamide in severe or resistant cases.
- Hypertension can be difficult to manage and may require angioplasty or surgery to stenosed vessels. There is no absolute contraindication to angiotensin-converting enzyme inhibitors though caution is needed in those with renal artery stenosis. β-blockers may be of value.
  ⚠ Vasodilators are potentially dangerous.
- Surgical management ranges from angioplasty to bypass procedures. These are best performed during the inactive phase of disease. Overall operative mortality is 4%, associated mostly with aneurysm rupture.

- The prognosis depends mainly on the presence of hypertension and aortic incompetence. The majority of patients (75%) will have some impairment of daily living, and 50% are permanently disabled. Mortality is low, 5- and 10-year survival rates reported as 80% and 90% respectively.
- The disease does not prevent successful outcome of pregnancy. Cytotoxic agents should be stopped and steroids kept to as low a dose as possible. Obstetric decisions can be made on their own merits and not because of coexistence of TA. The main complications are exacerbation of hypertension and congestive cardiac failure.

Polymyalgia rheumatica and giant cell arteritis

Polymyalgia rheumatica (PMR)

- The diagnosis of PMR is based essentially on clinical symptoms and signs. The criteria of Jones and Hazleman (1981) are succinct and practical (see Table 14.4).
- There may be apparent muscle weakness on testing which is due to pain rather than intrinsic muscle disease.
- PMR is rare in patients < 50 and the mean age of onset is 70. Prevalence > 50 years is 1 in 133, and ♀ are affected more than ♂ (ratio 2:1). There is also an association with higher geographical latitudes.
- Parainfluenza, parvovirus B19, *Mycoplasma pneumoniae* and *Chlamydia pneumoniae* infections have been shown to have a temporal relation to incidence peaks of PMR, although other studies have found no relationship.
- HLA DRB1*04 and DRB*01 are associated with disease susceptibility.
- Symptoms may start asymmetrically but soon become bilateral. Systemic features of malaise, weight loss, low-grade fever, and depression are common. Arthralgia and synovitis may occur. Up to 5% of patients with RA (see Chapter 5) have an initial PMR-like presentation.
- Pathological features of PMR are minor and include synovitis with a CD4+ T-cell infiltrate similar to that seen in giant cell arteritis (GCA) (see below).
- ⚠ The lack of specific clinical features, a specific laboratory test, and the presence of several conditions that can present with polymyalgic symptoms, leaves the clinician having to follow the working diagnosis closely (see Table 14.5).
- PMR and GCA have a close clinical relationship. One-half of patients with GCA have symptoms of PMR and up to 20% of patients with PMR have histological or clinical evidence of GCA. The pathogenesis for both conditions is not known. It could be considered they are components of a single syndrome, the expression of which depends on currently unknown factors.

Giant cell arteritis (GCA) (Table 14.6)

- GCA is a granulomatous arteritis of the aorta and larger vessels, with a predilection for the extracranial branches of the carotid artery. It is the commonest vasculitis in Europe.
- Annual incidence in USA studies is estimated at 18 per 100 000, but many cases may be subclinical.
- Like PMR the ♀:♂ ratio is 2:1
- Infectious and genetic associations are also similar to PMR with evidence of disease 'clustering'.
- GCA is more common in White Caucasians than Afro-Caribbean racial groups.
- Histology of the temporal artery shows an occlusive vasculopathy rather than thrombosis. Intimal proliferation is seen with a reduction in lumen diameter. Inflammation is patchy, making normal biopsies difficult to interpret (see text below).

Table 14.4 Criteria for the diagnosis of PMR

1. Shoulder and pelvic girdle pain which is primarily muscular in the absence of true muscle weakness

2. Morning stiffness

3. Duration of at least 2 months (unless treated)

4. ESR >30 mm/h or CRP >6 mg/ml

5. Absence of inflammatory arthritis or malignancy

6. Absence of muscle disease

7. Prompt and dramatic response to corticosteroids

Jones JG and Hazeleman BL. The prognosis and management of polymyalgia rheumatica. *Annals of Rheumatic Diseases*, 1981; **40**: 1–5.

Table 14.5 Conditions that can present with polymyalgic symptoms

1. Rheumatic disease in the elderly. Rheumatoid arthritis. Systemic lupus erythematosus

2. Inflammatory myopathy

3. Hypo/hyperthyroidism

4. Carcinoma. Myeloma

5. Chronic sepsis

6. Bilateral shoulder capsulitis

7. Osteoarthritis

8. Depressive illness

9. Parkinsonism

- Severe headache and scalp tenderness localized to the occiput or temporal area are common initial symptoms, present in 70% of cases. The temporal artery can be swollen, tender, and pulseless. Scalp necrosis has also been reported.
- Large arteries are affected in 15% of cases, leading to claudication, bruits, absent neck and arm pulses, and thoracic aorta aneurysm and dissection.
- Visual disturbance is usually an early finding. Visual loss can be transient; or permanent in 20%. Diplopia and ptosis may also be seen. Fundoscopy may show optic disc pallor, haemorrhages, and exudates. Optic atrophy is a late finding.
- Jaw and tongue claudication are other common sinister features.
- Malaise, fatigue, weight loss, fever, and anaemia are common.
- The ESR and CRP are characteristically ↑, but can be normal in up to 3% cases.
- ⚠ Histological proof of inflammation on temporal artery biopsy is not absolute. Studies suggest temporal artery biopsies in clinically diagnosed cases of GCA may only be positive in 30–40% of patients. It is important to obtain tissue as soon as possible after starting treatment. Ideally the biopsy tissue should be as long as possible allowing the histopathologist to take multiple sections, potentially improving the chance of detecting disease. There is no correlation between histological and clinical features in an individual patient. A negative result should not sway the clinician from treatment in a patient with a good history and physical and laboratory abnormalities.
- Doppler US of affected arteries shows hypoechoic areas with a 'halo effect'. US has a positive predictive value of 50%, a sensitivity of 86% and a specificity of 68%. It is a useful adjunct but not diagnostic.
- PET is useful in showing abnormal metabolic activity in arteries >4 mm diameter. Pure temporal arteritis would not show up using this method.

Treatment of PMR and GCA

- Both conditions require corticosteroid treatment. Dramatic responses are usually seen within 48 hours. Careful supervision is then required in slowly reducing the steroid dose with time.
- PMR usually responds to 15 mg/day oral prednisolone. There are no universal guidelines on tapering dosage. Most clinicians would continue 15 mg/day for up to 2 weeks and then reduce to 10 mg/day for 2–4 weeks before gradually tapering in 1 mg steps every 4–6 weeks.
- A ↓ in ESR and maintenance of remission are reasonable indicators of control of disease at each step in dosage reduction. However, relapse can occur at any stage and it is wrong to be guided merely by the ESR.
- Studies on IM prednisolone suggest cumulative steroid dosage may be 40–60% lower than in a conventional regimen. Only one-half of patients have ceased steroids after 2 years. Prophylaxis against osteoporosis should be given as bisphosphonate and calcium and vitamin D supplementation.

Table 14.6 Diagnostic criteria for GCA

Diagnostic scheme	Criteria
Jones and Hazleman (1981)	Positive temporal artery biopsy or cranial artery tenderness
	One or more of: visual disturbance, headache, jaw pain, cerebrovascular insufficiency
	ESR > 30 mm/h or CRP > 6 mg/ml
	Response to corticosteroids
American College of Rheumatology	Three or more of:
	Age at onset >50 years
	New headache
	Temporal artery tenderness or decreased pulsation
	ESR over 50 mm/h
	Abnormal artery biopsies showing necrotizing arteritis with mononuclear infiltrate or granulomatous inflammation usually with multinucleated giant cells

Jones JG and Hazeleman BL. The prognosis and management of polymyalgia rheumatica. *Annals of Rheumatic Diseases*, 1981; **40**: 1–5.

- The same principle of slow reduction in steroid dose applies to GCA. However, an initial dose of 30 mg/day of prednisolone is given for symptoms of headache, and 60–80 mg/day if there is visual disturbance. There is no particular evidence that patients benefit from methyl-prednisolone given IV in the setting of acute visual loss.
- AZA or MTX may be used as a steroid-sparing agent in cases where long-term high-dose steroid therapy seems likely, although evidence for their efficacy is lacking.

Wegener's granulomatosis (WG)

- WG is a worldwide disease with a variable incidence of 4–9 per million population, slightly more common in ♂ than ♀, and most often appearing in the fourth and fifth decades (see Table 14.7).
- Of unknown aetiology, WG is associated with systemic necrotizing vasculitis. There is a classic triad of upper airway, lung, and renal disease (generalized WG), but the condition is often limited to a granulomatous disorder of the airways with no evidence of systemic vasculitis. Likewise any paired combination of the three sites may occur.
- WG can follow a subacute, protracted course of unpredictable duration before transforming (if at all) to a systemic phase; rheumatic complaints, malaise, weight loss, fever, night sweats, eye, ear, skin, and central and peripheral nerve involvement being ominous signs of impending full pulmonary–renal syndrome.

The clinical features of WG

Ear, nose, and throat

- Up to 90% of patients have ear, nose, and throat involvement.
- Involvement characteristically begins in the upper respiratory tract and precedes symptoms of generalized disease for a long period of time.
  ⚠ The diagnosis may not therefore be made for some time. WG may, however, start with a pure small-vessel vasculitis and it is important to realize that such features may overlap with microscopic polyangiitis.
- The earliest nasal manifestations include obstruction from mucosal swelling, serosanguinous discharge, and epistaxis. In the later stages of the disease there may be tissue destruction with the classic 'saddle deformity' of the nasal bridge due to septal cartilage loss and occasionally erosion posteriorly towards the cranial vault with cavity formation.
- In the oral cavity and oropharynx inflammation can lead to ulceration, gingivitis, and laryngeal symptoms of hoarseness and stridor.

Table 14.7 The American College of Rheumatology 1990 classification criteria of Wegener's granulomatosis—diagnosis requires 2 or more of

1. Painful or painless oral ulcers ± a purulent/bloody nasal discharge
2. The chest radiograph may show nodules, cavities, or infiltrate
3. Microscopic haematuria or red cell casts may be found in urine sediment
4. Histological changes of granulomatous inflammation within arterial walls is seen on biopsy of involved tissue

- The outer and middle ear can be affected, the latter often causing conductive deafness. Features include chondritis of the ear lobe with 2° atrophy, serous/suppurative otitis media, mastoiditis, and occasionally a peripheral facial nerve (seventh cranial nerve) palsy.
- Sensorineural deafness may occur as a result of small-vessel vasculitis of the cochlea.
- It is thought that *Staphylococcus aureus* has a role in disease pathogenesis. Nasal carriage in WG patients is 3 times that of healthy populations. The exact mechanisms leading to disease are unclear.

Pulmonary disease
- 80% of cases have pulmonary disease.
- The tracheobronchial tree may be locally involved before any signs of generalized disease. Subglottic pseudotumours and/or stenosis cause stridor or dyspnoea. Lower bronchial stenosis may cause atelectasis and obstructive pneumonia. Multiple nodules with or without cavitation are found in the lungs of asymptomatic patients.
- ⚠ Transformation to the fulminant generalized disease is associated with alveolar capillaritis, haemorrhage, and haemoptysis, with infiltrates on the plain chest radiograph. The radiograph typically shows an alveolar or mixed alveolar–interstitial pattern; the distribution is often like that of pulmonary oedema and focal infection. Sometimes migratory shadows are also seen.

Renal disease
- Up to 90% of cases have renal involvement.
- In the generalized phase of the disease renal involvement can range from milder focal and segmental glomerulonephritis (GN) to fulminant diffuse necrotizing (rapidly progressive) and crescentic GN ⚠, which within a few days to weeks may lead to oligo/anuria and the need for dialysis. The milder form of the condition is most common, manifesting in the asymptomatic patient as a nephritic picture of microscopic haematuria, active sediment, and mild renal impairment.

Skin disease
- 40% of cases have skin disease.
- Features include palpable purpura due to a leucocytoclastic vasculitis, necrotic papules from necrotizing vasculitis, livedo reticularis, and pyoderma gangrenosum.

Rheumatic symptoms
- Rheumatic symptoms are observed in 60% of cases.
- Symptoms can range from mild myalgia (in 50% of the cases) and arthralgia to overt arthritis and myositis. 20–30% of rheumatic symptoms may be related to a non-erosive and non-deforming polyarthropathy. Over 90% of cases with rheumatic symptoms also have the generalized form of WG and therefore their symptoms form part of the constitutional symptoms associated with active vasculitis.

Nervous system
- About one-third of patients with WG have involvement of the nervous system. Mononeuritis multiplex and distal sensorimotor poly-neuropathy are the main lesions. Seizures and cerebritis are far less frequent events.
- Disseminated granulomatous lesions can spread to the retropharyngeal area and skull base with involvement of cranial nerves I, II, III, VI, VII, and VIII, diabetes insipidus, and meningitis.

Eye disease
- Granulomatous lesions may obstruct the nasolacrimal duct and cause protrusio bulbi with optic nerve compression from masses developing in the retrobulbar space. Rarely a purulent sinusitis may spread and cause 2° bacterial orbital infection.
- Manifestations in the generalized stage of WG include episcleritis (red eye), vasculitis of the optic nerve, and occlusion of retinal arteries, in addition to the granulomatous lesions described above.

Investigation of WG
- Laboratory investigation should include an assessment of the inflammatory markers ESR and CRP, both ↑ during active disease. The difficulty lies in interpretation in the presence of infection. Indeed suspicion of infection must always be at the forefront of investigations, particularly atypical infections such as tuberculosis and nocardia.
- The FBC might be expected to show a normochromic, normocytic anaemia with a leucocytosis and thrombocytosis.
- Investigation of renal function depends on the degree of involvement and should include urea, electrolytes, creatinine, and urinalysis initially with a view to 24-hour urine collection and more formal investigation as required.
- A positive cANCA is found in 90% of patients with generalized WG; 67% of those with limited WG. Levels correlate with disease in many patients and are not influenced by the presence of infection in the same way as the ESR and CRP. Consequently titres can be a good marker of disease activity, but treatment decisions should not be based on baseline or change in ANCA titre alone.
- Studies have reported the presence of antibodies to endothelial cells (AECA) in the sera of both patients with WG and polyarteritis. These may be important in the pathogenesis of vasculitis but as yet are of no useful diagnostic or management value.
- Assessment of lung disease following from the plain radiograph, sputum culture, and cytology, includes lung CT ± biopsy or bronchoscopy and lavage.
- The extent of sinus disease is best demonstrated with CT, MR of the sinuses and brain being useful in investigating intracerebral disease.

Treatment and prognosis in all the medium-vessel vasculitides is discussed at the end of this section.

Classical polyarteritis nodosa, microscopic polyangiitis, and Churg–Strauss syndrome

Classical polyarteritis nodosa

- Classical polyarteritis nodosa (PAN) is a rare systemic illness characterized by necrotizing inflammation of medium-sized arteries leading to aneurysm formation. There is no glomerulonephritis. It principally affects the viscera, mainly causing aneurysm formation, organ infarction and haemorrhage.
- There is a preponderance of ♂ (gender ratio 2:1), with the majority Caucasian.
- The condition is now considered uncommon in adults but is one of the more common vasculitides in childhood.
- Positive hepatitis B serology has been noted in 5–40% of cases in different series of patients with PAN. The exact link with hepatitis B is not understood. However, the prevalence of PAN appears to reflect the incidence of hepatitis B in the population. These patients also appear more likely to have nephrotic syndrome, which is otherwise rare in PAN.
- A positive ANCA is not seen in classical PAN.
- The clinical features are shown in Table 14.8. Patients often present with non-specific features of systemic disease comprising myalgia, arthralgia, weight loss, and fever. About 50% of cases develop a vasculitic rash, often with 'punched out' ulcers. GI and renal involvement is common; 50% in both cases. Non-specific abdominal pain, gut/gallbladder infarction, and pancreatitis are all features. Renal disease usually appears in the form of abnormal urinary sediment. Renal impairment is often mild and present in around 20% of cases. Isolated organ involvement is rare, but disease affecting the skin, testes, epididymis, breasts, uterus, appendix, and gallbladder has been reported.

Treatment and prognosis in all the medium-vessel vasculitides is discussed at the end of this section.

Microscopic polyangiitis (MP)

- This condition predominantly involves the kidneys. Unlike WG (see above), there is no granuloma formation, and unlike classical PAN most patients with microscopic polyangiitis (MP) present with or develop severe renal disease. The characteristic lesion is a focal, segmental necrotizing glomerulonephritis with fibrinoid necrosis and thrombosis of the glomerular tufts.
- Glomerular immune deposits are sparse, differentiating MP from conditions such as SLE (see Chapter 9) and Henoch–Schönlein purpura. Most biopsies also show tubular damage, the degree of which correlates more closely than glomerular damage with the severity of renal impairment.

Table 14.8 Clinical features at presentation (as % of cases) in classical polyarteritis nodosa, microscopic polyangiitis, and Churg–Strauss syndrome

Clinical feature	Polyarteritis nodosa	Microscopic polyangiitis	Churg–Strauss syndrome
Renal impairment	25%	90%	50%
Pulmonary disease	40%	50%	General 50%, asthma 100%
Fever	60%	40%	
Skin vasculitis	40%	50%	50%
Locomotor complaint	60%	50%	50%
Gastrointestinal disease	45%	20%	60%
Cardiovascular disease	15%	20%	45%
Peripheral neuropathy	10%	10%	60%
Ear, nose, and throat	10%	20%	
Ocular disease	10%	20%	

- In MP, a perinuclear pattern of staining for antineutrophil cytoplasmic antibody, p-ANCA, is found. This is in contrast with the c-ANCA detected in WG (see the introduction to this chapter).
- Like PAN the ♂ to ♀ ratio is 2:1, with the majority of patients being Caucasian. The mean age of presentation is 50 years.
- The clinical features of the disease are shown in Table 14.8. Over 90% of patients have renal disease, 80% microscopic haematuria (6% frank haematuria), and 80% proteinuria. Symptoms of lung disease are found in 50% of cases, usually as pleurisy, haemoptysis, or asthma. Frank pulmonary haemorrhage, akin to that seen in WG, develops in 5% of patients with MP. Peripheral neuropathies may also be seen.

Treatment and prognosis in all the medium-vessel vasculitides is discussed at the end of this section.

Churg–Strauss syndrome

- This condition is characterized by asthma (or often allergic rhinitis), eosinophilia, fever, and a systemic illness.
- Anaemia, weight loss, heart failure, recurrent pneumonia, and bloody diarrhoea are common as are skin lesions varying from purpura to granulomatous nodules, and peripheral neuropathy.
- Often a necrotizing arteritis with an eosinophilic infiltrate is found.
- The UK incidence is 3.1 per million.
- Although rare, significant renal involvement does occur and usually presents as microscopic haematuria plus proteinuria. Less often there may be renal failure with nephrotic syndrome. Like MP the predominant renal lesion (in 80% of renal disease) is a focal, segmental glomerulonephritis. The clinical features are shown in Table 14.8.

Treatment and prognosis in all the medium-vessel vasculitides is discussed at the end of this section.

Investigation of classical polyarteritis nodosa, microscopic polyangiitis and Churg–Strauss syndrome

- The initial diagnosis is often difficult, partly because of the overlap in the clinical spectrum, and particularly in the elderly and those with rapid development of renal failure, which in turn carries high mortality.
- ⚠ Often a high index of suspicion of vasculitis is needed with intent to treat being a higher priority than establishing the exact diagnosis initially.
- There is usually an acute phase response with a ↑ white cell count, and ↑ ESR and CRP. A biopsy of involved tissue is often helpful, e.g. skin, muscle, peripheral nerve, or kidney. An eosinophilia (>1.5 × 10^9/litre) is characteristic of Churg–Strauss syndrome (CSS).
- Microscopic haematuria and proteinuria may be found in all of the conditions.
- Deranged liver function tests with a raised serum alkaline phosphatase are a common finding (50% of cases) in MP.
- Low titres of rheumatoid factor, antinuclear antibodies, and immune complexes are found in a minority of patients with PAN. Their significance is uncertain.

- The value of ANCA has been discussed in the introduction to this chapter. The majority of patients (80%) with PAN and a minority of patients (20%) with MP have a negative ANCA. Serial changes in ANCA titres do not always predict disease activity. Correlation with disease activity is not close enough to justify changes to treatment.
- Where there is clinical suspicion of PAN it is reasonable to do renal and coeliac angiograms. The radiological findings include hepatic and renal artery aneurysms, segmental narrowing of arteries, and pruning of the peripheral vascular tree. Wedge-shaped infarcts may also be seen in the kidneys. Aneurysms may also be found in the cerebral and pulmonary vasculature. They are also an infrequent finding in WG and SLE.

Treatment and prognosis

The treatment of the conditions above are broadly similar. Large randomized controlled trials have until recently been difficult due to the rarity of these conditions, however multinational studies are ongoing which will help address key issues in management. Treatment is in two phases: induction and remission.

Induction

- Cyclophosphamide and corticosteroid remain the standard induction therapy.
- The introduction of corticosteroids ↓ mortality rate, but steroids do not fully control disease. Steroid dose should be kept to the lowest possible. Prophylaxis against osteoporosis should be given.
- Cyclophosphamide (CYC) may be given orally or IV. Pulsed IV therapy may have the added bonus of reducing exposure to this toxic agent by 50% in the induction of remission.
- The National Insitute for Health regimen of low dose oral cyclophosphamide(2 mg/kg/day), continued for at least 1y after remission, with prednisolone (1 mg/kg/day) dramatically improves induction, remission and survival.
- The European Vasculitis (EuVas) consensus group has advised up to 12 months treatment with oral CYC substituting with AZA following induction of remission. CYC has significant side-effects including cystitis, infections, and increased risk of bladder and haematological malignancies.
- Pulsed IV CYC is popular, the rational being that it reduces cumulative dose and toxicity. Evidence suggests that pulsed CYC is as effective at inducing remission as oral therapy, but perhaps less effective at preventing relapse. Pulsed regimens may also allow for a shorter duration of treatment.

Maintaining remission

- Once remission has been achieved with CYC (up to 90% of cases within 12 months), MTX or AZA can be used in a maintainance regimen. A recent study has shown MTX to be as effective as CYC in maintaining remission in early non-renal ANCA-associated vasculitis, however the relapse rate may be higher with MTX than CYC if MTX

is withdrawn too soon. It is advised to continue with MTX for > 12 months.
- MTX has been used as 1° therapy in limited non-renal vasculitis and efficacy is similar to CYC. It is not recommended as a therapy for induction for those with renal involvement or severe multisystem disease.

Other treatments
- Plasma exchange has been used with some effect in those with severe renal disease requiring dialysis.
- IV immunoglobulin has been found to have short-lived benefit.
- Mycophenolate has a been used successfully to maintain remission after induction with CYC. Its role needs to be evaluated further.
- Anecdotal reports have shown the benefit of infliximab in treatment of resistant vasculitis. Randomized trials are ongoing.
- PAN associated with hepatitis B should be treated with antiviral therapy in addition to immunosupressants to improve mortality.
- There is evidence that respiratory tract infections may trigger a relapse of WG. Co-trimoxazole in patients with stable disease on maintenance therapy may ↓ respiratory infection and relapse rate.

Prognosis

Prior to the introduction of corticosteroids, mortality was certain after a few months. Untreated Churg–Strauss syndrome had a 1-year survival of 4%, and most generalized WG patients died within 5 months. With current therapies, mortality has improved but morbidity remains considerable. 10-year survival for WG is now 75% and 55% for microscopic polyangiitis. Causes of death are likely to be due to complications of drug treatment (e.g. infection).

For a detailed analysis of the literature on induction of remission in ANCA positive disease the reader is referred to Jayne (2005)[1]

1 Jayne D. How to induce remission in the primary vasculitides. *Best Pract Res Clin Rheum*, 2005; **19**: 293–305.

Small-vessel vasculitis

The definition of small vessel vasculitis is open to different interpretations. Small vessel disease can be one feature of WG, microscopic polyangiitis, and Churg–Strauss syndrome. However, there are a range of clinical and pathological features that define a specific group of small-vessel vasculitides outlined in Table 14.9.

Leucocytoclastic vasculitis

- Histologically, leucocytoclastic vasculitis appears as a neutrophil infiltration in and around small vessels, with fragmentation of the neutrophils (leucocytoclasis), fibrin deposition, and endothelial cell necrosis. Immune complex deposition appears to be important in pathogenesis.
- Small-vessel vasculitis usually presents in the skin, although the microvasculature of any tissue may be affected, especially joints or kidneys. The division into leuco- and non-leucocytoclastic vasculitis is not absolute. Likewise, the clinical presentation of cutaneous vasculitis can vary considerably.
- The finding of leucocytoclasis should prompt a thorough review of drug treatment (e.g. sulphonamides, penicillin, thiazides), a search for infection (hepatitis B, human immunodeficiency virus, β-haemolytic streptococcus), a screen for autoimmune rheumatic disease, malignancy (in particular myelo- and lymphoproliferative diseases), inflammatory bowel disease, chronic active hepatitis, and cryoglobulinaemia (see below).

Allergic vasculitis

- Allergic vasculitis is the most common pattern of presentation in adults, both sexes being affected equally.
- Non-blanching haemorrhagic papules (palpable purpura), purpuric macules, plaques, pustules, bullae, and ulcers may occur, classically distributed maximally over the lower leg.
- A low-grade fever, arthralgia, and microscopic haematuria often accompany such presentation.
- Often the condition is self-limiting and identifiable causes should be managed as appropriate. Analgesia may be needed and systemic steroids may be required for acute organ disease, especially progressive renal impairment. AZA may be appropriate for refractory disease.

Table 14.9 Conditions associated with small-vessel vasculitis

Leucocytoclastic vasculitis	Allergic vasculitis (hypersensitivity angiitis): drugs, infection, inflammation, autoimmune disease, malignancy, Henoch–Schönlein purpura
	Urticarial vasculitis (hypocomplemen taemic vasculitis)
	Cryoglobulinaemia
	Hypergammaglobulinaemia
	Erythema elevatum diutinum and granuloma faciale
Non-leucocytoclastic vasculitis (localized skin disease)	Drugs (penicillins, thiazides)
	Nodular vasculitis (see 'panniculitis')
	Livedo vasculitis
	Pityriasis lichenoides

Henoch-Schönlein purpura

- This tends to be regarded as a special form of allergic vasculitis. It occurs most often in children but can affect adults of any age. IgA is usually detected in skin, gut, or renal biopsies.
- The classical presentation is with purpura, arthritis (50%), haemorrhagic GI disease (40%), and glomerulonephritis (50%). Corticosteroids given early may relieve joint and GI symptoms but there is little evidence that they prevent progression of renal disease or influence overall outcome. If renal function is rapidly deteriorating pulsed methylprednisolone and/or plasmapheresis may be of benefit.
- Amongst patients who present with a nephritic or nephrotic syndrome, 40% have hypertension on long-term follow-up, whereas 80% who present with just haematuria and/or proteinuria are normal.

Urticarial vasculitis

- Urticarial lesions with arthralgia are the commonest features of this condition, with ♀ outnumbering ♂ 2:1; the typical age of onset 40–50 years.
- Morphologically the skin lesions resemble ordinary urticaria and sometimes may be mistaken for erythema multiforme. The distinction tends to be length of time (the vasculitis lasting 2–3 days and ordinary urticaria 24 hours), and symptoms (vasculitis tending to be burning and painful).
- Although the term 'hypocomplementaemic vasculitis' has been applied in the past, this abnormality is by no means universal. Patients with low complement tend to develop more systemic features such as renal, GI, and pulmonary disease. Less common manifestations include lymphadenopathy, uveitis, and benign intracranial hypertension.
- Systemic antihistamines are widely used but tend to be disappointing.
- There are anecdotal reports of success with indomethacin, hydroxy chloroquine, colchicine, and dapsone.
- For the majority of patients the condition is chronic and benign. For those with end-organ damage, oral steroids, tapered to the lowest maintenance dose, are often required.

Cryoglobulinaemia

- Cryoglobulins are immunoglobulins that precipitate when cold. They are divided into three types: type I single monoclonal, type II mixed monoclonal and polyclonal, and type III mixed polyclonal.
- Mixed cryoglobulins are associated with autoimmune rheumatic diseases, infection, and lymphoproliferative disorders. ⚠ Hepatitis B and C virus infection should always be excluded; the latter in particular is strongly associated with essential mix cryoglobulinaemia.
- Mixed cryoglobulinaemia presents with purpuric skin lesions showing a leucocytoclastic vasculitis on biopsy, polyarthralgia (70%), weakness, progressive renal disease (55%), and hepatic inflammation (70%). It is uncommon. ♀ are affected twice as frequently as ♂ and in the sixth decade on.

- Rarer complaints include oedema, hypertension, leg ulcers, Raynaud's phenomenon, abdominal pain, neuropathy, and susceptibility to bacterial pneumonia.
- ⚠ The prognosis is worse with renal disease, the main causes of death being renal failure, systemic vasculitis, and infection.
- Treatment requires management of the underlying cause, otherwise per se it is unsatisfactory. High-dose steroids, chemotherapy, plasmapheresis, or a combination of all three may bring about limited improvement in renal function and skin lesions.

Hypergammaglobulinaemic purpura

- This is a rare, benign IgM condition presenting as long-standing leucocytoclastic purpura similar to the cutaneous features of Sjögren's syndrome (see Chapter 11).
- It should not be confused with Waldenström's macroglobulinaemia, a monoclonal IgM paraproteinaemia associated with lymphoma.

Erythema elevatum diutinum (EED) and granuloma faciale (GF)

- These are rare but distinctive forms of chronic localized leucocytoclastic vasculitis. There is no systemic involvement and the aetiology is unknown.
- EED is characterized by slowly enlarging oedematous purplish-brown plaques or blisters over the backs of the hands, elbows, or knees. They heal very slowly (months to years) with fibrosis. It may respond to dapsone.
- GF presents as single or multiple pink-brown, well-defined, smooth papules and plaques on the face. They persist for years. It is distinguished histologically from EED by the presence of eosinophils and a normal collagen beneath the epidermis. It may respond to intralesional steroids.

Non-leucocytoclastic vasculitis

- The differential diagnosis of nodular forms of cutaneous vasculitis embraces a wide range of disorders, including the panniculitides (see Chapter 18).
- Nodular vasculitis is regarded as a distinct group characterized by recurrent subcutaneous nodules usually found on the legs of young to middle-aged ♀. Patients are otherwise healthy. Streptococcal infection may be found but not tuberculosis (Bazin's disease). The condition resolves spontaneously but may take many years. Intra-lesional triamcinolone may help.
- Livedo vasculitis is characterized histologically by endothelial proliferation and intraluminal thrombosis leading to ischaemic damage. Antiphospholipid antibodies may prove to be relevant in the pathogenesis of this disorder. The lesions heal with white atrophic scars—atrophie blanche.
- Pityriasis lichenoides is a uncommon disorder of pink papules which enlarge rapidly and may become haemorrhagic before becoming necrotic and heal with scarring. It is usually self-limiting and may respond to ultraviolet B irradiation.

Kawasaki Disease

- This is a febrile, acute vasculitic illness of childhood. It is probably more common than rheumatic fever as the cause for rheumatic heart disease in children < 5 yrs of age and is associated with coronary artery aneurysms, myocarditis and MI. Other organs involved include liver, pancreas and kidney.
- It is seen most often in Japanese-Americans with a peak prevalence age of 18 months to 2 years, and is more common in $\male$, ratio 5:1.
- Fever is usually present for >5 days and associated with conjunctivitis, erythema and oedema (skin, lips and pharyngeal), and lymphadenopathy. Joint inflammation may also occur during the acute phase.
- Myocarditis may appear early but arterial aneurysm formation appears later, its risk of occuring ↑ after longer periods of being febrile (14–16 days).
- There are no specific blood tests. Acute phase markers are usually high and cultures negative.
- An ECG and Echocardiogram may show conduction defects and myocardial inflammation respectively.
- Treatment is supportive with the use of aspirin and anti-coagulation. The role for corticosteroids is unclear. Gamma-globulin should be considered. Cases should be referred immediately to a Paediatrician and may require the expertise of Paediatric Cardiothoracic surgeon also.

The crystal arthropathies

Gout and hyperuricaemia

The crystal arthropathies include gout, calcium pyrophosphate deposition disease (CPPD) or pseudogout, basic calcium phosphate (BCP) associated syndromes, and calcium oxalate arthritis. These conditions will be discussed in turn in this chapter.

Epidemiology of gout

- In its most general sense, gout is a group of conditions characterized by hyperuricaemia and uric acid crystal formation. These clinical conditions include arthritis, tophaceous gout, uric acid nephrolithiasis, and gouty nephropathy. In its more commonly assumed definition, gout refers to the acute inflammatory arthropathy caused by uric acid crystal deposition.
- Gout is a relatively common condition. Prevalence data from the United States on self-reported disease show figures of 13.6 per 1000 persons in adult ♂ and 6.4 per 1000 persons for ♀. In the United Kingdom, 250 000 people per year consult their general practitioners with a diagnosis of gout, with a ♂:♀ ratio of 4:1. It is more common in the middle aged and elderly. Gout is a significant cause of time off work and in 1999–2000 in the UK, 1.2 million working days were lost.
- The risk factors for gout mirror those for hyperuricaemia, and are shown in Table 15.1.

The clinical features of gout

- The first stage of the condition is usually asymptomatic hyperuricaemia.
- Clinically, the first symptom is most often an acute, self-limiting, monoarticular inflammatory arthritis; up to 60–70% of attacks first occur in the big toe. Other frequently involved joints include the ankle, foot, knee, wrist, elbow (olecranon bursa), and the small joints of the hands. The axial large joints and spine are rarely involved in early disease. Some 70–80% of individuals will have recurrent attacks within 2 years.
- In the later stages of untreated disease, acute attacks are more often polyarticular, with shorter periods of remission, joint damage and deformity, loss of mobility, chronic pain, and formation of tophi.
- Tophi are deposits of urate embedded in a matrix composed of lipids, proteins, and calcific debris. Tophi are usually subcutaneous, but rarely can occur in bone and other organs such as the eye. The classic sites for tophi are the pinna of the ear, bursa of the elbow, and knee, Achilles tendon, and the dorsal surface of the MCP joints. Tophi are usually painless, though the overlying skin may ulcerate and become infected. Those most at risk of tophi are patients with prolonged severe hyperuricaemia, polyarticular gout, and the elderly with primary nodal OA (see Chapter 6) on diuretics.
- Three renal syndromes are associated with gout. Current dogma states that urate crystals themselves produce only minor renal damage— 'urate nephropathy'—by inducing inflammation. However, 'uric acid nephropathy' is seen in the acutely ill, dehydrated patient often taking cytotoxics for a lymphoproliferative disorder. An acute obstructive uropathy ensues with oliguric renal failure. Finally, uric acid stones are common, even in the absence of hyperuricaemia. Patients with gout also have greater risk of non-urate stones.

Table 15.1 The causes of hyperuricaemia and risk factors for gout

Primary gout	Male gender
	Age <40 years
	Obesity
	Family history
	Alcohol use and purine rich foods
	Renal insufficiency
	Hypertension
Inherited metabolic syndromes	X-linked HPRT deficiency (Lesch–Nyhan) X-linked raised PRPP synthetase activity Autosomal recessive G6P deficiency (von Gierke's disease)
Uric acid overproduction	Cell lysis—tumour lysis syndrome, myeloproliferative disease, haemolytic anaemia, psoriasis, trauma Drugs—alcohol, cytotoxics, warfarin
Uric acid underexcretion	Renal failure
	Drugs—alcohol, salicylates, diuretics, laxatives, ciclosporin, levodopa, ethambutol, pyrazinamide
Lead toxicity	Renal impairment and altered purine turnover

HPRT = hypoxanthine guanine phosphoribosyl transferase—a salvage enzyme converting hypoxanthine back to precursors and therefore competing with its conversion to xanthine and then uric acid.

PRPP = phosphoribosylpyrophosphate synthetase—a component enzyme in purine ring synthesis.

G6P = glucose 6 phosphatase. G6P deficiency leads to increased activity of amido phosphoribosyl transferase and purine formation.

Investigation of gout

- Synovial fluid analysis remains the single most important diagnostic study. The diagnosis is made by the presence of typical, negatively birefringent, needle-shaped crystals seen with a polarized light microscope. The crystals may be extra- or intracellular. The absence of crystals does not rule out the diagnosis.
- Serum uric acid levels may be normal during an acute attack and may not reflect pre-attack levels. They cannot be used to exclude the diagnosis in an acute attack. Uric acid levels are of value in assessing the patient once the acute attack has subsided, either to establish the presence of hyperuricaemia or to monitor the effectiveness of therapies that ↓ serum urate.
- Radiographs are often normal during the early phase of the disease, except for the presence of soft tissue swelling. They are, however, useful for excluding other conditions such as trauma or infection (see Table 15.2). Later in the disease, radiographs may demonstrate tophi

near joints, tissue swelling, joint erosions, periosteal new bone formation, and joint deformity. Once these changes occur gout may be misdiagnosed as RA (see Chapter 5) in some cases.
- ⚠ 2° causes of hyperuricaemia should always be considered.

The management of gouty arthritis

- The efficacy of any public health improvement measure for the prevention of gout is yet to be proven. It is reasonable to suggest that avoiding excess weight gain and alcohol, controlling hypertension, and avoiding exposure to diuretics and lead, may have some effect on ↓ the incidence of the condition.
- The management of gout otherwise should be seen as two phases: treatment of the acute attack, and treatment of chronic or tophaceous gout. The principal therapies for acute gout are NSAIDs, colchicine, and steroids. Many treatments are empirical rather than evidence based.
- Traditionally indomethacin has been the NSAID of choice in acute gout, but has no advantage over other NSAIDs or Coxib. With treatment, symptoms should subside within 3–5 days.
- NSAIDs are contraindicated in renal insufficiency and should be used with caution in the elderly (who are often also taking aspirin) or those with GI risk factors. Evidence shows that NSAIDs ↓ pain, swelling, and duration of attack. There is no evidence for the use of selective COX-2 inhibitors, except etoricoxib, in gout.
- Colchicine can be very effective in acute gout, with a rapid onset of action. Oral colchicine, given at 0.5 mg 4 times per day for 5 days is very useful and ↓ the risk of abdominal pain and diarrhoea compared to standard doses listed in formularies. It is often given in addition to NSAIDs (although there is no evidence to support this) or where NSAIDs are contraindicated. The 5-day dosage may be repeated for an acute attack after 72 hours. IV colchicine is rarely used due to the potential for bone marrow suppression. There are no randomized controlled trials comparing colchicine to NSAIDs.

Table 15.2 Clinical conditions that can mimic gouty arthritis

CPPD disease (pseudogout)
BCP arthritis
Cellulitis
Infectious arthritis
Trauma
Rheumatoid arthritis
Psoriatic arthritis
Erythema nodosum
Reactive arthritis

- The true efficacy of oral and IM corticosteroids in acute gout remains to be proven. Steroid regimens range from oral prednisolone at tapering doses from 20–50 mg daily for an average of 10 days, to IM triamcinolone 60 mg once only. A study comparing IM triamcinolone with indomethacin found no significant difference in time to recovery. Intra-articular steroids are useful if only one or two joints are affected. In a case series from 1999, injection of triamcinolone acetonide into affected joints resolved all symptoms within 48 hours.
- The exact mechanism of action of ACTH injections in acute gout is unclear. One randomized controlled trial showed a faster response with a single dose of ACTH than indomethacin. There is no evidence that ACTH is superior to corticosteroids. ⚠ Corticosteroids should not be used if there is a possibility of septic arthritis.
- Drugs that ↓ serum uric acid levels are the standard therapy for prophylaxis against repeated gout attacks, but should not be started after just one isolated attack. Allopurinol, a xanthine oxidase inhibitor, is the drug most commonly used, and the drug of choice in the presence of renal insufficiency, nephrolithiasis, or tophi. The drug should not be started during an acute attack of gout, as it is likely to make the situation worse. Allopurinol is usually given as a once daily dose of 300 mg. Patients, however, may require doses anywhere between 100–900 mg daily to achieve normal serum uric acid levels. The dose should be adjusted down in renal impairment. The onset of action of allopurinol is rapid, with effects seen as early as 4 days to 2 weeks.
- The most common side-effect of allopurinol is a hypersensitivity reaction with rash and fever. ⚠ Rarely a severe reaction is seen with hepatitis, nephritis, and toxic epidermal necrolysis. In mild to moderate intolerance allopurinol can be reintroduced at very low levels, e.g. 10 mg, and built up slowly using desensitization regimens. Allopurinol can interfere with the metabolism of azathioprine and warfarin, augmenting their potential side-effects. During its introduction a patient may also experience an acute flare of gout. This may be treated with NSAIDs and/or low dose colchicine.

- Sulphinpyrazone is a uricosuric agent which, by definition, alters renal handling of urate and ↑ urate excretion. It is effective and well-tolerated, but contraindicated in patients with renal stones and ineffective in those with renal insufficiency.
- Benzbromarone is a uricosuric drug available in Europe. It is effective in patients with renal insufficiency.
- A randomized controlled trial comparing uricosuric and xanthine oxidase inhibitor treatment found no difference in frequency of acute attacks of gout.
- Some patients may respond to a combination of allopurinol and a uricosuric when either alone has been ineffective.
- In patients who are unable to take allopurinol or a uricosuric drug, daily low-dose oral colchicine may be useful in preventing attacks. It is usually given in doses of 0.5–1.0 mg/day. Serious side-effects can still occur at this dose. This low-dose regimen may also be useful as prophylaxis against acute flares during the introduction of allopurinol.
- Fenofibrate is an established treatment for many lipid disorders. It also has the ability to ↓ serum urate by ↑ renal uric acid clearance. It may have a role (off licence) in patients resistant or intolerant to other agents. It should be avoided in hepatic and biliary disease, hypothroidism and pregnancy. Side-effects may include arthralgia and myalgia.
- Patients with uric acid stones are best managed with adequate hydration, urinary alkalization (with bicarbonate or acetozolamide), and allopurinol. This regimen is also effective in preventing calcium oxalate stones.
- Finally, gouty tophi may occasionally be amenable to surgical removal.

Calcium pyrophosphate dihydrate (CPPD) disease

- CPPD disease is the second most common form of crystal arthropathy. Understanding of the pathophysiology of CPPD remains rudimentary, and consequently no specific therapies for this arthropathy exist.
- Several clinical syndromes are associated with CPPD and the features of the condition are heterogeneous, sometimes mimicking other rheumatic conditions. Definite associations with CPPD and chondrocalcinosis (calcification of fibro- and hyaline cartilage typically at the knee and wrist) include:
  - hypomagnesaemia
  - hypophosphatasia
  - haemachromatosis
  - Wilson's disease
  - hyperparathyroidism.

  Possible associations include:
  - gout
  - ochronosis
  - hypocalciuric hypercalcaemia
  - diabetes mellitus
  - X-linked hypophosphataemic rickets.
- These crystals are also found in the synovial fluid of patients with both acute and chronic arthritis. They are associated with advanced age, chondrocalcinosis, and a characteristic pattern of severe joint degeneration.
- There are several presentations of CPPD that afford at least some form of classification based on clinical features. It is not easy to categorize all cases, but the classification serves to point out the heterogeneity of the condition in both acute, chronic, inflammatory, and non-inflammatory arthritis (see Tables 15.3, 15.4).

Table 15.3 The clinical presentations of CPPD disease

Type	Description	Frequency	Features
A	Pseudogout	25%	Acute pain and swelling, often a monoarthropathy of the knee, wrist or shoulder. Rare in small joints
B	Pseudorheumatoid	5%	Polyarthritis. Synovitis. Joint flares out of phase with each other
C and D	Pseudo-osteoarthritis; C with attacks D without acute attacks	50%	Acute attacks on chronic symptoms
E	Asymptomatic	?	Incidental chondrocalcinosis
F	Pseudoneurotrophic	Rare	Severe joint destruction ± neuropathy
Others	Tophaceous CPPD deposits		
	Spinal CPPD: 'Crowned dens syndrome' deposits around the atlantoaxial joint. Spinal stenosis. Cervical myelopathy		
	Tendon and bursa deposits		

Laboratory investigations

- CPPD disease is defined by the presence of positively birefringent, rhomboid crystals on examination of synovial fluid under polarized light microscopy. The crystals may be intra- or extracellular.
- Radiographs of the affected joints may not be helpful in establishing the diagnosis. The presence of chondrocalcinosis ↑ the likelihood of CPPD disease. Radiographic clues that may help to distinguish CPPD from OA include:
  - axial involvement
  - sacroiliac erosions
  - cortical erosions of the femur
  - osteonecrosis of the medial femoral condyle.
- Patients under the age of 60 years should be screened for 2° CPPD disease, i.e. serum calcium, magnesium, alkaline phosphatase, ferritin, iron, and iron binding capacity.

Management of CPPD disease

- NSAIDs are the most commonly used therapy, but must be used with caution as the majority of affected patients are the elderly.
- Joint aspiration and intra-articular corticosteroids are of benefit in acute flares of pseudogout. The role of oral steroids remains unclear. There has been some resurgence of interest in ACTH given as per gout.
- Low-dose oral colchicine (1 mg per day) may reduce the frequency of acute attacks in pseudogout.
- Rest, splinting, and eventual joint replacement may be helpful.
- Other therapies that have been tried include:
  - oral magnesium carbonate
  - intra-articular glycosaminoglycan polysulphate (arteparon)
  - intra-articular ^{90}yttrium and corticosteroid
  - IM gold or hydroxychloroquine for type B pseudorheumatoid disease.

Table 15.4 Factors that may trigger acute pseudogout

Intercurrent illness, e.g. chest infection
Direct trauma to the joint
Surgery, especially parathyroidectomy
Blood transfusion and parenteral fluids
Institution of thyroxine replacement therapy
Joint lavage

Basic calcium phosphate (BCP) associated disease

- BCP crystals include hydroxyapatite, octacalcium phosphate, and tricalcium phosphate.
- These crystals are associated with several rheumatic conditions as shown in Table 15.5.
- The treatment of these conditions is as per CPPD disease (see previous section), with NSAIDs and colchicine principally.

Table 15.5 BCP associated conditions

Articular disease	Milwaukee shoulder syndrome (severe degenerative arthropathy, more common on the dominant side and in elderly women)
	Osteoarthritis (synovial fluid crystals found in up to 60% of OA patients)
	Erosive arthritis
	Mixed crystal deposition
Periarticular	Pseudopodagra Calcific tendonitis and bursitis

Calcium oxalate arthritis

- This is an unusual form of arthritis. The crystals are positively birefringent and bipyramidal on polarized light microscopy.
- Radiographs and laboratory tests are not diagnostic.
- Treatment is as for CPPD disease.
- Several conditions are associated with calcium oxalate arthritis (Table 15.6).

Table 15.6 Conditions associated with calcium oxalate arthritis

End-stage renal disease on dialysis
Short bowel syndrome
Diet rich in rhubarb, spinach, ascorbic acid
Thiamine deficiency
Pyridoxine deficiency
Primary oxalosis: recessive trait
early renal failure (age 20s)
arthritis
tendonitis

Metabolic bone diseases and disorders of collagen

Osteoporosis

- In the Western world osteoporosis causes considerable suffering in individuals over the age of 50 years. The disorder can be defined as a ↓ in bone mass and strength resulting in an ↑ risk of fracture. Unlike osteomalacia, the ratio of matrix to mineral deposit in bone is normal in osteoporosis, there generally being less of it.
- The WHO defines osteoporosis on the basis of bone density. Normal bone density lies >−1 standard deviation (SD) *below* the young adult mean value. Thereafter the disease is categorized as low bone mass (osteopaenia) if it is between −1 and −2.5 SD below the mean; osteoporosis if −2.5 SD or more below the mean; and severe if the latter includes low-trauma or spontaneous fractures.
- The risk of osteoporotic fracture is greater in ♀ than ♂ and in both sexes varies with site (see Table 16.1).
- The age-adjusted incidence of hip fractures has been ↑ steadily. In the United Kingdom > 80% of hip fractures occur in ♀ over the age of 65 years. There were 46 000 hip fractures in England and Wales in 1985 and current estimates (Advisory Group on Osteoporosis 1994) suggest that 60 000 occur annually. In the United States there were 238 000 hip fractures in 1986. Recent estimate places the cost of in-patient and community care at £680 million and $8 billion for the United Kingdom and United States respectively.

Pathogenesis and classification

- During childhood and adolescence, growth and modelling lead to an ↑ in the size, shape, strength, and composition of bone. Growth ceases with the closure of the growth plates (epiphyseal cartilage). However, remodelling and mineral homeostasis continue throughout life with bone resorption and deposition coupled by the interaction between osteoclasts and osteoblasts respectively.
- Peak bone mass, or maximal bone density, is usually achieved in the third decade. Peak bone mass is determined by both genetic (e.g. vitamin D receptor gene polymorphism, oestrogen receptor–cytokine interaction), and environmental factors. Indeed, changing lifestyle and behaviour patterns in adolescence has been suggested, but not yet proven, as an effective way of ↑ peak bone mass.
- After the age of 35, and presumably due to ↓ osteoblast activity, the amount of bone laid down is less than that resorbed during each remodelling cycle sequence. The net effect is an age-related ↓ in bone mass. Trabecular and cortical bone mass decline by approximately 6% and 3% per decade, in ♀ and ♂ respectively.
- Further bone loss occurs at the time of menopause with declining ovarian function and levels of oestrogens. Up to 15% of bone mass can be lost over the 5-year period immediately post-menopause. A further 15% of bone mass can be lost if vitamin D deficiency coexists.

- The mechanism of age-related bone loss is unknown. Several possibilities exist:
  - ↓ intestinal calcium absorption.
  - ↓ synthesis of 1,25-dihydroxyvitamin D (due to ↓ renal 1 α hydroxylase).
  - the net effect of above two situations is chronic parathyroid stimulation and the increase in parathyroid hormone (PTH).
  - ↓ osteoblast function.
  - fatty infiltration of the bone marrow and loss of precursor cells and locally generated growth factors.
- Major risk factors for osteoporosis are:
  - race (White or Asian > Afro Caribbean)
  - age and gender (as above)
  - positive family history, particularly maternal hip fracture
  - previous 'fragility' fracture
  - long-term use of corticosteriod therapy
  - malabsorption disorders
  - endocrinopathies.
- Other established risk factors include:
  - low body mass index (BMI <16)
  - short fertile period (late menarche, early menopause including early ovarian failure, hysterectomy and oophorectomy)
  - nulliparity
  - ↓ physical activity
  - low intake of calcium (< 240 mg daily)
  - excessive alcohol intake
  - smoking
  - malignancy (multiple myeloma).

Table 16.1 Risk of osteoporotic fracture with site

Fracture site	Overall lifetime risk of fracture (%)	
	Men	Women
Hip	6.0	17.5
Vertebral	5.0	15.6
Distal forearm	2.5	16.0
Any of above	13.1	39.7

Table 16.2 Classification of osteoporosis

Major type	Causative factor(s)	Details
Primary (physiological)	Post-menopausal Age-related	
Idiopathic		
Juvenile onset		
Secondary	Endocrine	Hyperparathyroidism
		Hypopituitarism
		Thyrotoxicosis
		Hypogonadism
		Cushing's syndrome
		Insulin-dependent diabetes
	Drugs	Corticosteroids
		Excess thyroxine replacement
		Heparin
		Anticonvulsants
		Cyclosprin A
	Haemopoietic	Multiple myeloma
		Lymphoma
		Leukaemia
		Mastocytosis
		Gaucher's disease
	Inflammatory diseases	Rheumatoid arthritis
		Ankylosing spondylitis
	Congenital	Osteogenesis imperfecta
	Immobilization	
	Idiopathic hypercalciuria	
	Osteoporosis of pregnancy	

Table 16.3 The causes of juvenile idiopathic osteoporosis

Type	Causative factor(s)
Primary	Calcium deficiency
	Idiopathic
	Osteogenesis imperfecta
Secondary	Endocrine (see Table 16.2)
	Intestinal:
	malabsorption
	biliary atresia
	type I glycogen storage disease
	Inborn errors of metabolism—homocystinuria
	Leukaemia
	Congenital cyanotic heart disease

Idiopathic osteoporosis

- Idiopathic osteoporosis defines occurrence of the condition in pre menopausal ♀ or ♂ under the age of 60 years, with no 2° cause. The ♀:♂ ratio is 10:1. Most cases are found to have 'low bone turnover' with low rates of bone formation. Some cases have 'high bone turnover' with hypercalciuria; these cases may respond to antiresorption drugs such as calcitonin and bisphosphonates.
- ⚠ The difficulty with this group of patients is knowing who, with borderline low bone density (−2.5 to −3.0 SD below the mean) in the absence of other risk factors, to treat. For the majority in this age group the risk of fracture remains low as although the bone density is below the mean for age the absolute bone density will be relatively good. Anti-catabolic (anti-resorptive) agents are unlikely to significantly shift the risk of fracture.

Juvenile idiopathic osteoporosis (JIO)

- Juvenile osteoporosis (JIO) is an uncommon disorder that occurs before, or at onset of puberty. It affects the sexes equally. The cause is unknown and there are no consistent biochemical abnormalities (see Table 16.3).
- The child presents with pain, non-traumatic fractures around the weight-bearing joints, and collapsed vertebrae. No specific treatment is available and for most, bone mass ↑ to normal values as puberty progresses; however, in some cases fractures may lead to deformity. Supportive physical therapy should be made available.
- In the same way that height and weight charts are used to assess childhood development, there may be a role for serial bone density measurement in children with known low bone mass, as a surrogate assessment of appropriate development.

Corticosteroid-induced osteoporosis (CIO)

- ⚠ CIO is as a major concern. Large numbers of people take long-term corticosteroid therapy for a number of different reasons and there needs to be an awareness of the condition amongst physicians of all disciplines. Treatment should be offered to all patients taking prednisolone for a period likely to be 3 months or more. The risk is present at doses as low as 2.5 mg daily although data would suggest it increases considerably for doses > 5mg daily.

- There is conflicting evidence as to the effect of inhaled corticosteroid on fracture risk. Patients on maximal doses of inhaled corticostroids should be assessed for additional risk factors for osteoporosis and may require prophylaxis. Studies to date would suggest that underlying lung disease and associated morbidity are greater risk factors for falls and fractures than inhaled steroid treatment and their induction of bone loss per se.

- The pathogenesis of CIO is controversial. Corticosteroids can affect calcium and phosphate metabolism both directly and indirectly in bone, kidney, and the intestine. Possible mechanisms are shown in Table 16.4.

Table 16.4 Possible pathogenesis of corticosteroid-induced osteoporosis

Mechanism	Site	Effect
Reduced bone formation	Osteoblasts	Reduced activity
		Reduced recruitment
		Reduced collagen synthesis
		Reduced growth hormone
		Reduced cytokine levels
	Adrenal–testis	Reduced gonadal hormones
Increased bone resorption	Adrenal–testis	Reduced gonadal hormones
	Parathyroid	Increased PTH
	Intestinal	Reduced calcium absorption
		Reduced sensitivity to vitamin D
	Renal	Reduced calcium resorption
	Muscle	Decreased muscle load

Primary hyperparathyroidism

Primary hyperparathyroidism is a relatively common disorder with an adult prevalence of about 0.2% in the fifth to seventh decades of life. It is 3 times more common in ♀ than ♂, this arising from an ↑ incidence after the menopause. Most patients with mild hyperparathyroidism remain asymptomatic, the condition being diagnosed following investigation of a ↑ serum calcium on biochemical screening. The management of this condition will be discussed, later in this chapter.

Hypogonadism

- Hypogonadism due to any cause may lead to an ↑ risk of osteoporotic fracture.
- Causes of amenorrhoea include 1° ovarian failure, use of oestrogen antagonists (e.g. in the management of endometriosis), hyperprolactin-aemia, anorexia nervosa, and low body mass index (e.g. elite sports-women).
- Causes of ↓ testosterone levels include Klinefelter's syndrome, hypo-gonadotrophic hypogonadism, hyperprolactinaemia, anorexia nervosa, and testicular dysfunction following mumps orchitis.

Hyperthyroidism

Hyperthyroidism leads to osteoporosis as a consequence of high bone turnover, enhanced osteoclast recruitment, and ↑ bone resorption.

Malignancy

Malignant infiltration and replacement of marrow tissue occurs in multi-ple myeloma, lymphoma, leukaemia, systemic mastocytosis, and diffuse bone metastases. Mechanisms differ, for example:

- Overproduction of osteoclast-activating cytokines (such as IL-1 and TNF) in myeloma.
- Local synthesis of 1,25-hydroxyvitamin D by malignant cells in lymphoma.
- Overproduction of heparin, histamine, and prostaglandins that stimulate osteoclasts in mastocytosis.

Other factors

Potential factors that may cause generalized osteoporosis in inflammatory disorders, such as RA and AS, include the systemic effects of inflamma-tory products, alterations in sex hormones, altered calcium metabolism, changes in load bearing, and the effect of drugs used in treatment. Immo-bilization per se leads to a net loss of bone (rates as high as 5% per month in the first 6 months).

Investigation of osteoporosis and low-trauma fracture

- ⚠ Low-trauma fracture in those aged 50–75 years should be investi-gated to exclude the possibility of osteoporosis. The three most common sites of fracture are the wrist, vertebrae, and hip. Many now consider a low-trauma fracture in a person >75 years of age as strongly suggestive of osteoporosis and would treat without measuring bone mass (National Institute for Clinical Excellence guidance, UK, 2005). Assessment and investigation for possible underlying 2° disease is still required.

- Plain radiographs are an insensitive method of assessing bone mass. The high correlation between bone mineral density (BMD) and bone strength and therefore bone fragility has led to the development of several techniques for assessing BMD.
- The standard technique for measuring BMD is dual energy X-ray absorptiometry (DEXA). It is quick, has high resolution, precision and accuracy, and can assess the lumbar spine, femoral neck, wrist, and whole body. DEXA gives two readings, the 'T' and 'Z' scores. The T score is the individual's bone mineral density compared with the mean bone density achieved at peak bone mass for the same sex (and, more recently, race). The Z score is the individual's bone mineral density compared with the mean bone density for someone of the same age and sex (and, more recently, race). Most analyses and studies have focused on the T score. The score is recorded as a + or − figure above or below the mean. For every one standard deviation (SD) below the mean there is a two-fold ↑ in the risk of fracture, i.e. an individual three SD below the mean has an 8-fold risk of fracture compared with a 'normal' individual of the same age, bearing in mind also that baseline risk ↑ with age in the 'normal' population.
- Quantitative CT allows volume measurements and can distinguish between cortical and trabecular bone in vertebrae. It is, however, costly and entails a high radiation exposure.
- Ultrasonography is a non-invasive technique that is currently being correlated with DEXA. US can be performed at the heel (calcaneus) and patella. Correlation seems poor and its role in clinical diagnostics remains unclear.
- Since the advent of non-invasive techniques, transiliac bone biopsy is no longer essential unless there is the need to diagnose osteomalacia as the underlying cause. Bone biopsy may be used as a tool in research, in particular for the quantification of rates of bone turnover.
- Routine biochemical and haematological tests are usually normal in osteoporosis. Investigation of the newly diagnosed osteoporotic person should include a screen for malignancy and metabolic bone biochemical abnormalities. This at least would include an ESR, U&E, LFT, serum immunoglobulins, calcium and phosphate. Measurement of the sex hormones should also be considered.

- Biochemical markers of bone turnover are available but their precise clinical role has not been established. These include:
  - bone formation: serum bone alkaline phosphatase, osteocalcin (bone gla protein), type 1 procollagen peptides.
  - bone resorption: fasting urine calcium and hydroxyproline, urine collagen cross links (deoxy)pyridinoline, serum tartrate-resistant acid phosphatase.
- These markers may be helpful in comparing 'high bone turnover' with 'low bone turnover' cases in established osteoporosis, and in monitoring the effects of and compliance with treatments.

Management of osteoporosis and low-trauma fractures

Prevention

Bone mass at any one time will be determined by 'peak bone mass', rate of bone loss with ageing, and, with ♀, the rate and duration of post-menopausal bone loss. Genetic factors cannot be manipulated but nutritional and environmental factors may. Pharmacological intervention in 'at-risk' individuals is good prevention practice. Currently this would include those in the age group 50–65 with a T score of <–3.0, or with a T score <–2.5 with other risk factors (especially fragility fracture), and those >65 with a T score of <–2.5 regardless of presence of additional risk factors.

Calcium

- Calcium supplementation is sensible in those who have a low-calcium diet (poor in dairy products, green leafy vegetables, nuts, dried fruits, etc.). There is conflicting evidence about whether supplements have any effect on preventing bone loss and therefore risk of fracture per se in the young adult.
- Calcium supplementation in prepubertal children enhances the rate of ↑ in bone mineral density but whether this translates into higher peak bone mass is unknown.
- In post-menopausal women, calcium supplements can lead to a ↓ rate of loss of total-body bone mineral density.
- There is a role for calcium and vitamin D supplementation in the elderly osteoporotic; it can help prevent cortical bone loss and subsequent vertebral fractures.
- At present the use of calcium supplements is recommended for:
  - definite osteoporosis
  - poor calcium diet (< 400 mg intake per day)
  - supplement to any anti-catabolic (anti-resorptive) treatment in the elderly.

Exercise

There is some evidence to suggest that physical activity ↓ the rate of bone loss around the menopause, although the level and type of activity remains unclear. The activity must, however, be weight-bearing. There is little impact of exercise in ↑ bone mass once osteoporotic, though it may aid in preventing further loss.

Hormone replacement

- Oestrogen replacement therapy is an effective way of preventing post-menopausal bone loss. The addition of a progestogen allows endometrial shedding and minimizes the risk of hyperplasia and neoplasia. The minimum oral dose of oestrogen required is 2 μmg/day, and conjugated oestrogen 0.625 mg/day. Gels and transdermal/depot treatments should be started at around 3 mg/day or 50 μg/day respectively.
- Most studies would suggest a relative risk of breast cancer of 1.3–1.4 in $\female$ > 60 years and on HRT for > 10 years. There is no evidence that progestogens protect against this risk.
- HRT is administered with caution in individuals with hypertension.
- Post-menopausal HRT is also cardioprotective, partly through lipid lowering effects.
- Evidence would suggest that the use of HRT increases the risk of deep vein thrombosis. The absolute risk is small, about 20 per 100 000 per year excess cases. This risk is lost on cessation of HRT.

Treating established disease

- Virtually all the treatments listed below have demonstrated in the order of 40–50% reduction in risk of fragility fracture, either vertebral or at the hip in post-menopausal women with established osteoporosis.
- Bisphosphonates are now the most commonly used of all agents available in the treatment of established osteoporosis. They are potent inhibitors of bone resorption (anti-catabolic). Cyclical disodium etidronate (400 mg daily for 2 weeks, every 3 months), alendronate (10 mg daily or 70 mg weekly), risedronate (5 mg daily or 35 mg weekly), and ibandronate (2.5 mg daily or 150 mg *monthly*) are the agents currently available. Etidronate is often packaged as Didronel PMO®, containing 2 weeks' supply of etidronate and 10 weeks' calcium supplementation.
- In general, bisphosphates are well-tolerated but should be used with caution in renal impairment and history of oesophageal reflux/hiatus hernia. Symptoms of nausea and reflux can be lessened by taking these medications with plenty of water and avoid lying down for at least 30 minutes afterwards. These agents should also be taken on an empty stomach as absorption is poor. Compliance rates with therapy are variable with reports from the United States of < 30% but reports in the United Kingdom of > 80% at 2–4 years' duration of therapy. Calcium supplements should be taken alongside bisphosphonate therapy unless otherwise contraindicated.
- Calcium (800–1000 mg) and vitamin D supplements (400–800 IU) are recommended in the elderly and those whose diet is poor in them.
- HRT may be used as described above. Selective oestrogen receptor modulaters (SERMs) such as raloxifene may become more popular in the future as alternatives to HRT.
- Calcitonin may be as effective as HRT in abolishing post-menopausal bone loss. It may, in the long-term, prove to be a useful alternative to HRT for those to whom HRT is contraindicated or unacceptable. Nasal spray and s/c formulations are available. Cyclical calcitonin is also useful for its analgesic effect early after osteoporotic fractures.

- Strontium ranelate (Protelos) has been shown to both increase osteoblastic bone formation and reduce osteoclastic bone resorption. Given at 2 g daily orally, it may be used as first line therapy or in those intolerant of Bisphosphonates. Its indication for use is currently post-menopausal osteoporosis, studies having shown 36–41% reduction in fracture risk (hip and vertebral) against placebo. Further research into its efficacy in osteoporosis is on-going.
- Strontium, by its incorporation into bone structure, gives false high readings on DXA scanning, making assessment of change in BMD following therapy difficult to interpret at present.
- Teriparatide is a parathyroid hormone analogue and an anabolic agent now available for use in severe osteoporosis. It is given as a s/c injection daily for 18 months. Animal studies raise concern over an increased risk of renal malignancies. In the UK there are specific guidelines for the use of teriparatide. Patients should fulfill the following criteria and have failed (either intolerant of, or fractured despite 18 months of) a bisphosphonate:
  - age 65 or over
  - T-score < –4.0
  - or T-score < –3.0 with 2 or more fragility fractures and 1 age-independent risk factor.
- △ Acute back pain due to vertebral collapse is discussed in Chapter 20.

A Flow chart for the management of fractures in osteoporosis is provided (Fig. 16.1).

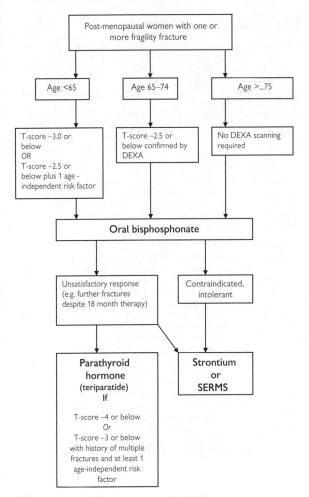

Fig. 16.1 Treatment pathways for post-manopausal women with one or more fragility fracture (based on NICE, UK guidelines 2005)

Osteomalacia and rickets

- Osteomalacia and rickets are characterized by defective mineralization of bone and cartilage and the accumulation of unmineralized bone matrix (osteoid), i.e. there is, unlike osteoporosis, a ↓ in the ratio of mineralized bone to matrix.
- Rickets is the term used for this defect in growing children before the closure of the epiphyses.
- There are many causes of osteomalacia but essentially they all occur due to either a deficiency or resistance to vitamin D, or a non-PTH related defect in renal handling of phosphate (see Table 16.5).
- Both vitamin D_2 (ergocalciferol) from vegetables in the diet, and D_3 (cholecalciferol) from animal tissues and de novo synthesis in skin, are metabolized in the liver to 25-hydroxyvitamin D and thence in the kidney to 1,25-dihydroxyvitamin D_3. The latter affects calcium metabolism by acting on the parathyroid glands (negative-feedback loop on PTH stimulation of renal vitamin D hydroxylases), gut (positive absorption of calcium and phosphate), and bone (both bone resorption and osteoblast activation with bone formation).

Clinical and laboratory findings

- Classical symptoms are bone pain and tenderness, bone deformity (depending on age of onset), and a proximal muscle weakness with a 'waddling gait'. Muscle enzymes and biopsy are normal. Proximal myopathy is not a feature of X-linked hypophosphataemic rickets.
- The hypocalcaemia of osteomalacia is usually silent but some individuals develop parasthesia and tetany. Rarely it is severe enough to cause cardiac dysrhythmia, convulsions, or psychosis.
- Children may be hypotonic and apathetic with growth retardation and delayed walking. On weight-bearing, bones become bowed, and there is irregularity of the metaphyseal–epiphyseal junction, usually at the wrist and costochondral junctions. The latter gives rise to the feature 'rachitic rosary'. An indentation may also arise along the attachment of the diaphragm to the softened ribs (Harrison's groove). Rapid growth of the softened skull leads to cranio-tabes, parietal bone flattening, and frontal bossing. Dentition is also delayed and poor.
- Many bony deformities persist despite treatment (unless due to simple dietary deficiency and treated early) and may require surgery, e.g. tibial/fibial osteotomy to correct lower limb alignment.

Table 16.5 The classification of osteomalacia

Abnormal vitamin D metabolism	Reduced availability	Poor diet
		Inadequate exposure to sun
		Malabsorption
	Defective metabolism	Hepatobiliary disease
		Chronic renal failure
		Anticonvulsant drugs
		Vitamin D-dependent rickets type I
		X-linked hypophosphataemia
		Oncogenic hypophosphataemia
	Receptor defects	Vitamin D-dependent rickets type II
Altered phosphate homeostasis	Malabsorption	
	Renal phosphate loss	X-linked hypophosphataemia
		Fanconi syndrome
	Defective mineralization	Aluminium and fluoride toxicity
		Bisphosphonate toxicity
		Hypophosphatasia
		Fibrogenous imperfecta ossium

- The classical radiographic change of osteomalacia is the pseudo fracture (Looser's zone), found most often at the following sites:
  - ribs and clavicles
  - outer border of the scapulae
  - pubic rami
  - femoral neck
  - metatarsals.

They appear as incomplete, radiolucent fracture lines perpendicular to the cortex, with poor callus formation.

- Laboratory investigations of vitamin D deficiency demonstrate a ↓ serum calcium and phosphate, ↑ serum alkaline phosphatase, ↑ urinary phosphate and ↓ urinary calcium excretion, ↓ levels of 25-hydroxyvitamin D, and a mild 2° hyperparathyroidism. The latter may cause a mild hyperchloraemic acidosis due to renal bicarbonate loss. If this acidosis is severe then it suggests a renal tubular defect (see later in this chapter).
- Levels of 1,25-dihydroxyvitamin D may be normal and are therefore not helpful. If the serum calcium and 25-hydroxyvitamin D levels are normal as well, then the defect is likely to be renal handling of phosphate or end-organ resistance. If doubt remains as to the diagnosis of osteomalacia, a transiliac bone biopsy can be taken.

Features and treatment of abnormal vitamin D metabolism

- Vitamin D deficiency through poor diet intake is rare unless combined with ↓ exposure to sunlight. It is a phenomenon seen most often in the housebound elderly, and in immigrant Asian populations.
- Bone pain and muscle weakness respond quickly to replacement therapy though laboratory and radiological features may take longer to return to normal. Limb deformity can be prevented if simple vitamin D deficiency is treated early. Vitamin D_2 (ergocalciferol) at physiological doses of 200–400 IU/day (5–10 mg) daily can prevent disease. In severe disease it may be better to give a high loading dose daily for one month initially at doses of 2000–5000 IU/day.
- Intestinal disorders that lead to fat malabsorption can cause vitamin D deficiency, as vitamin D is fat-soluble. Cortical bone loss is usually irreversible in this group. Prevention of further damage is best achieved by annually monitoring levels of serum 25-hydroxyvitamin D and, if levels are low-to-normal or less, replacement with ergocalciferol or calcitriol and calcium. Calcium should be supplemented at doses of 800–1000 mg/day for adults.
- Chronic renal failure and renal osteodystrophy are discussed in the section on parathyroid disease and related disorders later in this chapter. Essentially two problems arise as a consequence of renal failure: the first a ↓ in production of 1,25-dihydroxyvitamin D, and second poor phosphate excretion and subsequent hyperphosphataemia. The latter worsens hypocalcaemia that in turn leads to parathyroid hyperplasia and 2° hyperparathyroidism.

- Type I vitamin D-dependent rickets is a rare autosomal recessive disease. Defective 25-hydroxyvitamin D 1 hydroxylase enzyme activity leads to low levels of 1,25-vitamin D. Children are often affected with rickets before the age of 2 years, and fail to respond to normal levels of vitamin D replacement. Treatment is most effective with physiological doses of calcitriol or 1-calcidol (up to 6 µg/kg, maximum 60 µg/day for 3–6 months).

- Type II vitamin D-dependent rickets is a rare receptor defect disorder. About 70% of patients will have alopecia and this is an important prognostic feature when discussing likely outcome of treatment. In patients with normal hair, a remission can be achieved with high doses of vitamin D (as above). In patients with alopecia a 10-fold increase in vitamin D dosing is often required and about 50% will not respond.

Features and treatment of altered phosphate homeostasis

- Osteomalacia from phosphate depletion is rare and usually occurs as a consequence of abuse of phosphate-binding antacids over many years. Histologically it appears the same as vitamin D deficiency disease, although biochemically serum calcium is usually normal and vitamin D ↑. Treatment is with phosphate supplements and avoidance of antacids.

- X-linked hypophosphataemic rickets (also known as 'familial hypophosphataemic rickets') is a disorder of vitamin D resistance. It is important to diagnose early as treatment can prevent deformity. It manifests itself as short stature and rickets in the homozygous ♂, with variable growth and expression of bone deformity in the ♀. Dental delay occurs but dentition is usually normal. Proximal myopathy is not a feature of this condition. Laboratory tests show a ↓ serum phosphate, normal serum calcium and PTH, and a low/normal 1,25-dihydroxyvitamin D. Urine phosphate excretion is ↑ in the absence of abnormal acidification, glycosuria, or aminoaciduria. A combination of calcitriol (0.125–1.5 µg/day) and phosphate (25 mg/kg/day in infants, and 1–3 g elemental phosphorus in adults) is the most effective therapy. The induction of hypercalcaemia is a risk and the serum calcium should be monitored regularly every 2 weeks for a couple of months on induction of therapy and thereafter approximately every 3 months.

- Renal tubular acidosis (RTA) and Fanconi syndrome may be associated with osteomalacia and rickets. In RTA there is a disorder of bicarbonate handling leading to ↓ plasma bicarbonate, metabolic acidosis, and an inappropriate urine pH. Type I, distal tubular RTA occurs as a result of failure to secrete hydrogen ions (see Table 16.6).

- Type II, proximal RTA is a consequence of bicarbonate wasting. Type II RTA is often associated with Fanconi syndrome. The development of rickets in both forms of RTA is 2° to hypophosphataemia. The acidosis should be treated and vitamin D supplements given.
- Fanconi syndrome is associated with a number of acquired and inherited disorders. These include multiple myeloma, amyloidosis, heavy metal toxicity and disorders of carbohydrate metabolism. The net effect of the proximal renal tubular defects is glycosuria, aminoaciduria, phosphaturia, and hypophosphataemia. Treatment of the bone disease is with phosphate and 1-calcidol supplements.
- Oncogenic hypophosphataemic osteomalacia is a phenomenon seen with some tumours (usually mesenchymal). The proposed mechanism is the production of a humoral factor that affects proximal renal tubular handling of phosphate. The bone disease regresses after removal of the tumour. A similar condition occurs in fibrous dysplasia and neurofibromatosis. Treatment involves phosphate and calcitriol supplements.

Table 16.6 Some causes of type I, distal RTA

Hereditary	Primary	
	Renal	Medullary sponge Polycystic kidney
	Fructose intoterance	
	Ehlers-Danlos syndrome	
Acquired	Rheumatic	SLE Sjögren's syndrome Sarcoidosis
	Renal	Obstruction Pyelonephritis Transplantation
	Endocrine	Hyper/hypothyroidism Hyperparathyroidism Hyperprolactinaemia
	Hepatic	Chronic active hepatitis Liver cirrhosis
	Tuberculosis	
	Lithium toxicity	
	Cryoglobulinaemia	

Parathyroid disease and related disorders

This section will discuss hypercalcaemia in adults and children and its relation to musculoskeletal disorders. Hyper- and hypoparathyroidism, and renal osteodystrophy are considered. For further information on vitamin D and phosphate imbalance the reader is referred to the previous section on osteomalacia and rickets.

Hypercalcaemia

- The clinical picture of hypercalcaemia can range from the asymptomatic to an acute medical emergency.
- Calcium plasma concentrations are normally balanced between the homeostatic mechanisms operating in the gut, skeleton, kidneys, and extracellular fluids. Hypercalcaemia arises most often as a result of excessive loss of calcium from bone but may also occur due to excessive gut absorption. The excessive bone loss combined with a failure of the kidneys to handle high loads of calcium, and a failure of bone to reclaim minerals quickly enough, leads to the imbalance. Accelerated bone loss (osteoclast stimulation) may be driven by several causes including parathyroid hormone (PTH) and cytokines interleukin-1 (IL-1), TNF, and transforming growth factor (TGF). PTH also induces calcium reabsortion from the kidneys.
- The clinical presentation of moderate to severe hypercalcaemia includes:
  - joint, bone, muscle pain
  - muscle weakness
  - dehydration and polyuria
  - lethergy
  - fatigue
  - acute confusional state—unconsciousness
  - abdominal pains and vomiting
  - renal colic pains
  - electrocardiogram findings—short QT interval, etc.
- Hyperparathyroidism and malignancy are the most common causes of hypercalcaemia, accounting for 90% of all cases. A thorough history and examination is required when considering the cause of serum calcium (see Table 16.7).

Table 16.7 Some cause of hypercalcaemia

Common	Primary hyper-parathyroidism	
	Malignancy	Lytic metastases: TNF, IL-1
		Ectopic PTH and TGF-α
		Ectopic 1,25 vitamin D
Uncommon/rare	Drugs	Thiazide diuretics
		Lithium
		Aminophyline
	Granuloma	Sarcoidosis
		Tuberculosis
		Histoplasmosis
	Endocrine/metabolic	Thyrotoxicosis
		Pheochromocytoma
		Excess vitamin A or D
		Renal failure
	Immobilization	

- Treatment options depend on the level of serum calcium, the presence of symptoms, renal impairment, and the underlying cause. For example borderline ↑ serum calcium in an asymptomatic individual with a mildly ↑ PTH may simply warrant observation in the absence of renal impairment or vitamin D deficiency. ⚠ On the other hand an individual with severe hypercalcaemia, dehydration, and renal impairment 2° to a treatable malignancy would require urgent aggressive management.
- Dehydration is very common. Early rehydration is very important and often given for 24–48 h prior to review of serum calcium levels and the instigation of further therapies such as bisphosphonates and loop diuretics (see Table 16.8).

Hypercalcaemia in infancy and childhood

- Chronic hypercalcaemia of infancy may not be associated with the more common clinical features mentioned above. More often there is a failure to thrive, abdominal pain, and irritability. Acute hypercalcaemia is very rare in children.
- Conditions to consider are listed in Table 16.9.

Parathyroid disorders
Primary hyperparathyroidism

- Primary hyperparathyroidism (1°HPT) is a relatively common condition with an incidence of 1 in 1000. It occurs at all ages though is much more common after the age of 60 with a ♀ to ♂ ratio of 3:1. It is unusual in childhood and should raise the possibility of familial multiple endocrine neoplasia (MEN) type I or type II.

- A single benign adenoma accounts for 80% of cases of 1°HPT. Generalized gland hyperplasia accounts for 15–20% of cases. Parathyroid carcinoma is very rare.
- The condition is associated with bone, renal, GI, and neuromuscular complications. Bony problems can be seen on plain radiographs and range from mild subperiosteal bone resorption to full 'osteitis fibrosa cystica' with bone cysts, 'brown tumours', bone resorption of the distal phalanges and clavicles, patchy osteosclerosis (classic 'rugger jersey' spine), and multiple lytic lesions of the skull. These changes may often, however, be non-specific.
- Renal stones are a common complication. GI manifestations include peptic ulceration and pancreatitis. The myopathy of 1°HPT is rare and more often a syndrome of fatigue and weakness is seen.
- 1°HPT is diagnosed by assaying PTH levels. The assays are sensitive and able to distinguish between non-parathyroid tumour secreting PTH and parathormone.

Treatment
- Medical management includes adequate rehydration and avoidance of high calcium intake. In the UK there are no specific agents on the market for lowering PTH. However, clinical trials with calcimimetic agents (stimulate calcium receptors with consequent inhibition of PTH secretion) and in particular cinacalcet hydrochloride are ongoing and may be effective in 1°HPT. At the time of writing, cinacalcet has completed phase III trials and in some countries will soon enter the market.
- Some individuals (especially the elderly) have physiological mild elevation of PTH due to vitamin D deficiency with normal calcium levels. Vitamin D should be replaced and the serum calcium and PTH levels monitored after 8–10 weeks.
- Parathyroidectomy should be offered to individuals with moderate-to-high serum calcium and/or symptoms and complications of the condition, the latter regardless of whether serum calcium levels are 'borderline' raised or not. US imaging, thallium/technetium scans, MR, and CT are all useful ways of establishing the position of an adenoma. However, exploration by an experienced surgeon is equally effective.

Secondary and tertiary hyperparathyroidism
Secondary hyperparathyroidism (2°HPT) occurs as a consequence of abnormalities in serum calcium and homeostatic 'sensing' of calcium levels. With time, PTH secretion becomes autonomous and the abnormality is then called tertiary hyperparathyroidism. This is most often seen in conditions such as end-organ renal disease and vitamin D resistance. Calcimimetics may have an important role to play in controlling 2°HPT but at present parathyroidectomy is the best treatment option. Vitamin D replacement to lower PTH secretion does not appear to be effective in patients with otherwise normal vitamin D levels.

Table 16.8 Treatment of hypercalcaemia

General principles	Rehydrate with normal saline 4 litres in 24 h if needed
	Correct hypokalaemia and hypomagnesaemia
	Mild metabolic acidosis need not be treated
Specific treatment	Loop diuretics when hydrated
	Bisphosphonates (pamidronate)
	Calcitonin
	Glucocorticoids (haematological malignancies)

Table 16.9 Conditions which may be responsible for hypercalcaemia in infancy and childhood

Williams' syndrome	A spectrum of aortic valve stenosis and facial dysmorphism ('elfin' facies). Radioulnar synostosis impedes growth in 25% of cases. There is a deletion of the elastin gene on chromosome 7; pathogenesis otherwise is unknown	
Idiopathic infantile hypercalcaemia	Similar milder appearance to Williams' syndrome can be seen. There are also features of inguinal hernias, hypertension, strabismus, and kyphosis	
Familial hypocalciuric hypercalcaemia	See later in this section	
Neonatal primary hyperparathyroidism		
Other	Fat necrosis	
	Sarcoidosis	
	Jansen syndrome (metaphyseal dysplasia)	
	Overdosing of milk/vitamin D	

Familial hypocalciuric hypercalcaemia (FHH) or familial benign hypercalcaemia (FBH)

- This condition is common but most often asymptomatic. It is inherited as an autosomal dominant with high penetrance. Radiographs, PTH, and renal function are usually normal. Although parathyroid gland hyperplasia occurs, parathyroidectomy is invariably unsuccessful at lowering serum calcium levels.

- The two indications for parathyroidectomy are neonatal severe hyperparathyroidism and adult relapsing pancreatitis. Use of diuretics, oestrogens, or phosphate to regulate serum calcium has been unsuccesful. Patients should therefore be followed without intervention unless complications arise.
- In pregnancy the three situations to be aware of are:
  - asymptomatic hypercalcaemia in the affected offspring of a carrier.
  - severe neonatal hypercalcaemia in affected offspring of an unaffected mother (intrauterine 2° hyperparathyroidism which usually resolves spontaneously).
  - hypocalcaemia in the unaffected offspring of an affected mother (fetal parathyroid supression).

Familial hyperparathyroid syndromes

Up to 10% of cases of hyperparathyroidism may have a hereditary syndrome. The most common of these is multiple endocrine neoplasia (MEN). Type I, autosomal dominant and equal in both sexes, is associated with pancreatic and pituitary adenomas, and adrenal hyperplasia. Type IIA, autosomal dominant Sipple's disease, is characterized by pheochromocytomas and medullary carcinoma of the thyroid.

Parathyroid hormone resistant syndromes

- Pseudohypoparathyroidism (PHP) occurs as a result of resistance to PTH by target tissues. The biochemical consequences are hypocalcaemia, hyperphosphataemia, and ↑ PTH.
- Cyclic AMP (cAMP) mediates many actions of PTH. Administration of bioactive PTH to normal individuals leads to ↑ urinary excretion of cAMP. The abnormal response to this test in individuals with PHP classifies them either type I—no increase in urine cAMP with bioactive PTH—or type II—normal increase in urine cAMP but abnormal phosphate handling.
- The net effect is features similar to those of hypoparathyroidism of any cause (such as congenital parathyroid absence, or surgical removal).
- Common symptoms include:
  - neuromuscular irritability (due to associated hypocalcaemia)
  - muscle cramps
  - pseudopapilloedema
  - extrapyramidal signs
  - mental retardation
  - cataracts
  - coarse hair/alopecia
  - abnormal dentition
  - Personality disturbance.
- PHP type Ia (Albright's hereditary osteodystrophy (AHO)) manifests as short stature, round facies, obesity, brachydactyly, and s/c ossification. Albright observed that some individuals have these features without PHP. The term pseudopseudohypoparathyroidism was coined. This group have a normal serum calcium and PTH/cAMP test.
- Cases with PHP type I but who lack features of AHO are classified type Ib. They often have the skeletal abnormalities seen in cases of hypoparathyroidism.

- In type II PHP there is a normal cAMP response but an abnormal phosphate response in the kidney.
- The mainstay of therapy is the maintenance of serum calcium and phosphate levels. The complication of calcium and vitamin D supplements is the ↑ risk of renal stones due to hypercalciuria. One gram a day of calcium is recommended and products rich in phosphate (e.g. dairy foods) should be avoided. Hydroxyvitamin D supplements are valuable but serum calcium and phosphate levels should be checked weekly for 4–6 weeks up to steady state and then every 3–6 months.

Renal osteodystrophy

- The kidneys regulate calcium/phosphate balance, are a target organ for PTH, and produce 1,25-dihydroxyvitamin D (calcitriol). Renal osteodystrophy is the net effect on bone that occurs due to derangement of calcium homeostasis in chronic renal failure. Renal bone disease is classified as 'high turnover' or 'low turnover' depending on whether serum PTH levels are ↑ or low/normal respectively. Low turnover, adynamic osteodystrophy, is related to excess bone aluminium deposition in dialysis patients and is also seen in diabetes mellitus and corticosteroid therapy and as part of ageing.
- Hyperphosphataemia, hypocalcaemia, impaired calcitriol production, and skeletal resistance to PTH all contribute to 2°HPT in chronic renal failure. Serum PTH varies too widely in the condition to be useful in assessing treatment. Serum alkaline phosphatase is ↑ and is a useful marker though it does not distinguish between 'high' and 'low' turnover states.
- The clinical manifestations of renal osteodystrophy are shown in Table 16.10.

The management of renal osteodystrophy

- Good dietary control of phosphate can maintain normal calcium levels, but low-phosphate diets are often unacceptable and normal phosphate levels are best achieved with binding agents, e.g. calcium carbonate or calcium acetate.
- Small doses of calcitriol (vitamin D) may help to lower serum PTH levels. Some individuals may be sensitive to calcitriol and serum calcium levels may ↑. Most patients require doses of 0.25–0.5 µg daily; children may require higher doses.
- Parathyroidectomy is indicated in persistent symptomatic hypercalcaemia, ectopic calcification, and severe bone pain.

Table 16.10 The clinical manifestations of renal osteodystrophy

Clinical feature	Comment
Bone pain	Common
Skeletal deformity	Common. Affects appendicular and axial skeleton
	Children: onset <3 years, rachitic; onset <10 years, bowing of long bones, widened metaphyses, pseudoclubbing, slipped epiphyses
	Adults: lumbar scoliosis, kyphosis, distorted thorax
Growth retardation	
Proximal muscle weakness	
Ectopic calcification	Soft-tissues. Visceral. Vascular—if severe, individuals may develop ischaemic necrosis

Ectopic calcification and ossification
- Ectopic calcification can arise from any one of a number of causes of hypercalcaemia or hyperphosphataemia. These include renal failure, hyperparathyroidism, and sarcoidosis. Dystrophic calcification is also a feature of SScl (see Chapter 12), DM (see Chapter 13), and 1° calcinosis.
- Ectopic ossification can be seen post-trauma and following a myositis. It is also a feature of several rare conditions including pseudo-hypoparathyroidism and myositis ossificans progressiva. Early signs of muscle ossification are best detected with MR scanning. Later ossification it easily visible on plain radiographs. Treatment is difficult but includes physiotherapy to maintain suppleness and possibly heparins or bisphosphonates to halt bone formation.

Paget's disease of bone

- Paget's disease is a chronic disorder of acclerated bone resorption and formation resulting in deformity in size and shape of bone as well as fragility despite apparent 'thickening' of bone.
- The condition is common (about 5% of the population over the age of 55) in the United Kingdom, the United States, Australia, and New Zealand, with a ♂ to ♀ ratio of 3:2. It is uncommon in Asia, and non-White races.
- Very little is known of the molecular basis of Paget's disease. There is evidence to suggest that it may be triggered by exposure to a slow virus. Paramyxovirus antigens found in bone cells, and compatible with measles, respiratory syncytial virus, and canine distemper have all been implicated.
- The clinical features of Paget's disease are shown in Table 16.11.

Investigation and treatment

- Serum alkaline phosphatase, a measure of bone formation, is the most useful marker and may be ↑ as much as 30 times above normal. Occasionally, in limited Paget's, the enzyme is normal. This should not be a deterrent to treating painful lesions. The differential diagnosis of ↑ bone alkaline phosphatase includes metastatic bone disease, osteomalacia, hyperparathyroidism, and hyperphosphatasia.
- Urine hydroxyproline excretion is also ↑. Hydroxyproline is a breakdown product of collagen and a marker of bone resorption. Other markers of bone turnover are available but most remain experimental and are not needed for the diagnosis and treatment of Paget's disease.
- There is a wide variation in radiographic appearance of the condition but the main features are sclerosis, bone expansion, and coarse, disorganized, trabecular bone.
- Isotope bone scanning is a sensitive investigation for defining the extent of lesions.
- Many rare hereditary dysplastic conditions are associated with bone sclerosis. These include osteopetrosis, Engelmann's disease, and pycnodysostosis. These conditions are beyond the scope of this book.
- Sclerosis is also a feature of many other conditions including metabolic disease (fluorosis, hypervitaminosis D, parathyroid disease, renal osteodystrophy), malignancy (lymphoma, myeloma, skeletal metastases), infection, sarcoidosis, and tuberous sclerosis.

Table 16.11 Clinical features of Paget's disease of bone

Clinical feature	Details
Pain	Deep, boring pain, possibly correlated to blood flow
Bone expansion and deformity	Hands or feet 10% of cases
	Pelvis 75%
	Lumbar spine 50% of cases
	Femur 35% of cases
	Sacrum 35% of cases
	Skull 35% of cases
	Tibia 30% of cases
	Radius 15% of cases
Fractures	
Heat	
Neurological syndromes	Deafness (sensorineural or conductive)
	Tinnitus
	Headache
	Brainstem/cerebellar compression
	Spinal cord/root compression
	Cranial nerve entrapment
High-output cardiac failure	Rare—occurs when > 40% of the skeleton is involved
Malignant osteosarcoma	Seen in 0.1% of cases, esp. if disease present for > 10 years
Immobilization hypercalcaemia	Serum calcium levels are nearly always normal
Gout	
Retinal angioid streaks	

- Thermographic improvement and pain reduction are correlated with effective treatment of Paget's; thermographic observations probably demonstrate the phenomenon of ↓ (from ↑) in bone and periosseous blood flow after treatment.
- There are several indications for treatment of Paget's disease:
  - pain arising from Pagetic sites
  - deforming disease
  - skull disease

- complications: progressive neurological syndrome, fractures, hypercalcaemia, high-output cardiac failure, serum alkaline phosphatase (over twice upper normal).
- Pagetic and related osteoarthritic pain may be reduced by simple analgesics but pure pagetic bone pain responds poorly to this. In most cases now the choice of treatment falls between bisphosphonates and calcitonin. These drugs are discussed in the section on osteoporosis.
- Etidronate may be given for 6 months at a dose of 5 mg/kg/day. Vitamin D supplements may minimize the mineralization defects that can occur with even low doses of etidronate. Oral tiludronate 400 mg daily for 3 months has been licensed for the treatment of Paget's disease in the United Kingdom. IV pamidronate may also be used and many in current practice offer a single dose infusion of 30–90 mg (dependent on renal function) to symptomatic patients, with follow-up and measurement of serum alkaline phosphatase after 3 months. Transient 'flu-like' symptoms of fever, myalgia, and arthralgia often occur after the first dose of IV pamidronate. Risedronate may also be given at 30 mg daily for one month.
- S/c or IM calcitonin may also be used in Paget's disease. The disadvantages are common symptoms of nausea and diarrhoea, relapse on therapy, and expense. Nasal spray calcitonin may be useful but the therapeutic effect is probably weaker than with newer bisphosphonates. Typical dosing for salmon calcitonin would be a 10 IU test dose followed by 50–100 IU daily, reducing to 50 IU 2–3 times per week once a symptomatic response is achieved (usually after 4–8 weeks). If there has been no symptomatic response after 3 months, calcitonin therapy should be stopped.
- Plicamycin (mithramycin) is potent and marrow, hepatic, and renal toxicity are seen. The drug has been largely superseded by bisphosphonates.
- There is no consensus on whether or when to treat Pagetic joints per se prior to joint replacement.

Miscellaneous diseases of bone

Osteochondritis and osteonecrosis

- The osteochondroses are a heterogeneous group of disorders, defined by their radiological appearances. In a few instances, radiological osteochondritis may be an incidental finding, not associated with symptoms and may represent a normal developmental variant. Usually, however, it is painful, occurs in the growing skeleton between the ages of 3–16 years, and is more frequent in ♂ and in the peripheral skeleton. Some cases are due to infarction (osteonecrosis) of subchondral bone. For others the aetiology is unknown.
- Osteonecrosis (synonyms: avascular necrosis, ischaemic necrosis, aseptic necrosis) occurs at several sites and is associated with as many eponyms (see Table 16.12). Bone infarction and subsequent pain occurs in susceptible areas because of limited collateral circulation and low perfusion pressure, e.g. in the femoral head. First, bone and adjacent marrow becomes necrotic. Granulation tissue then advances into the dead bone, which is resorbed. Osteoblasts then lay down new osteoid. Advanced osteonecrosis leads to secondary osteoarthritis, severe disability, and eventually the need for joint replacement. Whether or not core decompressive surgery should be performed in the acute phase of the condition remains open to debate. The use of MR to assess the extent of osteonecrosis may become helpful in selecting cases for early surgery.
- Aetiological factors for osteonecrosis include trauma, sepsis, radiation, thermal, and electrical injury. Caisson's disease is an obliterative endarteritis of the femoral head caused by expanding nitrogen gas in divers who decompress too quickly. Haematological causes include haemophilia, coagulopathies, and haemoglobinopathies. Endocrine causes include Cushing's syndrome and glucocorticoid use (high dose >60 mg/day over a period of months). There is an ↑ susceptibility to the condition in several rheumatic conditions including RA (Chapter 5), SLE (Chapter 9), SScl (Chapter 12), and vasculitis (Chapter 14). Finally, a miscellaneous group of associations with osteonecrosis include alcohol abuse, organ transplantation, dialysis, HIV infection, pancreatitis, chronic liver disease, hypertriglyceridaemia, and pregnancy.
- Osteonecrosis complicates 20% of cases of intracapsular hip fracture.
- Fat embolism may account for some cases, e.g. in alcoholism and Cushing's disease.
- Asymptomatic osteonecrosis in SLE may be as high as 35% (it is symptomatic in 5–10%).

Table 16.12 The osteochondroses

Skeletal area		Disease eponym	Mechanism
Upper limb	Basal phalanges	Thiemann	Trauma
	Second metacarpal head	Mauclaire	Trauma
	Lunate	Kienbock	Osteonecrosis
	Carpal navicular	Prieser	Trauma
	Humeral capitellum	Panner	Trauma/osteonecrosis
Lower limb	Second metatarsal base	Freiberg	Osteonecrosis
	Fifth metatarsal base	Iselin	Trauma
	Tarsal navicular	Köhler	?Trauma/normal variant
	Talus	Diaz	Trauma-related
	Calcaneal	Sever	Traction apophysitis*
	Apophysis of tibial tubercle	Osgood–Schlatter	Traction apophysitis*
	Proximal tibia	Blount	–
	Inferior patella pole	Sinding–Larsen–Johansson	Traction apophysitis*
	Femoral epiphysis	Legg–Calvé–Perthes	Osteonecrosis
Axial skeleton	Vertebral epiphysis	Scheuermann	Repeated trauma

*Due to repetitive overloading of tendons, usually from sports.

- Osteonecrosis is diagnosed and classified radiologically: (Arlet and Ficat classification): I = normal; II = osteoporosis, cysts, sclerosis giving mottled appearance; III = subchondral bone collapse; IV = abnormal bone contour and joint space loss. Bone scintigraphy, CT, and MR are more sensitive. MR can identify early changes in bone marrow before bone necrosis and has greatest specificity once bone changes occur.
- Legg–Calvé–Perthes' disease is osteonecrosis of the femoral epiphysis and occurs in the age range 3–8 years, most frequently in ♂ (ratio 4:1 ♂ to ♀). It is bilateral in 10–20% of cases. Symptoms include an insidious onset of limp and pain in the groin or referred to the knee/thigh which is relieved by rest. Limitation of hip internal rotation and abduction (due to adductor spasm) is typical. Leg length inequality suggests bone collapse. There may be spontaneous resolution,

especially in younger patients, in whom conservative management is indicated.

- Osgood–Schlatter's disease is probably due to repetitive trauma at the site of patellar tendon insertion into the tibial tubercle, typically in athletic adolescents, especially ♂ aged 14–16 years. Pain on exercise usually eases with rest. The diagnosis is made clinically and on demonstrating an enlarged fragmented tibial tubercle on a lateral view radiograph. Bilateral knee views helps to distinguish normal from abnormal.

- Scheuermann's disease, though not consistently defined, is thought to be a vertebral epiphyseal osteochondritis that occurs in adolescence. Though an incidental radiographic finding it is also associated with diffuse spinal pain which is more likely to be present if the osteochondritis is thoracolumbar (25%) rather than thoracic (75%) and the child is an athlete or very active. It can present with painless dorsal kyphosis with compensatory lumbar lordosis and lateral spine radiographs show irregularity of vertebral end-plates, anterior vertebral wedging, and kyphosis.

- Sinding–Larsen–Johansson's disease occurs as a consequence of over-loading of the patella at its secondary centre of ossification producing a traction apophysitis at the patella lower pole. Though not exclusive to the group, it is a typical sports-related injury in adolescent athletes who jump, e.g. high-jump, basketball. Treatment is with simple analgesia or NSAIDs, and rest.

- Köhler's disease is osteonecrosis of the tarsal navicular. Changes may represent a developmental variation in ossification and it presents with a painful limp. Weight bearing is more comfortable on the outside of the foot and the navicular is tender.

- Freiberg's disease, osteonecrosis of the metatarsal (usually the second) head following trauma, is most common in adolescent ♀. Pain is local-ized and worse on weight bearing with swelling sometimes detectable.

Osteochondritis dissecans

- This is usually a solitary lesion of the medial femoral condyle. A fragment of articular cartilage and subchondral bone becomes demarcated and may form an intra-articular loose body. The cause is unknown but may be due to abnormal ossification or trauma. Similar features may occasionally be seen at the elbow, hip, and talus.

- The condition is seen most often in ♂ adolescents. Symptoms are mainly acute onset pain, an effusion, and limited movement of the joint.

- Plain radiographs will show a well-circumscribed, sclerotic lesion.

- In young patients before skeletal maturity there is a good chance of healing. After the epiphyses have closed, however, there is more risk of a loose body and secondary osteoarthritis. Arthroscopy can assist in assessing the degree of damage and removing loose bodies. Surgery ranges from drilling the lesion *in situ* to encourage healing, to bone osteochondral allografts.

Osteoid osteoma

- This is a benign osteoid-forming tumour that can be an elusive cause of bone pain, radiculopathy, or arthritis in children and adults. It is uncommon and accounts for 10% of benign bone neoplasia. It is 2–3 times more common in ♂ than ♀ and the incidence is highest in the second and third decades of life. More than two-thirds of lesions occur in long bones and especially the femur and tibia.
- Pain is the primary symptom and may be referred.
- The typical lesion is seen on plain radiography as an isolated, well-defined area of sclerosis with a radiolucent nidus often containing speckles of calcium. Isotope bone scanning is a sensitive method of isolating a lesion and CT is valuable for localizing the nidus before surgical resection.
- Most individuals will respond, in part, to aspirin or NSAIDs. Provided the nidus is completely resected, surgery is curative.

Fibrous dysplasia

- This condition manifests as sporadic isolated or multifocal fibrous bone cysts and occurs most often in the second to third decade of life in isolated (mono-ostotic) disease, and before the age of 10 years in multifocal (polyostotic) disease.
- McCune–Albright syndrome is a triad of fibrous dysplasia, hyper pigmented 'café-au-lait' patches, and endocrine abnormalities.
- Laboratory tests are usually normal.
- There is no specific treatment. Some lesions regress. Fractures heal in the normal way. Girls with McCune–Albright-associated precocious puberty may respond to the aromatase inhibitor testolactone.

Molecular abnormalities of collagen and fibrillin

- Collagen and fibrillin are major connective tissue proteins with important mechanical functions. This section will deal briefly with osteogenesis imperfecta, Ehlers–Danlos syndrome, and Marfan syndrome.
- There are a number of types of collagen and a number of gene mutations leading to subtypes of collagen diseases. In this respect we will focus only on commoner aspects of these uncommon conditions, although the reader should be aware that joint hypermobility syndrome (akin to Ehlers-Danlos hypermobility type) is probably far more common than most clinicians realize and therefore under-diagnosed.

Osteogenesis imperfecta (OI)

- OI (also known as brittle bone disease) is a spectrum of conditions ranging from stillbirth to asymptomatic signs. The pathogenesis centres around abnormalities of type I collagen that is found not only in bone but also ligaments, teeth, sclerae, and skin.
- Ligament laxity, joint hypermobility, easy bruising, and poor dentition are common features. The differences between the four types of OI are shown in Table 16.13.
- Generalized osteopenia, deformity, and fractures are common bone and radiographic findings. The differential diagnosis in children includes juvenile osteoporosis, Cushing's disease, and homocystinuria.
- There is no effective medical therapy for OI. Patients may need surgery in late childhood/adulthood for deformities, and good dental hygiene.
- ⚠ Children may present with multiple injuries that lead the clinician to consider child-abuse as a source for these—absolute care must be taken in ensuring neither OI or another collagen disorder is present before considering further action.

Marfan syndrome

- Marfan syndrome is characterized by long extremities (span/height ratio >1.03), long fingers and feet (arachnodactyly) with a hand/height ratio >11% and hand/foot ratio >15%, tall stature (with upper segment/lower segment ratio <0.89), pectus deformity of the chest wall (increasing risk of chest infections), high-arched palate, mandibular hypoplasia, lens dislocations and myopia, and joint laxity.
- ⚠ There is a predisposition to mitral valve prolapse and acute aortic root rupture. All patients should have an echocardiogram and thoracic CT/MR to assess the aortic valve and arch.
- It is an autosomal dominant condition with complete penetrance and prevalence of 1 in 25 000.
- A subgroup similar to Marfan syndrome but without vascular fragility exists. The condition is called congenital contractural arachnodactyly.
- Numerous gene mutations have been found for both conditions, both linked to abnormalities of the protein fibrillin type I and II.

Table 16.13 Clinical and biochemical abnormalities in OI

Type	Clinical features	Inheritance	Defect
I	Normal bone growth. Normal dentition. Hearing loss in 50%. Blue sclerae	Autosomal dominant	Decreased production of type I procollagen
II	Lethal. Stillbirths	Autosomal dominant. Autosomal recessive (rare)	Rearrangement of collagen IA/2A genes
III	Often deformed growth at birth and worsens. Poor dentition common. Hearing loss common. May have blue sclerae	Autosomal dominant or recessive	Mutations in alpha-1 and alpha-2 collagen chains
IV	Often bone deformity and short stature. Poor dentition common. Hearing loss uncommon. Normal sclerae.	Autosomal dominant	Mutations in the alpha-2 chains

- The main aim of follow-up and assessment of these individuals is the early detection and referral of cardiac valve and aortic disease. There are currently no medical therapies available for cardiac disease. Musculoskeletal symptoms should be managed in much the same way as outlined in the section below on joint hypermobility syndrome.

Ehlers–Danlos syndrome

- This is a clinically heterogeneous condition characterized by skin fragility, ligament laxity, short stature, spinal deformity, vascular fragility, and (rarely) retinal detachment. △ Retinal detachment and a history of early onset OA should lead the clinician to consider the diagnosis of Stickler's syndrome, a Collagen 1 abnormality.
- There are at least 9 genetic subtypes of Ehlers–Danlos syndrome (EDS), of which at least 5 have defined biochemical abnormalities. The classification, genetic abnormalities and clinical features of EDS are shown in Table 16.14. Various inheritance patterns are found dependent on the subtype of EDS. Hypermobility type EDS is the most common of these conditions and probably synonymous with JHS (see text below).
- The clinician should be very sure they have confidently excluded vascular (type IV) EDS as this is associated with significant mortality.
- Therapy for these conditions centres on graded exercise and joint and skin protection. Some individuals require joint splints. Spinal deformity may need bracing or surgery and retinal disease requires ophthalmic expertise.
- Vascular rupture is a major concern in vascular type (type IV). This may occur even in the absence of documented aneurysms. This risk should always be taken into account during surgery or pregnancy, indeed as should tissue fragility in general for all subtypes.
- Tissue vulnerability should always be at the forefront of planning any surgical intervention.
- Patients are often also resistant to local anaesthetics—the cause unclear. Failing to recognize this phenomenon can lead the clinician to inadvertently accuse the patient of being 'sensitive' or anxious without realizing that they truly do not get a full effect from the anaesthetic.
- Difficulties may arise during pregnancy—patients may get additional joint pain from ↑ body weight, early rupture of membranes and premature birth, cervical incompetence and spontaneous abortion, excessive tissue trauma during delivery, and musculoskeletal complications in the post-natal period due to lifting and caring for the newborn.
- The diagnosis is primarily clinical. Genetic testing can be done by looking for abnormalities of collagen types I, III, and V. At present such facilities are not available in the UK and most centers rely on expert units in the Netherlands and Belgium. A skin biopsy is required.

Table 16.14 Clinical features and genetics of EDS

Type	Inheritance	Genetic defect	Common Clinical picture
Classical (type I and II)	AD	Abnormal pro-alpha 1 and 2 encoded by COL5A1 and A2 gene	Hyper lax skin. Profound bruising and scarring
Hypermobility (Type III)	AD	Not known. ? Tenascin X insufficiency	See BJHS, Table 16.16
Vascular (Type IV)	AD	Abnormal pro-alpha 1 encoded by COL3A1 gene	Characteristic facies—wide spaced eyes, lobeless ears. Vascular rupture
Kyphoscoliosis (Type VI)	AR	Deficiency of lysyl hydroxylase	Severe hypotonia. Scoliosis. Scleral fragility
Atherochalasia (Type VII subtype)	AD	Abnormal pro-alpha 1 and 2 encoded by COL1A1 and A2	Severe dislocations. Skin laxity. Bruising. Hypotonia
Dermatospraxis (Type VII subtype)	AR	Deficiency of procollagen 1 peptidase	Severe, sagging skin. Bruising. Hernias
Rare forms:			
X-linked (Type V)	X-linked	?	Milder version of Classical type
Periodontal (Type VIII)	AD	?	Classical with gum fragility
Type X	?AR	?	Milder version of classical type with platelet aggregation

AD-autosomal dominant; AR-autosomal recessive

Benign joint hypermobility syndrome (BJHS)

- Joint hypermobility can be associated with a multisystem clinical picture and may be associated with diffuse chronic pain.
- Hypermobility is usually considered present if a person satisfies four or more manoeuvres in the nine-point Beighton hyper-mobility score (Table 16.15).
- BJHS is excluded in the presence of Marfan syndrome or Ehlers–Danlos syndrome (excluding hypermobility (Type III)). It may be synonymous with EDS hypermobility type.
- The revised (Brighton 1998) criteria for BJHS are shown in Table 16.16. BJHS is diagnosed in the presence of two major, one major and two minor, or four minor criteria. Two minor criteria will suffice where there is an unequivocally affected first-degree relative. The criteria serve to demonstrate the range of clinical findings in the condition.

Treatment of hypermobility syndrome

- Although hypermobility diminishes with age, the symptoms tend to continue and may worsen.
- It is important to remember that older patients may have been previously more mobile and that the Beighton score may not be an appropriate measure. A history of joint laxity should be sought.
- Hypermobility extends beyond the joints highlighted in the Beighton scale. The clinician should look at the fingers, shoulders, neck, hips, patello-femoral joint, and skin laxity.
- Analgesics are often unhelpful for chronic pain but have their place in acute symptoms. Pain and fatigue cause significant morbidity.
- Joint stabilizing exercises with particular reference to core stability, posture and proprioception are beneficial, as may be advice on avoiding overuse injuries and practical ways of managing day-to-day activities. A global approach to joint stability and function, as opposed to just treating regional symptoms, is effective.
- 'Pain management' should be considered in chronic pain cases. This might include for example, cognitive behavioural therapy and the process is similar to that used in fibromyalgia (see Chapter 18).
- The role of serotonergic/noradrenergic agents in these patients is unclear. In part there may be effective control of depression, however, there may also be direct analgesic properties to these agents.
- Neuroleptic agents for neuropathic pain have not been studied in this group of patients. However, gabapentin or pregabalin and other similar agents may have a role.

Table 16.15 Beighton hypermobility rating

	Subject has the ability to:	Right	Left
1.	Passively dorsiflex the fifth metacarpo-phalangeal joint to ≥90°	1	1
2.	Oppose the thumb to the volar aspect of the ipsilateral Forearm	1	1
3.	Hyperextend the elbow ≥ 10°	1	1
4.	Hyperextend the knee ≥ 10°	1	1
5.	Place hands flat on the floor without bending the knees	1	
	Possible total score	9	

Table 16.16 The Brighton (1998) criteria for benign joint hypermobility syndrome

Major criteria	A Beighton score of 4 out of 9 or greater (current or historical)
	Arthralgia for > 3 months in four or more joints
Minor criteria	A Beighton score of 1, 2, or 3 out of 9
	Arthralgia in one to three joints or back pain, either for longer than 3 months, spondylosis/spondylolisthesis
	Dislocation/subluxation in > one joint, or one joint on > one occasion
	Soft tissue rheumatism in three or more sites
	Marfanoid habitus
	Abnormal skin: straie, hyperextensibility, papyraceous scars
	Eye signs: drooping eyelids, myopia, antimongoloid slant
	Varicose veins, hernias, uterine/rectal prolapse

Rare chondrodysplasias and storage disorders

There are > 150 distinctive chondrodysplasias representing autosomal dominant, recessive, and X-linked patterns of inheritance. The first identified mutations were found in the collagen 2A1 gene, and are associated with premature osteoarthrosis. Such conditions include achondrogenesis, Kniest syndrome, spondyloepiphyseal dysplasia, and the Stickler syndrome. Clinical features in the latter three conditions include premature joint destruction, joint/bone deformity, short stature, and progressive myopia (with or without retinal detachment). Stickler syndrome patients are also prone to hernias and cardiac valvular and conduction disorders.

Storage diseases associated with progressive skeletal dysplasia include:
- Mucopolysaccharidoses, e.g. Hurler, Hunter, Scheie
- Mucolipidoses
- Sphingolipidoses
- Gaucher's disease
- Fabry's disease.

The detail and complexities of these conditions is beyond the remit of this book.

Infection and rheumatic disease

Introduction

Infectious agents have been linked directly and indirectly (through organism-specific and autoimmune responses) to a number of acute and chronic inflammatory rheumatic diseases. This chapter will introduce some examples of inflammatory mechanisms (see Table 17.1) and infectious agents (see Table 17.2) linked to rheumatic disease, and then discuss septic arthritis, osteomyelitis, Lyme disease, and rheumatic fever in turn.

Viral pathogens are discussed further in the chapters on the appropriate rheumatic disease. However, protozoal, helminthic, and fungal infections, and details of cell-mediated and immune reactions to infection are beyond the scope of this book.

Table 17.1 Pathogenesis of rheumatic disease associated with infection

Inflammatory process	Basic process	Example	Susceptibility
Local infection at musculoskeletal sites	Infection. Tissue inflammation and direct damage	Pyogenic septic arthritis	Structural damage to joint replacement Diabetes, complement and immunoglobulin deficiencies
Pathogen and pathogen-specific immune response	Infection and organism-specific response. Immune response to intact organism or fragments, probable immune complex-mediated tissue injury	Syndromes associated with viral hepatitis, e.g. Sjögren's syndrome	Not generally established
Pathogens, immune response, and autoimmunity	i. Cross-reactive immune response ii. Infection inferred but not established autoreactivity	Rheumatic fever Rheumatoid arthritis Juvenile idiopathic arthritis Systemic lupus erythematosus	Certain MHC class I and II genes Receptor genes MHC class I and II genes T-cell receptor genes

Table 17.2 Some pathogens associated with arthritis

Class	Examples	Disorder
Bacteria	*Staphylococcus* and *Streptococcus*	Non-gonococcal arthritis
		Septic monoarthritis
		Osteomyelitis
	Neisseria spp	Gonococcal arthritis
	Brucella	Septic monoarthritis
		Spondylarthropathy
	Chlamydia	Reactive/Reiter's
Mycobacteria	*M. tuberculosis*	Osteomyelitis
		Spinal disease
		Monoarthropathy
Atypical mycobacteria	*M. avium* complex *M. malmoense*	Septic arthritis in immuno-suppressed patients
Spirochaete	*Borrelia burgdorferi*	Lyme disease
Viruses	Parvovirus B19	Fifth disease
	Rubella	Polyarthropathy
	Hepatitis B	Polyarteritis nodosa
	Hepatitis C	Cryoglobulinaemia
		Sjögren's syndrome
	HIV	Polyarthralgia and myopathy
		Vasculitis
		Sjögrens-like disease
Protozoa	Toxoplasma	Polyarthritis
	Giardia	Oligoarthritis
		Small-vessel vasculitis
	Trypanosoa	Myopathy
Helminths	Toxocara	All cause myositis and arthritis
	Dracunculus	
	Schistosoma	
Fungi	Histoplasma	Cause monoarthropathy
	Cryptococcus	

Pyogenic non-gonococcal and gonococcal arthritides

- Septic arthritis caused by a pyogenic bacterium is a medical emergency. Incidence in the general population is 2–10 per 100 000, rising to 30–70 per 100 000 in those with autoimmune rheumatic disease or prosthetic joint replacements.
- Bacteria can reach a joint through the blood, by direct penetration through the skin, or by local spread from a contiguous infected site.
- Haematogenous spread is by far the most common route for pyogenic joint infection.
- Joints damaged by chronic arthritis (e.g. RA, OA) and prosthetic joints are at ↑ risk of infection. Immunodeficiency states and diabetes are added risk factors. Septic monoarthritis is uncommon in childhood.
- The most common pathogens are *Staphylococcus aureus, Streptococcus* spp and *Neisseria gonorrhoeae* in adults. Up until the development of the 'Hib' vaccine, *Haemophilus influenzae* type b was one of the most common pathogens to affect children. The clinical features and natural history of gonococcal and non-gonococcal arthritis are sufficiently distinct to discuss them separately (see Table 17.3).
- Unusual organisms may be involved in patients with a current history of IV drug abuse, or those who are immunosuppressed.

Management of pyogenic joint infection

Three principles determine outcome: prompt diagnosis, immediate institution of appropriate antibiotics, and adequate drainage of joint.

- Apart from clinical suspicion, specific tests for infection should include joint aspiration, Gram stain, and culture of synovial fluid; blood cultures, probably three sets over consecutive days; skin/rash swabs, and oral and urethral swabs. Surgical drainage may also be required.
- Polymerase chain reaction studies of synovial fluid or tissue may be useful when other cultures have grown no identified organism.
- Plain X-rays in early disease may be unhelpful or show only soft tissue swelling. In later untreated disease, joint space narrowing and erosion will be seen. Ultrasound may show a joint effusion.
- An affected joint should be rested, non-weight-bearing until the inflammation and pain have subsided enough to allow passive mobilization. Mobilization should be encouraged as soon as possible.
- An empirical 'best fit' treatment whilst awaiting results of cultures is IV penicillin and a cephalosporin. Liaison with local microbiology departments will ensure practice is in line with local protocols. If a urinary or GI pathogen (*Enterococcus* spp.) is suspected then the cephalosporin should be replaced with gentamicin initially, and in older patients with underlying disease (or intravenous drug users) consider vancomycin first line rather than penicillin. *Pseudomonas* spp. responds to ceftazidime or ciprofloxacin. Fusidic acid is often given in combination with other treatments as it has good bone penetration.

Table 17.3 Clinical features of gonococcal and non-gonococcal arthritis

Gonococcal arthritis	Non-gonococcal arthritis
Causative agents: *Neisseria gonorrhoeae* *Neisseria meningitidis*	Causative agents: *Staphylococcus aureus* (50% of cases) *Staphylococcus epidermis* (15% of cases) *Streptococcus pyogenes/pneumoniae* (20% of cases) Gram-negative bacteria (10% of cases) anaerobes (5% of cases)
Most often in young, healthy adults	Most often in the very young, old, or underlying joint or medical condition
♀>♂	♂>♀
Hip disease uncommon	Hip disease common (20% of cases)
Migratory polyarthritis common	Polyarthritis uncommon
	Monoarthritis very common
Rash, skin blisters/pustules, tenosynovitis common	Extra-articular manifestations common
Synovial fluid analysis: Gram's stain is positive in 25% culture +ve, 50% lactate normal	Synovial fluid analysis: Gram's stain is positive in 60% culture +ve, 90% lactate raised
Rapid response to therapy	Often slow response, may require surgery
Full recovery in most cases	10% mortality; one-third residual damage

- In general, IV antibiotics are continued for 7 days until the swelling subsides and blood cultures become negative. Thereafter, uncomplicated cases will complete a 4 week course with oral antibiotics. Prolonged courses of up to 6 weeks may be required in severe cases until swelling subsides, inflammatory markers normalize and cultures become negative.
- There is no evidence comparing long and short courses of antibiotics.
- Two further complications warrant mention. First the infected prosthetic joint; in most cases this must be removed together with a prolonged antibiotic course. Orthopaedic colleagues should be alerted to the situation immediately. Second is the chronic synovial swelling that can hamper recovery from purulent gonococcal arthritis. These effusions eventually resolve and may be assisted by NSAIDs.
- Under no circumstances should a joint be injected with corticosteroid if intra-articular infection is suspected, or if there is superficial infection over the skin covering a joint, e.g. cellulitis/psoriasis. Likewise, there is no benefit from intra-articular antibiotics; indeed these drugs may cause a chemical synovitis.

Management of septic bursitis

- The two most common sites of bursal infection are the olecranon and prepatellar bursae. These are usually managed with serial aspiration and oral antibiotics. Those who do not respond will need IV antibiotics ± incision and drainage.
- Osteomyelitis is an occasional complication of chronic infected bursitis.

Mycobacterium tuberculosis

- Until 1985 the USA and Europe saw a decline in the number of tuberculosis (TB) cases. The appearance of acquired immune deficiency syndrome halted that trend. More recently the recurrence of TB has become an important complication of new disease modifying anti-rheumatic therapies with immunosuppressive effects.
- It is estimated that one-third of the world's population is infected with TB. In developed countries <5% of cases of TB develop infection of bone or joints.
- Tuberculosis of bone is usually a low grade and slow progressive infection associated with a variable degree of local and systemic symptoms such as fatigue, weight loss or night sweats. The onset is insidious and usually mono-articular or mono-osseous. Predisposing factors include pre-existing arthritis, alcoholism, prolonged use of corticosteroids, and immune suppression.
- TB can affect any part of the musculoskeletal system. The spine is a common site, whether within a vertebral body, disc, or a paravertebral 'cold', abscess. Spinal cord compression due to vertebral destruction and/or soft tissue swelling due to a abscess is a serious complication and must be treated as an emergency, with review by a neurosurgeon. Spinal stabilization procedures carry a good prognosis in preventing neurological sequelae. Mono-articular disease is seen most often in the weight-bearing joints of the hip, knee, ankle or sacro-iliac joint, in that order. The wrist and shoulder are rarer though well-recognized sites for disease. Osteomyelitis may affect any long bone and is associated with either solitary or multifocal cysts. Poncelet's disease is a feature of active visceral infection; the inflammatory joint/soft-tissue disease is a 'reactive polyarthritis/tenosynovitis'.
- The diagnosis of TB is best made by identifying acid-fast bacilli from a lesion or by histopathological changes in excised tissue. Occasionally a high level of clinical suspicion, in the absence of other identified pathology, will lead the physician to treat empirically. Standard anti-TB regimes should be used for prophylaxis or treatment and surveillance for 1 year after the end of treatment is recommended. Surgical intervention may be necessary; this may take the form for example of tissue-biopsy, debridement of necrotic tissue, or stabilization of a joint or long bone.

Atypical mycobacterial infection

- Patients with autoimmune rheumatic disease on immunosuppressant medication are at risk of developing atypical infections.
- These infections are usually chronic in nature and can mimic an inflammatory flare of rheumatic disease, which can make diagnosis difficult. *M. malmoense* has been described causing tensoynovitis and septic arthritis of the knee. *M. avium* complex and *M. chelonae* osteoarticular infections have also been described.
- Atypical infections should be considered in patients with autoimmune rheumatic disease who present with musculoskeletal symptoms that do not settle with conservative treatment.

Osteomyelitis

- This term is now used to describe any infection involving bone or marrow.
- A number of general, local, and systemic factors need to be taken into account when managing osteomyelitis (see Table 17.4).
- Important pathogens to consider are tuberculosis, pseudomonas, and salmonella.

Investigations

- No single laboratory investigation is reliable enough to be used routinely for the diagnosis of osteomyelitis. An ↑ white cell count and ESR are often not seen despite infection. The CRP is usually ↑. Imaging plays an important part in establishing the diagnosis. Whether a particular imaging technique is successful at picking up osteomyelitis depends partly on the stage of the infective process.
- Once the pathogen has reached bone, a suppurative reaction and marrow oedema occurs. This can be seen using MR imaging. The next stage, vascular congestion, ischaemia, thrombosis, and soft tissue swelling, is readily detected by CT. After 2–3 weeks bone reactions including new periosteal bone formation and decalcification can be seen on plain films.
- Plain films should always be taken if the clinical setting is appropriate, even in assumed early disease, as they may be highly informative.
- Vertebral osteomyelitis is often seen early on plain films. There may be erosion of the vertebral body or disc, and paravertebral abscesses and vertebral collapse are common complications.
- Isotope bone scanning may be helpful in localizing an area of abnormality. ^{99}Tc^{m}-labelled scans are, however, not specific and the negative predictive value is often greater than the positive predictive value in this scenario. ^{67}Ga- or ^{111}I-labelled leucocyte scans are often helpful in localizing infection.

Treatment

- Initial treatment in the acute phase is the same as that for septic monoarthritis (see above). In general, antibiotics are needed for 6 weeks though chronic infection may require long-term (in excess of 3 months) low-dose treatment. In addition to the common IV antibiotics discussed above, rifampicin and clindamycin are often used. They have good bone penetration and excellent activity against Gram-positive bacteria. Rifampicin should not be used alone because of single-agent bacterial resistance. The drug may also turn body fluids red. Clindamycin should be used cautiously in the elderly because of the association with development of *Clostridium difficile* colitis.
- Surgery is required early in the acute phase especially if there is an abscess or spinal involvement. Chronic osteomyelitis implies that dead bone is present and this will require surgical debridement.
- Hyperbaric oxygen has also been used successfully in the treatment of air embolism, osteonecrosis, myonecrosis, and burns patients with infection.

Table 17.4 Factors relevant to the management of osteomyelitis

Factors	Examples
General	Age: neonates tend to harbour S. aureus, enterobacteriaceae, and Beta-haemolytic streptococci. In children > 4 years, H. influenzae is common, and in adults S. aureus
	Bone: long bones (especially lower limb) are more susceptible than short bones. Pelvic and cranial bones are infrequently involved
Local	Chronic lymphoedema
	Venous stasis
	Arterial disease with poor flow
	Scars
	Sensory neuropathy
	Prosthetic material
Systemic	Malnutrition
	Renal and liver failure
	Immunodeficiency
	Diabetes
	Malignancy
	Extremes of age
	Chronic hypoxia
	Parenteral drug use

Lyme disease

- Lyme disease is a tick-borne infection caused by the spirochaete *Borrelia burgdorferi*.
- Cases of Lyme disease have been reported from most states in the United States as well as throughout Europe, the former USSR, China, and Japan.
- The highest incidence is in children under the age of 15 years and middle-aged adults, with seasonal variation, being most common in the summer months of June and July.
- The tick vector, *Ixodes*, is found on rodents mainly and in wooded, brush, or grassy areas. A history of potential exposure in an endemic country within the last 30 days is an important fact to establish in considering the diagnosis. There need not be a clear history of a tick bite.
- The diagnosis is approached clinically, partly based on epidemiological history as well as classical clinical features (see Table 17.5), and confirmed with laboratory tests.

Laboratory investigations

- Confirmation of Lyme disease may be by:
  - isolation of the spirochaete from tissue or body fluid
  - detection of diagnostic levels of IgM or IgG antibodies in the serum or CSF
  - detection of changes in antibody levels between acute phase and convalescent paired sera.
- False-positive results occur in other infections such as syphillis and treponema, as well as in RA and SLE. Western blotting is available as a confirming test, distinguishing between true seroreactivity and false positivity.
- If the serological status is negative then the diagnosis is unlikely and an alternative should be sought.

Treatment

Treatment of Lyme disease is summarized in Table 17.6.

Table 17.5 The clinical features of Lyme disease

System affected	Symptoms
Skin	Erythema migrans (EM). Begins as a red macule/papule expanding over days or weeks to a large round lesion often with partial central clearing. The lesion should measure 5 cm or more. There may be smaller secondary lesions*
	An expanding lesion is often accompanied by general symptoms: fever, fatigue, arthralgia, myalgia, headache
	Months later a chronic lesion, acrodermatitis chronicum atrophicans (ACA), can appear (violaceous infiltrared plaques or nodules)
Musculoskeletal system	Recurrent, brief attacks of joint swelling in one or a few joints (may become chronic—60% of untreated cases weeks to years after infection).
	A post-Lyme syndrome of fatigue, arthralgia and myalgia has been reported. Ongoing infection has been diffcult to prove and this may represent a fibromyalgia/chronic pain syndrome.
Nervous system	Lymphocytic meningitis
	Cranial neuritis (especially facial nerve palsy)
	Radiculoneuropathy (differential Guillain–Barré)
	Encephalomyelitis
Cardiovascular	Acute second- or third-degree atrioventricular conduction defects often associated with myocarditis. Resolve in days to weeks
	Carditis—rare and remits spontaneously

* A similar lesion occurring within hours of a tick bite is usually a hypersensitivity reaction and does not qualify as EM.

Table 17.6 The treatment of Lyme disease

Clinical feature	Treatment
Skin disease	Amoxycillin 500 mg thrice daily for 3 weeks or doxycycline 100 mg twice daily for 3 weeks or cefuroxime 500 mg twice daily for 3 weeks
Septic arthritis	As above except may require treatment for up to 30 days
Neurological disease	Meningitis—IV penicillin, cefotaxime, ceftriaxone/imipenem
Carditis	As oral/IV doses above
Acrodermatitis	Phenoxymethyl penicillin 3 g daily for 3 weeks

Rheumatic fever

- Rheumatic fever is a delayed, non-suppurative sequel to a pharyngeal infection with Lancefield group A β-haemolytic streptococci.
- There is a latent period of 2–3 weeks before the appearance of an illness characterized in one of three classical ways. A symptomatic pharyngitis is seen in 60% cases, migratory arthritis (typically of the large joints), carditis and valvulitis, and central nervous system disease (chorea).
- Whilst the infection is often self-limiting, chronic and progressive damage to cardiac valves occurs leading to cardiac decompensation and death.
- Although there has been a dramatic decline in the United States and Europe, the disease still occurs in these areas, and is common in developing countries. There are an estimated 10–20 million cases per year in these areas, with an annual incidence of 100–200 per 100 000.
- Associations have been described with HLA DR2, 3, and 4.

The clinical features may be summarized in the revised 'Jones' criteria (Table 17.7).

Clinical manifestations and treatment of rheumatic fever
Arthritis
- Joint involvement is more common and often more severe in teenagers and young adults. It tends to start in the large joints of the lower limbs and migrate. Arthropathy tends to occur early and the pain can be severe in the absence of objective signs of inflammation. It lasts 2–3 weeks and is self-limiting.
- NSAIDs are the main treatment for the condition.
- Where one draws the line between the phenomenon of post-streptococcal reactive arthritis (seen in the absence of carditis) and rheumatic fever is difficult. Most patients will fulfil the Jones criteria and therefore should be considered as having rheumatic fever.

Table 17.7 The revised Jones criteria for the diagnosis of acute rheumatic fever (diagnosis requires 2 major, or 1 major and 2 minor criteria)

Major manifestations	Carditis
	Polyarthritis
	Chorea
	Erythema marginatum
	Subcutaneous nodules
Minor manifestations	Fever
	Arthralgia
	Previous rheumatic fever or rheumatic heart disease
Laboratory tests	Raised ESR or CRP
	Normochromic normocytic anaemia
	Prolonged P–R interval on ECG
Supporting evidence	Raised ASO titre*
	Positive throat cultures for group A streptococci
	Recent scarlet fever

* ASO = antistreptolysin O antibodies (titres peak at about 4 weeks, which is about 2 weeks into the clinical onset of rheumatic fever; they fall off rapidly over the following 2–3 months).

Cardiac disease

- Rheumatic heart disease is the most severe outcome of acute rheumatic fever. It remains the major cause of acquired valvular heart disease in the world. The mitral valve (stenosis) is involved more so than the aortic valve. When left unchecked, cardiomegaly and cardiac failure secondary to valvular disease develops.
- Carditis may also occur and is associated with cardiomyopathy and conduction defects including second- or third-degree heart block.

Chorea

- Sydenham's chorea (St Vitus dance) is a neurological disorder consisting of abrupt, purposeless movements, muscle weakness, and emotional disturbance. The hands and face are usually the most obviously affected parts. The movements are not present during sleep but do occur at rest, and may be more marked on one side of the body.
- Chorea may be the sole feature suggesting rheumatic fever (beyond observing new cardiac murmurs) and may occur weeks to months after onset of an arthropathy.

Skin

- The subcutaneous nodules of rheumatic fever are firm and painless. They are located over bony surfaces or near tendons, and are present for 2–4 weeks only, and more often in patients with carditis.
- Erythema marginatum is an evanescent, non-purpuric rash, usually affecting the trunk and proximal part of the limbs, but sparing the face. Because the rash often appears to make a ring, it is also called 'erythema annulare'. The lesions come and go in a matter of hours and heat may make them appear, or become worse. Again, it is more common in association with carditis. They resolve spontaneously.
- Erythema nodosum is rare.

Investigations

- There is no diagnostic investigation.
- Raised inflammatory markers are seen, often with a mild anaemia.
- Serial rises in anti-streptolysin O titres may be seen if measured every 14 days.
- Chest radiograph and ECG to look for conduction defects/cardiomegaly.

Treatment of rheumatic fever

- The mainstay of treatment is an anti-inflammatory agent, usually aspirin.
- If carditis is present, steroids should be started (2 mg/kg/day oral prednisolone for 1–2 weeks tapering over a further 2 weeks).
- Penicillin should be taken for 10 days, even in the absence of ongoing pharyngitis.
- Chorea can be treated with haloperidol 1–2 mg/kg/day, often given with prednisolone, although there is little evidence that this gives added benefit.
- Recurrence is most common within the first 2 years; however, recurrence rates seem to be ↓, and the risk of recurrence ↓ with age at first attack.
- Prophylaxis in those who have had rheumatic fever should probably continue for life, though some clinicians would recommend up to 10 years with antibiotic therapy to cover any dental or invasive procedure. Prophylaxis can be given either as oral penicillin V, 250 000 units twice daily, or as penicillin G, 1.2 million units IM once every 3–4 weeks. Erythromycin at 250 mg daily may be used if there is an allergy to penicillins. The future may bring new streptococcal vaccines.

Miscellaneous conditions

Behçet's syndrome

- Behçet's syndrome is a systemic vasculitis of unknown aetiology. It is most common in the Mediterranean basin, the Middle East, and the Far East.
- The usual onset of the syndrome is in the third or fourth decade.
- Onset is rare in children and after the age of 45 years.
- The ♂: ♀ ratio is approximately equal but the syndrome tends to run a more severe course in men and the young.
- Based on registries the prevalence is about 1 in 300 000 in Northern Europe, 1 in 10 000 in Japan, and 40 in 10 000 in Turkey.
- The syndrome is classically associated with HLA B5—its presence associated with greater disease severity. However, there are geographical variations. Patients from Mediterranean countries and Japan show this association with B5 whereas, with the exception of those with eye disease, United States and United Kingdom patients do not. In patients of Israeli origin there is an association with HLA B51.
- The full-blown syndrome might be easy to identify but there are conditions that mimic the incomplete picture, namely reactive arthritis, Steven–Johnson syndrome, and inflammatory bowel disease with skin and eye complications.
- There are no laboratory findings specific to the condition. The ESR and CRP are often only moderately raised.

Clinical features and their management

Skin and mucosa involvement (see Table 18.1)
- Oral aphthae are almost always present, frequently the first manifestation of the syndrome, and may precede any other features by several years. They are indistinguishable from ordinary ulcers, but tend to be multiple, more frequent, and may heal with scarring.
- Genital ulceration in ♂ is most prominent over the scrotum (90%). Urethritis is not seen unless there is a meatal ulcer. In the ♀ the labia are commonly affected. Cervical ulcers are rare.
- Skin lesions may be nodular (resembling erythema nodosum), acneiform, or vasculitic.
- The pathergy reaction, a hyperreactivity of the skin to a needle prick, is peculiar to this syndrome and pyoderma gangrenosum. After skin puncture with a needle, a papule or pustule forms in 24–48 h. The reaction is seldom found in patients from Northern Europe or the United States, but is positive in 60% and 70% of patients from Japan and Turkey respectively.
- Mild oral and genital ulceration may respond to topical colchicine 1.5 mg/day. More severe disease may require AZA 2.5 mg/kg/day or thalidomide 50–300 mg daily. Non-steroidal anti-inflammatory drugs can help pain control.

Eye disease
- This is a serious complication and a negative prognostic factor. Eye disease is more common in ♂ and patients <25 years of age.

Table 18.1 The clinical findings in Behçet's syndrome

Lesion	Prevalence (%)
Aphthous ulcers	97–100
Genital ulcers	80–90
Skin lesions	80
Eye lesions	50
Arthritis	40–50
Thrombophlebitis	25
Neurological disease	1–15
Gastrointestinal disease	0–25

- Disease is bilateral in 90% of cases and is usually a chronic relapsing panuveitis. The presence of a hypopyon (cells in the anterior chamber) is almost always associated with severe retinal vasculitis after which there is almost always some structural damage despite treatment. The extent of this damage determines the course of eye disease in Behçet's syndrome.
- Topical steroids and mydriatics with close supervision may be sufficient in mild disease, but severe disease requires the addition of AZA 2.5 mg/kg/day and/or cyclosporin A 5 mg/kg/day to the topical regimen.

Musculoskeletal system involvement
- Joint involvement is seen in about 50% of patients. It is usually mono- or oligoarticular but can be symmetrical, the latter common at the wrist and elbow, mimicking RA.
- Chronic synovitis is rare, self-limiting, non-erosive, non-deforming, arthropathy being the normal pattern of disease.
- In general, knees, ankles, wrists, and elbows are involved (in descending order of frequency).
- Back pain is rare.
- Pain may respond to NSAIDs. Inflammatory disease often requires the introduction of AZA 2.5 mg/kg/day or sulphasalazine 2–3 g/day.

Cardiovascular and pulmonary involvement
- Endocarditis, myocarditis, pericarditis, coronary vasculitis, and ventricular aneurysms can all occur but are rare.
- Venous involvement is one of the main features of Behçet's syndrome. Thrombophlebitis occurs in 25% of all patients. Limb venous thrombosis is often observed. ⚠ Occlusion of the suprahepatic veins, Budd–Chiari syndrome, carries a high mortality.
- Pulmonary embolism is quite rare despite high rates of thrombophlebitis. It might be explained by the difference in architecture of thromboses seen in Behçet's syndrome and normal (e.g. postoperative) thromboses. The former tends to adhere throughout its length to the vein wall; the latter tends to have a long, non-adherent and potentially embolic tail.

- Arterial lesions can occur anywhere. Aneurysms may develop and rupture. This is frequently fatal.
- The pulmonary pathology of Behçet's syndrome is related to arterial vasculitis. Aneurysms, thromboses, and infarcts are found.
- Aspirin and NSAIDs can be used to relieve the symtoms of phlebitis. Aneurysms and arterial occlusion require cytotoxic therapy with cyclophosphamide 2.5 mg/kg/day and prednisolone 1 mg/kg/day; surgery may also be indicated. There remains debate as to whether to use heparin or oral anticoagulants for the thrombophlebitis. In practice it is most likely they will be used in the setting of acute vessel obstruction.

Neurological involvement

- Prospective surveys suggest a prevalence rate of 5% for neurological disease in the condition.
- Pyramidal signs are the most common, followed by cerebellar and sensory symptoms and signs. The most common site is the brainstem. Meningeal irritation and dementia may also feature. As is the case with eye disease, central nervous involvement is often more severe in ♂.
- In contrast to other vasculitides, peripheral neuropathy is unusual.
- CNS disease should be treated with IV methylprednisolone, and cyclophosphamide should be considered.

Gastrointestinal involvement

- Whilst seen in up to one-third of patients in Japan, gastrointestinal disease is rare in patients from the Mediterranean basin.
- The basic pathology is mucosal ulceration, seen most often in the ileum and caecum. The course is one of relapse and remission, with a distinct tendency to perforation.
- Ulceration may respond to prednisolone 0.5–1 mg/kg/day and/or sulphasalazine 2–6 g/day. Clearly in the event of, for example, severe malaena or perforation, surgery may be necessary.

Renal involvement

- This is seen much less than might be expected in a systemic vasculitis. There are occasional reports of glomerulonephritis. Amyloidosis usually presents with nephrotic syndrome.
- About 5% of ♂ develop epididymitis. Treatment is symptom control.

Treatment of Behçet's

- Thalidomide, dapsone, and colchicine have all been used with some degree of effect on orogenital ulceration.
- Warfarin should be used in the usual way for thrombotic episodes.
- Interferon-α has been used to ↓ aphthous ulcers and skin lesions.
- There have been several case reports describing rapid efficacy of anti-TNF-α agents.
- The condition has a high morbidity; a 20-year follow-up study estimated a mortality of 10%.

Sarcoidosis

- Sarcoidosis is a multisystem disease of unknown aetiology, characterized by the presence of multiple, non-caseating granulomas in involved tissue.
- It occurs worldwide, but the prevalence, clinical features, and outcome varies. It is seen more often in developed versus underdeveloped, Western versus Eastern, and in Northern versus Southern European countries. Sweden and Denmark have prevalence rates of 60 per 100 000: the United Kingdom 20 per 100 000. In the United States, sarcoidosis is 10–15 times more prevalent in the African/Caribbean population than in Caucasians. There is also an ↑ incidence of sarcoidosis in families. Recently studies have suggested a link between HLA B8, DR3, and acute sarcoidosis with arthritis.
- Acute sarcoidosis presents with rapid onset fever, erythema nodosum, and hilar lymphadenopathy. This condition has a high rate of remission and a good prognosis, the chest radiograph clearing within 1 year in 60% of cases.
- Chronic sarcoidosis is less common and has a subtle, insidious, progressive, and highly variable clinical course (see Table 18.2).
- Sarcoidosis is rare in childhood, and usually indolent. If arthritis occurs it is usually before 5 years of age and associated with eye and cutaneous disease.

Musculoskeletal manifestations of sarcoid

Joints

- Distinctive patterns of arthropathy are seen in both acute and chronic sarcoidosis. In acute disease, a transient flitting arthralgia can precede the emergence of fever, etc. The arthritis is usually symmetrical and can persist for 1–4 months on average, and in association with erythema nodosum (EN). Effusions are common at the knees and ankles. After recovery, acute sarcoidosis only occasionally recurs.
- Chronic arthritis is uncommon in sarcoidosis, particularly monoarthritis and involvement of the spine. Again, knees and ankles appear to be most often involved with inflammatory disease, characterized by acute exacerbation with synovial thickening and effusions. Unlike acute sarcoidosis, a history of EN is unusual. Chronic polyarthritis is also more frequent in ♀ than ♂. It may progress to joint deformity and destruction.

Bones

- Bone involvement occurs in 5% of all patients with sarcoidosis. Bone cysts are seen most often in the hands and feet and are most frequently seen in patients with persistent disease and/or lupus pernio. Cysts are often asymptomatic and found by chance on plain radiographs. Clinically they can present in the phalanges with 'sausage-like' swollen digits.
- Other radiological features include thickening of cortical bone, acrosclerosis, and joint destruction.

Table 18.2 Clinical manifestations in chronic sarcoidosis

Organ/system	Clinical features
Lung	Parenchymal disease in > 90% of cases
Skin	Lupus pernio, plaques, and nodules
Ocular	Uveitis, conjunctivitis, sicca
Lymphatics	Lymphadenopathy, splenomegaly
Bone marrow	Infiltration
Hepatic	Failure, granulomata, portal hypertension
Renal	Nephrocalcinosis, granulomata, glomerular disease
Cardiac	Arteritis, cardiomyopathy, conduction abnormalities
Nervous system	Central and peripheral neuropathy. Intracerebral lesions. Meningitis. Seizures
Granulomata	Endocrine and reproductive organs. Gastrointestinal tract. Salivary/lacrimal glands. Nose, tonsils, and larynx

- Occasionally lytic lesions appear in vertebral bodies, leading to back pain and crush fractures. Lytic lesions may also be seen in the skull bones and long bones.

Muscles

- Often asymptomatic, in the early stages of acute sarcoidosis granulomatous muscle involvement is common (50–80%). It may present as proximal pain, tenderness, and weakness. Involvement may be focal with a granulomatous mass or diffuse and symmetrical myopathy, the latter leading to progressive weakness and atrophy.
- Electromyography looks similar to that of polymyositis.

Investigations and treatment of sarcoidosis

- The red cell count is usually normal. Leucopenia can be seen in up to one-third of cases, and eosinophilia in one-quarter. Thrombocytopenia is a relatively common problem.
- The ESR may be ↑ in the acute phase, particularly if EN is present.
- Reports of hypercalcaemia vary widely from 2–60%. The level tends to fluctuate and the reasons for such wide variation remain unclear.
- Liver function tests may be deranged.
- One-third of patients have significant proteinuria.
- Epithelial cells found in the granulomas produce angiotensin-converting enzyme (ACE). Serial measurements of this enzyme can be useful in monitoring the course of the disease.
- As sarcoidosis can resemble other diseases such as lymphoma and tuberculosis, it is advisable to obtain histological confirmation of the diagnosis. Peripheral tissues such as skin or salivary glands may be helpful. Transbronchial lung biopsy is widely used and highly sensitive and selective.

- Acute, transient disease requires rest and NSAIDs. Occasionally, in severe acute sarcoidosis, corticosteroids may be required.
- Most patients with chronic disease will require steroid therapy, the decision to treat more often related to systemic involvement than articular disease.
- No therapy is required for asymptomatic osseous or cystic bone disease, or asymptomatic muscle disease. The place for steroids in chronic sarcoid myopathy remains uncertain.

Miscellaneous skin conditions associated with arthritis

Panniculitis

Panniculitis refers to inflammation within the subcutaneous fat. It is a dynamic inflammatory process involving neutrophils, leucocytes, and histiocytes that ends in fibrosis, and, sometimes, granulomatous change.

The are four categories of panniculitis, based on histopathology:

- Septal panniculitis
- Lobular panniculitis
- Mixed type septal and lobular
- Panniculitis with vasculitis.

Septal panniculitis

This includes erythema nodosum (EN) and Vilanova's disease (subacute nodular migratory panniculitis). EN is a common, acute, and self-limiting condition found typically over the anterior tibial surface. It usually heals within 4–6 weeks without scarring, though a rare form can cause ulceration and a migratory form can occur for several years (more often in women of average age 45 years). The causes and associations of EN are shown in Table 18.3.

Lobular panniculitis

Listed below are a number of conditions that cause lobular panniculitis.

- *Weber–Christian disease*: a relapsing, febrile, nodular non- suppurative disorder. There may be multiple recurrent nodules plus fever, and arthralgia, myalgia, and abdominal pain are common. Any area of the body containing fat can become involved, e.g. mesentery, heart, lung, liver, kidney. There is a 10–15% mortality. Investigations may show:
  - typical histological features on biopsy
  - ↑ ESR
  - anaemia
  - leucopenia
  - leucocytosis
  - ↓ complement.
- *Lipogranulomatosis*: this group of conditions tends to occur in children. Multiple lesions, often on the extremities, resolve with subcutaneous atrophy.
- *Post steroid use*: the pathogenesis of this rare condition is not understood. It seems to be limited to children, occurs on withdrawal of corticosteroids, and may clear up on steroid readministration.
- *α1-antitrypsin deficiency*: may respond to doxycycline.
- *Pancreatitis*.
- *Calcifying panniculitis* is a feature of chronic renal failure. It is not the same as metastatic calcification. The prognosis is poor even with good calcium-phosphate balance. Parathyroidectomy may help.
- *Lipodermatosclerosis*: this condition may be a result of venous insufficiency and thrombophlebitis. It may respond to intralesional corticosteroid or low-dose aspirin.

Table 18.3 Aetiological causes of EN

Cause	Examples
Infection	Streptococcal
	TB/leprosy
	Yersinia/Salmonella
	Histoplasmosis
	Blastomycosis
	Psitticosis
Drugs	Penicillin
	Sulphonamides
Pregnancy	
Diseases	Sarcoidosis
	Inflammatory bowel disease
	Collagen vascular disease (SLE, scleroderma, dermatomyositis)
	Malignancy (rare)
	Sweet's syndrome

- *Lupus profundus* is a rare manifestation of chronic cutaneous SLE, occurring in <3% of cases of SLE. The lesions are usually tender and may ulcerate and calcify. The lesions commonly occur on the face, upper arms, and buttocks, and may underly an area of discoid lupus. The lesions do not seem to follow the course of the systemic disease. It may respond to steroids.
- Factitial.

Panniculitis with vasculitis
This is seen in small-vessel and medium-vessel vasculitis. The reader is referred to Chapter 14.
Treatments include:
- Treatment of the underlying disease or agent
- NSAIDs
- Bed rest and limb elevation
- Antimalarials
- Steroids
- Dapsone
- Colchicine
- Azathioprine
- Cyclosporin.

Neutrophilic dermatoses

The neutrophilic dermatoses are a group of non-infectious disorders characterized by the presence of an angiocentric, vessel-based, 1° neutrophilic inflammatory cell infiltrate. The disorders can be divided into those that cause vessel wall destruction (vasculitis) and those that do not. Table 18.4 lists the causes of non-infectious neutrophilic dermatoses. The majority of diseases are discussed in detail in their own chapters in this book. This section will discuss Sweet's syndrome, and pyoderma gangrenosum.

Sweet's syndrome

- This condition is rare and occurs more often in ♀ than ♂ (ratio 3.7:1), between the ages of 30–70 years. It has occasionally been reported in children. The pathogenesis is unknown.
- The characteristic features are myalgia, fever, arthralgia, and painful erythematous plaques (occasionally nodules resembling erythema nodosum). Untreated the lesions resolve over 6–8 weeks but new lesions appear recurrently and chronically. The condition is usually an acute, steroid-responsive, self-limiting disorder. If longer-term treatment is required, steroid dosage may be reduced by the addition of an NSAID, dapsone, colchicine, or possibly methotrexate.
- A 2° cause for the condition should be sought (see Table 18.5).

Pyoderma gangrenosum

- This is an uncommon, ulcerative, cutaneous condition associated with several systemic diseases (see Table 18.6).
- The lesion is charaterized by an erythematous, violaceous border overhanging a central area of ulceration and necrosis. The lesions start as discrete pustules, most often on the legs, and are often extremely painful, healing with scars.
- There is no specific treatment. An underlying disease should be sought. Treatments include topical sodium cromoglycate or 5-amino salicylic acid, oral sulphonamides, dapsone, and cortico-steroids (oral and systemic).

Table 18.4 Non-infectious neutrophilic dermatoses

Group	Examples
Non-angiocentric	Psoriasis
	Reactive arthritis
	Acne fulminans
Angiocentric and vessel destruction	Leucocytoclastic vasculitis
	Polyarteritis nodosa
Angiocentric no vessel destruction	Sweet's syndrome
	Pyoderma gangrenosum
	Bowel-associated Dermatosis–arthritis
	Behçet's disease
	Rheumatoid arthritis
	Ulcerative colitis
	Familial Mediterranean fever

Table 18.5 The associations with Sweet's syndrome

Associations	Examples
Haematological malignancy	Leukaemia
	Lymphoma
	Myelodysplastic disorders
Solid tumours	Breast
	Gastric
	Genitourinary
	Colon
Infectious diseases	HIV
	Hepatitis
	Tuberculosis
	Salmonella
Inflammatory bowel disease	Ulcerative colitis
	Crohn's disease
Rheumatic diseases	Rheumatoid arthritis
	Systemic lupus erythematosus
	Sjögren's syndrome
	Behçet's disease

Table 18.6 Diseases associated with pyoderma gangrenosum

Association	Examples
Rheumatic diseases	Seronegative spondylarthropathy
	Rheumatoid arthritis
	Osteoarthritis
	Psoriatic arthritis
	Systemic lupus erythematosus
	Wegener's granulomatosis
	Sarcoidosis
	Takayasu's arteritis
Haematological diseases	Leukaemia
	Myelofibrosis
	Gammaglobulinaemia
	Polycythemia rubra vera
Gastrointestinal diseases	Inflammatory bowel disease
	Chronic active hepatitis
	Primary biliary cirrhosis
Other	Solid tumours
	Diabetes mellitus
	C7 complement deficiency

Multicentric reticulohistiocytosis
- This is a rare systemic disease, primarily a disorder of adults in their fifth decade. It is recognized clinically by the combination of papular and nodular skin lesions and a severe destructive polyarthritis.
- The disorder is distinct from the solitary nodule lesion of the reticulocytoma in that the latter is not associated with systemic disease. Multicentric reticulohistiocytosis may involve any organ system.
- The arthritis may mimic a RA pattern. Often the distal interphalangeal joints are involved and the destruction may give a picture similar to arthritis mutilans.
- The skin lesions occur in approximately 90% of cases. Histologically, the infiltrate consists of multicentric giant cells and histiocytes from the monocyte-macrophage lineage. The lesions are usually numerous, non-pruritic, skin coloured (or yellow/brown), and range in size from millimetres to several centimetres in diameter. They occur most often on the dorsum of the hands and on the face (at the nose, corner of the mouth, and ears). Extensive facial involvement may lead to a 'leonine' facies.
- About 25% of cases have xanthelasma.

- One-third of cases have constitutional symptoms/signs such as weight loss or fever.
- Approximately 25% of cases have been reported to have malignant (mostly solid tumour) disease. The investigation of the condition therefore requires a thorough screen for rheumatic and malignant disease.
- The are no specific laboratory markers. Histology is helpful. Biopsies may be taken from skin or inflamed synovium.
- The differential diagnosis includes:
  - rheumatoid or psoriatic arthritis
  - sarcoid dactylitis
  - xanthoma
  - histiocytosis X—a disorder of children
  - histiocytoma or tendon sheath giant-cell tumour—usually solitary.
- As a rule the condition 'waxes and wanes' and tends to 'burn out' after 5–8 years.
- The prognosis is dominated by the presence of an underlying malignancy. There is consensus that cyclophosphamide or chlorambucil is the treatment of choice. Corticosteroids do not seem to have any major impact on the skin lesions, though they can help joint inflammation. MTX has also been reported as successful in some cases.

Chronic regional pain syndrome

This syndrome is characterized by variable dysfunction of the musculoskeletal, skin, neurological, and vascular systems. It may occur in a variety of situations with a number of clinical manifestations varying around central core features. As such several terms have evolved, describing the same phenomenon:

- Reflex sympathetic dystrophy syndrome or Algodystrophy
- Sudeck's atrophy
- Shoulder–hand syndrome
- Transient osteoporosis
- Regional migratory osteoporosis
- Post-trauma painful osteoporosis

Complex regional pain syndrome (CRPS) has 2 types; type 1 is symptoms in the absence of nerve injury, and type 2 ('causalgia') in the presence of nerve injury.

Epidemiology

- CRPS is a common disorder. It affects both sexes equally and occurs at any age in all races and geographical regions. Typically the syndrome involves the distal part of a limb, e.g. forearm or foot.
- The early clinical features of the condition include:
  - pain
  - soft tissue swelling (may be synovitis if over a joint)
  - reticular/livedo rash
  - warmth over affected part occasionally there may be localized
  - sweating and piloerection.
- The pain has several particular characteristics and is often described as 'burning'. The features include:
  - allodynia—an otherwise innocuous stimulus produces pain
  - hyperalgesia—↑ pain perception to a given stimulus
  - hyperpathia—delayed over-reaction, often after repetitive cutaneous stimulus.

The net effect is abnormal tenderness to even minor stimuli.

- Trauma (whether accident, burn, surgery, etc.) is the most common triggering event. The event may have even seemed trivial or minor at the time.
- Several neurological conditions may act as triggers, including, for example, hemiplegia and meningitis. Peripheral nerve root injury may also lead to the syndrome.
- Pregnancy, tumours, and prolonged immobilization have also been linked as possible triggering factors. However, 25% of cases have no clear trigger.
- It is important to try and identify psychosocial stresses.
- The signs and symptoms of pain, swelling, etc. (see above), are traditionally placed as 'stage I' of the condition. In most cases the symptoms persist and fluctuate, though they may just gradually resolve. Stage II is a period of dystrophic change. This tends to occur several months after onset of the disorder. The affected region becomes cool, pale, and often cyanosed in colour with abnormal sensation (dysaesthesia).

There is a ↓ in hair and nail growth, osteopenia develops, and eventually atrophy (stage III) of skin and subcutaneous tissue occurs; at this point the condition becomes difficult to treat and reverse. Most cases tend not to progress beyond stage I, or at most early stage II.

Investigations

- There is no abnormality of acute-phase reactants nor biochemistry, except (and not suggested as a test in this context) evidence of bone demineralization manifest as raised urine hydroxyproline excretion.
- Although essentially a clinical diagnosis, CRPS does have some radiological and nuclear medicine imaging characteristics. No technique is diagnostic. Plain radiographs, DEXA, and MR may show features of osteoporosis.
- Thermography can demonstrate changes in cutaneous temperature.
- Perhaps of most value, and high specificity, is the triple-phase technetium scintigraphy study, showing three phases of abnormal early regional blood flow, blood pool, and late bone uptake respectively.

Management

- Success in treatment of this condition probably hinges on focusing on the whole individual and not the regional symptoms, and making an early and accurate diagnosis. Attention to anxiety, psychosocial stressors, pain behaviour, and sleep disturbance is important. The patient often requires repeated reassurance and counselling. The aim should be to resume premorbid levels of activity if possible. In this respect, early intervention with physiotherapy and hydrotherapy should be considered.
- Tricyclic antidepressants can help correct sleep disturbance and increase the pain threshold.
- TENS may help pain control and allow entry into a physical activity programme.
- In severe cases, regional sympathetic or ganglion blocks can control pain sufficiently to start more vigorous physiotherapy or exercise programmes.
- Some clinicians have also had success with corticosteroids and with pamidronate. There are no controlled trials of this or any other therapy mentioned above.

Relapsing polychondritis

- This is an uncommon multisystem disorder of unknown aetiology, characterized by episodic and sometimes progressive inflammation of cartilage leading to destruction and fibrosis.
- Common sites of involvement include the ear, nose, larynx, joints, heart, and eyes (cornea and sclera) (see Table 18.7).
- The disease predominantly affects Caucasians in the fourth to fifth decades of life.
- Approximately 30% of cases have an underlying systemic rheumatic or autoimmune disease such as RA, systemic lupus, Sjögren's syndrome, thyroiditis, or ulcerative colitis.
- There are no specific laboratory tests. The diagnosis is made on clinical grounds.

Treatment of relapsing polychondritis

- There are no controlled trials and the condition is rare. Intervention is based on anecdotal experience.
- Mild symptoms may be controlled with NSAIDs alone. Dapsone may also be of value. Corticosteroids (high doses, 1 mg/kg daily) may control systemic disease, particularly respiratory complications. In severe cases of, for example, vasculitis or renal disease, azathioprine or cyclophosphamide should be considered. Some cases may require temporary or permanent tracheostomy if laryngeal involvement is severe.

Table 18.7 Extent of organ involvement in relapsing polychondritis

Organ	Clinical feature	Prevalence (%)
External ear		85
Arthritis	Non-deforming and non-erosive	75
Nose		60
Eye	Episcleritis, uveitis, retinal vasculitis	50
Respiratory tract	Dysphonia, dyspnoea, stridor	50
Internal ear		40
Skin	Erythema nodosum vasculitis, Behçet- like ulceration	25
Kidney	Glomerulonephritis (poor prognosis)	20
Heart	Pericarditis, aortic valve incompetence, heart block	10
Blood vessels	Aneurysms	8

Miscellaneous disorders of synovium

Pigmented villonodular synovitis (PVNS)

- The term PVNS is used for a group of conditions that are characterized by the exuberant proliferation of synovial cells and supporting tissues of the joint, tendons, and bursae.
- The condition is rare (estimated 2 cases per million population).
- As the name implies, there is a villous and nodular proliferation. This is non-malignant and associated with iron and fat deposition. Repeated small haemorrhages and lipid deposits stain the synovium a red-brown and yellow respectively.
- The cause of the condition remains unknown though some studies have proposed a link with chronic repetitive trauma or haemarthroses.
- Experimental models and clinical experience with patients with bleeding disorders have, however, not reproduced the condition.
- The classic presentation is with a monoarthritis. Any age may be affected though it tends to occur more often in both sexes in the third or fourth decade. The knee is the most commonly affected joint and 'diffuse' disease, as opposed to 'localized' disease on clinical grounds, is more aggressive and more likely to recur.
- Insidious onset of pain and swelling in the absence of trauma, with a serosanguinous synovial fluid aspirate and a characteristic synovial biopsy are the basis for a diagnosis of PVNS. There are some important conditions to consider in the differential diagnosis:
  - malignant synovioma
  - synovial haemangioma
  - synovial chondromatosis
  - tuberculous arthritis
  - amyloidosis
  - haemophilia.
- Imaging may be helpful. Plain radiographs are often normal though may show soft tissue swelling that can be radiodense with haemosiderin deposition. Calcification, however, is not a feature of PVNS and would suggest a malignant lesion or perhaps chondromatosis (see below).
- Erosions and subchondral cysts (also on non-weight-bearing surfaces) can be seen. Loss of joint space can occur late in the condition. Typically this is not associated with juxta-articular osteoporosis or osteophyte formation. MRI can be highly suggestive of PVNS if there is sufficient haemosiderin and fat deposition in the lesion.

Treatment of PVNS

- Localized forms of PVNS are treated by marginal excision of the lesion.
- The prognosis is good.
- Diffuse forms of PVNS tend to be progressive and recurrent. Treatment techniques have included synovectomy, radiation therapy, arthrodesis, and arthroplasty. No one technique has particularly good results; however, there is only limited experience and little long-term follow-up.
- The most commonly reported treatment is surgical synovectomy.

Synovial chondromatosis

- This condition is characterized by chondrometaplasia of the sub-synovial connective tissues. The joint is filled with a thickened white/blue nodular synovium.
- The cause is unknown, the disorder uncommon, and the process non-malignant. It tends to occur more often in middle-aged men and has never been reported in prepubertal childhood.
- Clinically the condition resembles PVNS (above) but tends to be slowly progressive and sometimes self-limiting with regression. Plain radiographs may show punctate calcification outlining the joint margin.
- The diagnosis should be confirmed on synovial biopsy. In rare cases there may be transformation to a chondrosarcoma.
- Treatment is surgical and usually managed with arthroscopy, removing loose bodies and/or the synovial membrane.

Amyloidosis

- A number of disorders and clinical settings are associated with the extracellular deposition of the proteinaceous, fibrillar material, amyloid. The low solubility of amyloid and relative resistance to proteolytic enzymes contributes to the irreversible and often progressive course of amyloidosis.
- Despite morphological similarities (including the formation of a beta pleated sheet), amyloid is a heterogeneous group of proteins. Present in all types of amyloid fibrils is, however, a carbohydrate moiety in the form of glycosaminoglycans and proteoglycans. Most forms of amyloid also contain the extrafibrillar protein, amyloid-P (protein AP).
- The different amyloid proteins are often related to distinct clinical forms of amyloidosis. At the present time at least 17 proteins have been characterized. The detail of these proteins is beyond the scope of this book. However, two types are important as manifestations of a response to chronic systemic inflammation; amyloid-L (AL) and amyloid-A (AA).
- Protein AL consists of monoclonal immunoglobulin light chains and is seen in idiopathic and myeloma-associated amyloidosis. The clinical features of AL and AA are shown in Table 18.8.
- Protein AA (derived from serum amyloid A (SSA), an acute phase apolipoprotein) is associated with conditions such as secondary 'reactive' amyloidosis and FMF (see Table 18.9).
- The mechanisms by which the various precursor proteins are converted to insoluble amyloid fibrils, the reasons for the predilection of certain proteins for particular organs and tissues, and the reasons why not all cases of a particular chronic inflammatory disorder develop amyloid are not clear. The most studied mechanisms are those associated with the reactive AA type amyloidosis.
- Reactive AA amyloidosis is mainly associated with long-standing infectious or non-infectious inflammation, and less frequently with cancer. In the context of rheumatic disorders AA amyloidosis is mainly seen in:
  - Adult RA
  - JIA
  - AS.
- There are several rheumatic conditions that are rarely associated with AA amyloidosis. In these conditions there is a relatively low level of the acute-phase protein SAA. These conditions include:
  - SLE
  - systemic sclerosis
  - SS.

Table 18.8 The clinical features of AL and AA amyloidosis

	Organ/condition	Comment
AL amyloidosis	Heart	Death occurs in 50% of cases from: restrictive cardiomyopathy, congestive heart failure, conduction disturbances
	Lungs	90% develop cough and dyspnoea
	Skin	40% of cases: papules, nodules, tumours
	Neuropathy	10% of cases get carpal tunnel syndrome
	Macroglossia	
	Vasculopathy	
	Amyloid arthropathy	
	Autonomic disturbance	
Common to AL and AA	Weakness	
	Fatigue	
	Weight loss	
	Renal	Nephrotic syndrome/renal failure—major cause of death in AA*, cause of death in one-third of AL patients
	Gastrointestinal tract	Malabsorption, obstruction, diarrhoea, hepatosplenomegaly*

*In AA amyloid the spleen, liver, and kidneys are often involved first.

Investigations

- The diagnosis of amyloidosis is made by tissue biopsy (usually rectal or abdominal subcutaneous fat), and alkaline Congo red stain showing the amyloid deposits as apple green/yellow under the polarizing microscope.
- The strong calcium-dependent affinity of protein AP for amyloid fibrils is also used diagnostically in radiolabelled serum amyloid protein (SAP) scintigraphy. This technique may localize amyloid and could be of value in assessing degrees of response to treatment.
- Other laboratory tests include DNA analysis to detect the genetic variants of proteins known to make up the hereditary amyloidoses.

Treatment of amyloidosis

- The condition is progressive and there is no cure. Marked heterogeneity of the hereditary amyloidoses makes counselling difficult too. The processes by which the disorder may be controlled include liver transplantation for lysosomal amyloidosis and bone marrow transplantation.
- In the rheumatic diseases, cytotoxic drugs such as chlorambucil and melphalan (often in combination with corticosteroids) have improved the prognosis in RA and JIA patients.

Familial Mediterranean fever

- This condition has been in the literature since the early 1900s and was more recently characterized in the 1960s.
- Most cases (80%) present before the age of 20 and it is very rare to present with a first attack after the age of 40.
- Abnormalities of the gene coding for the protein pyrin (on chromosome 16) have been identified and constitute the only test specific for the diagnosis of FMF. FMF is an autosomal recessive disorder. It most frequently affects people of eastern Mediterranean descent, especially Armenians, Arabs, and Sephardic and Ashkenazi Jews.
- The most common symptoms of abdominal pain and pleuritis are related to serositis, present in up to 95% of cases. 75% of cases develop an arthritis that may be erosive and is most often isolated to a single joint. A rash with dermal neutrophil infiltration (rathar than a vasculitis) is common and looks not unlike erysipelas.
- Amyloidosis can occur in up to 40% of cases and does not appear to be associated with severity or frequency of attacks of FMF. Patients may develop renal failure, proteinuria, or malabsorption.
- Treatment includes NSAIDs for pain and continuous colchicine (1–2 mg daily). Up to 65% of cases can achieve complete remission with this regimen. A further 30% can achieve partial remission. All remaining cases should stay on 2 mg colchicine daily to help prevent amyloidosis. Concern over long-term use of prophylactic colchicine in FMF has not been borne out, the benefits of controlling the condition outweighing any complication. It is, however, recommended that amniocentesis be a routine part of antenatal treatment to exclude colchicine-related chromosomal aberrations. Corticosteroids are usually unhelpful.

Table 18.9 The clinical features of Familial Mediterranean fever

Clinical feature	Comments
Short attacks of high fever (39–40°C)	Repeated and unpredictable
Painful inflammation	Abdomen—90% of cases (may develop adhesions)
	Chest—45% of cases. Often febrile pleurisy
	Joints—most often monoarthropathy, especially the knee with acute onset pain and swelling with resolution over 1–4 weeks. Aspetic necrosis
	Skin—erysipelas-like erythema, often below the knee to the dorsum of the foot
	Other—orchitis, mild splenomegaly
AA amyloidosis	Renal—early, terminal renal failure Cardiac, hepatic, gut—see Table 18.8
Autosomal-recessive inheritance	Virtual ethnic restriction: Sephardi Jews, Ashkenazi Jews, Armenians, Anatolian Turks, Arabs

Tumour necrosis factor-associated periodic syndrome (TRAPs)

- This term covers a group of conditions similar to FMF but occurring in non-Mediterranean areas and associated with mutations in the TNF receptor superfamily type 1A.
- The onset is in the second decade and presents with rash, fever, abdominal pain, disabling arthralgia, and myalgia.
- 20% of patients develop amyloid AA.
- Colchicine is not efficacious. Corticosteroids may reduce the length and severity of attacks. Etanercept has been used successfully in some patients.

Fibromyalgia and chronic widespread pain

- Chronic widespread pain (CWP) is a common finding present in 5–10% of the general population. In the absence of diffuse degenerative or inflammatory rheumatic disease the two most common conditions found in association with CWP are fibromyalgia (FM) and joint hyper-mobility syndrome (JHS) (see Chapter 16).
- Compared to the point prevalence of CWP (10%), chronic regional pain is 25%.
- CWP affects ♀ more than ♂ with a ratio of 1.5:1, and is defined as pain for >6 months in 2 or more sites both above and below the pelvis.
- Treatment of CWP is similar to that for FM and JHS and discussed below.
- Fibromyalgia has two cardinal features: CWP and diffuse tenderness at discrete anatomical sites (see Table 18.10 and Chapter 2).
  In addition a range of symptoms that include fatigue, mood, and sleep disturbances add to the morbidity. It is a diagnosis of exclusion.
- Using the classification criteria for FM (see Table 18.10), prevalence rates range from 0.5–4% with a ♀:♂ ratio of 10:1.
- FM cases tend to aggregate within families.
- FM is also found in up to 25% of patients with RA (see Chapter 5), AS (see Chapter 8), SLE (see Chapter 9). It is also commonly found in the hypermobility syndrome (see Chapter 16) and overlaps sympto-matically with this condition and chronic fatigue syndrome in many ways. Care must be taken to avoid misdiagnosing CWP/FM as the only cause for pain when there is autoimmune rheumatic disease present.
- FM is a controversial condition and its existence as a distinct entity remains uncertain. Its aetiology is multifactorial, with neurological, psychological, and behavioral factors important in its development.
- Psychological stresses may precede the onset of FM and CWP.
- Both FM and CWP are often associated with other somatic symptoms such as chronic fatigue, irritable bowel syndrome, multiple chemical sen-sitivities, and headache syndromes. △ Other causes of fatigue should always be excluded e.g. hypothyroidism, hypoadrenalism, anaemia etc.
- Alterations in hypothalamic–pituitary axis function in response to stress have been explored, but no differences between FM and controls have been found.
- Both CWP and FM are associated with alterations in peripheral and central pain processing. Painful stimuli are detected at lower levels in affected patients. Allodynia (pain in response to non-painful stimuli) found in these conditions is thought to be due to central sensitization and an 'amplification' phenomenon.
- FM patients have been found to have ↑ levels of substance P in the CSF—this may be a marker for these conditions, but not a routine clinical test! CSF levels of noradrenaline and serotonin metabolites are ↓ in FM. These transmitters are involved in descending spinal cord pain inhibitory pathways, and the observed reduction may be responsible in part for central sensitization.

Table 18.10 ACR 1990 criteria for diagnosis of fibromyalgia (FM)

History of widespread pain:
Pain is considered when all of the following are present:
Pain in the left and right side of the body, pain above and below the waist, axial skeletal pain, pain present for 3 months

Pain in at least 11/18 tender point sites on digital palpation with 4 kg pressure*. One point is given for each side of the body at the following 9 sites:

1.	Occiput: at the suboccipital muscle insertions
2.	Low cervical: at the anterior aspects of the inter-transverse spaces at C5–C7
3.	Trapezius: at the midpoint of the upper border
4.	Supraspinatus: at origins above scapula spine near medial border
5.	2nd rib: at 2nd costochondral junction
6.	Lateral humeral epicondyles: 2 cm distal from epicondyles
7.	Gluteal: in upper outer quadrants
8.	Greater trochanter: posterior to trochanter
9.	Knees: at medial fat pad proximal to joint line

*Positive tender point when subject says palpation was painful, 'tender' is not considered painful.

Fibromyalgia said to be present when both criteria are satisfied.
FM is not excluded by the presence of another disorder.

Treatment

- It is of paramount importance to consider carefully the way in which an explanation is given as to the nature of the condition. Many patients have suffered disappointment and blows to self-esteem and confidence. It may take some time and may be best approached over several visits. Many will be seeking a physical cause for the pain and may misinterpret discussion about pain amplification and its treatment as 'labelling' their condition as psychological. The label 'psychological' is in itself also legitimate medically but to the layperson it often stirs ideas of 'mad', 'all in the head' or 'malingerer'.
- It is important to assess the effect of symptoms on the patient's life, and to develop a good rapport so that psychosocial issues can be discussed. Chronic fatigue can be very disabling.
- The emphasis in the explanation should be reassurance that there is no serious underlying inflammatory/systemic condition or damage to the joints and muscles. Reassure that other conditions are absent and that no further investigations are needed.
- Although exercise may cause a short-term increase in pain, a prolonged exercise programme may well help.

- Pacing of activities is also important, avoiding patterns of periods of over-activity when feeling well, followed by periods of inactivity due to pain and fatigue afterwards. Pacing is one key component of Cognitive Behavioural Therapy, a chronic pain programme that, alongside aerobic rehabilitation, may be of significant benefit to patients with FM, CWP and JHS. This multidisciplinary approach (psychologists, physio-therapists, occupational therapists, doctors) has been tried with some success but remains incompletely studied.
- Education of family and partners is invariably helpful and often essential.
- NSAIDs and corticosteroids are not effective as the pain is not due to inflammation or tissue damage, and may cause increased morbidity due to side effects. Morphine should be avoided. Many patients will have tried analgesics with little effect. This in itself can fuel anxiety as to the cause and severity of their underlying condition as well as frustration and lack of confidence in their doctor.
- Tricyclic antidepressants such as amitriptyline (10–50 mg nocte) are often helpful in improving quality of sleep, ↓ morning stiffness and alleviating pain. Patients should be warned of side-effects such as dry mouth and that they may take 3–4 weeks to take effect. Patients are often also wary of being given an antidepressant. An explanation that it is being used as an analgesic is important to improve adherence. Amitriptyline is one of a group of drugs that ↑ 5-hydroxytryptamine.
- Amitriptyline is often combined with tramadol successfully.
- The efficacy of selective serotonin reuptake inhibitors (SSRI) is contro-versial. The use of fluoxetine, sertraline, or citalopram improves mood, but are less effective than tricyclics in treating pain, fatigue and sleep disturbance.
- Venlafaxine (serotonin and noradrenaline reuptake inhibitor) in high dose is effective in treating multiple symptoms in FM. Low dose treat-ment is ineffective.
- Sedative hypnotics such as zopiclone may be used to improve sleep.
- Both CWP/FM are conditions with relapses and remissions. Most patients will have ongoing symptoms. Patients with appropriate coping strategies, improvements in psychosocial stressors, and good social support networks are more likely to have a better outcome.

Common upper limb musculoskeletal lesions

*For a detailed view on the differential diagnosis of the entire range
of upper limb lesions, see Chapter 2*

Subacromial impingement (SAI) shoulder disorders

This may be due to a number of different disorders, the generation of shoulder pain from specific rotational or elevation movements of the arm owing to abnormalities of subacromial structures or of the rotator cuff mechanism. For diagnostic work-up and steroid injection of the shoulder see Chapter 2.

- SAI is the commonest type of presentation of shoulder pain in adults.
- Pain is often referred to the upper arm.
- The causes include acute rotator cuff tendonitis (may be calcific), subacromial bursitis, rotator cuff tear with cuff instability and impingement, glenohumeral instability owing to a number of different lesions (e.g. labral tear, synovitis 2° to crystal arthritis).
- Inferior acromial osteophytes/ACJ OA can accompany any subacromial lesion and are risks for recurrent rotator cuff disease.
- Long-term rotator cuff disease can lead to 'cuff arthropathy' with OA of the glenohumeral joint and significant chronic morbidity.
- In children or young adults with SAI, consideration of an underlying glenohumeral (instability) lesion is mandatory.
- Some but not all patients give a history of acute injury.

Steps important in making a diagnosis

- Rule out adhesive capsulitis and referred neck and subdiaphragmatic pain referral on clinical grounds, and characterize by doing impingement tests, realizing that clinical testing is not specific (see Table 19.1).
- Decide if there is a significant rotator cuff tear present as simple treatment steps (see below) might then not work. If there is any doubt, then image the shoulder.
- An AP X-ray can show specific changes (see Plate 2) that identify underlying glenohumeral or bony pathology. Consider specific ACJ views.
- If available request MR to rule out subtle GH pathology. Some labral tears are missed by T1+T2 weighted MR sequences alone—consider IV MR arthrogram. MR characterizes sites of cuff inflammation and is more sensitive than US in identifying cuff tears.

Conservative management of cuff/SA bursal inflammation

- Avoid overhead arm activities.
- Trial a full-dose regular NSAID for 2 weeks.
- If confidant of no cuff tear then consider giving subacromial long-acting steroid (e.g. triamcinolone acetonide 40 mg, see Plate 13) and local anaesthetic injection (e.g. 5 ml 1% lignocaine). Approach laterally or posteriorly.
- Consider physiotherapy from an experienced shoulder physiotherapist 1–2 weeks later if the cuff muscles are weak.
- Consider a second injection after 6 weeks.

- Failure to progress after 3 months conservative treatment requires investigation with a view to considering arthroscopic subacromial decompression.

Table 19.1 The range of disorders presenting with a subacromial impingement pattern of pain. Clinical testing, though it can be elaborate, has been shown repeatedly in studies not to be as specific as the original literature appeared to suggest.

Condition	Diagnosis made by
Supraspinatus/cuff tendonitis	MR or US
Subacromial bursitis (e.g. trauma, RA, gout, CPPD)	US/MR
Rotator cuff tear (partial or full)	MR or CT arthrogram
Long head of biceps tendonitis	Clinical, US/MR
OA ACJ (impingement of osteophytes on cuff)	Clinical, X-rays, MR
Glenohumeral instability 2° to labral trauma (e.g. SLAP lesion), arthritis GH joint	MR
Enthesitis (e.g. deltoid origin at acromion) in SPAs	Clinical, US
Lesion at suprascapular notch (e.g. cyst, tophus)	MR

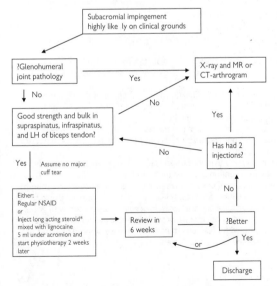

Fig. 19.1 Pragmatic algorithm for managing subacromial impingement pain
* Use 20–40 mg triaminolone acetonide (e.g Kenolog) or methylprednisolone acetate.

Adhesive capsulitis (AC)

Pain and restriction of the shoulder with active and passive movements of the joint in the absence of intrinsic disorder of the joint is highly suggestive of AC. The aetiology is unknown but it involves capsular and coracohumeral ligament contractures. The condition is more common in ♀ than ♂, typically affecting ♀ age 40–60 years and more common in diabetes (4 times). It is bilateral in 15%. Recurrence is unusual. If left alone symptoms of pain usually resolve within 2 years, though long-term restriction of shoulder movement is identifiable in a large minority.

Making the diagnosis

- Do not confuse AC with SAI disorders, where often passive movement done by the examiner can demonstrate good range of shoulder movements with less pain than with active movements. With AC the restriction remains, despite the examiner moving the joint.
- Clues to the diagnosis from examination include marked restriction of external rotation judged by rotating 'tray-holding' arms outwards; also, with abduction the scapular moves very early (normally it doesn't until 30° of abduction has been completed).
- If the presentation is delayed (>6 months) then a 2° SAI may have evolved as movement has been regained somewhat following the initial 'frozen' stage.

Principles of management

- Do not confuse AC with SAI disorders, though the 2 lesions can co-exist. The natural history and prognosis of AC and SAI disorders are not the same.
- Rule out associated conditions: diabetes, hypothyroidism, lung carcinoma, myocardial infarction, stroke, protease inhibitor use for HIV infection.
- Control pain during the initial painful–stiff phase of the condition. Consider NSAIDs, intra-articular steroid injections (e.g. 40 mg triamcinolone acetonide + 5–10 ml 1% lignocaine/saline), suprascapular nerve block, or a short course of prednisolone 30 mg/day for 3 weeks[1].
- Mobilize with physiotherapy early but be aware this may be limited by poor pain control.
- There is no good evidence for efficacy of these therapies or evidence that one intervention is better than another.
- Consider surgery if conservative management is failing after 6 months. Surgical procedures focus on releasing contracted/fibrotic tissue of the anteroinferior capsular structures. Procedures associated with good results (all studies open non-controlled series) include arthroscopic or open release with MUA or arthroscopic release alone. The latter has been combined with steroid injections.

---

1 Buchbinder R, Hoving JL, Green S et al. Short course prednisolone for adhesive capsulitis: a randomised, double blind, placebo controlled trial. Ann Rheum Dis 2004; **63**:1460–9.

Lateral epicondylitis (tennis elbow)

This condition is common, affecting 1–3% of the adult population, typically in the age group 40–60 years. The dominant arm is most affected. It is rare in elite tennis players though up to 40% of social players get it at some time. About 90% of all patients seen in clinical practice do not get this from playing tennis!

It is thought to be due to cumulative trauma overuse disorder from mechanical overloading. If chronic it can lead to tendon degeneration and osseous changes. Poor prognosis is associated with manual work, high level physical strain at work, and high baseline pain and distress.

Making the diagnosis

- The main differential diagnoses are: elbow joint lesions, referred neck pain and enthesopathies (e.g. DISH or enthesitis linked to spondylarthropathies—see Chapter 8).
- Pain is elicited by resisted force in pronation e.g. handshakes, turning doorknobs, carrying bags.
- There is tenderness at the lateral humeral condyle with pain elicited by resisted finger and wrist extension. Pain often extends down the extensor side of the forearm.
- Ask about psoriasis, inflammatory bowel disease, inflammatory spinal/buttock pain (e.g. AS), recent infection with chlamydia, or food poisoning (e.g. salmonellosis). These are all SpA-related features (see Chapter 8). SpAs are chronic, relapsing/remitting conditions. The many features do not necessarily occur simultaneously.
- Enthesopathies, tendon tears, and joint lesions may be diagnosed by an experienced musculoskeletal sonographer.
- MR may miss mild epicondylitis/enthesitis and appearances are not specific. MR is more useful for ruling out tendon tears and joint lesions. Do not use MR of the elbow to discriminate elbow lesions from referred neck pain.

Principles of management

- Systematic review identifies 7 different treatments to have shown some degree of evidence for working, but that laser therapy and pulsed EM field therapy is ineffective[1]. Extracorporeal shock wave treatment does not work better than placebo.
- Steroid injections around the epicondyle and onto the periosteum are frequently used. RCT evidence of efficacy is lacking but pain control with one injection indicates a good prognosis.
- A failure of conservative treatment requires imaging with MR/US.
- Surgery needs to be considered where the diagnosis has been confirmed and conservative management has failed (see Fig. 19.2).

1 Trudel D, Duley J, Zastrow I, et al. Rehabilitation for patients with lateral epicondylitis: a systematic review. J Hand Ther 2004; **17**: 243–66.

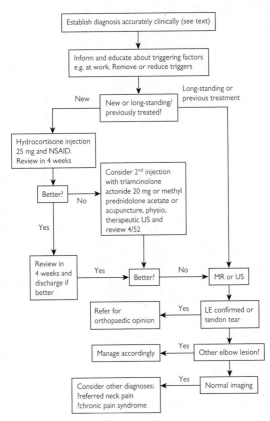

Fig. 19.2 Pragmatic algorithm for managing lateral epicondylitis (LE)

Back pain

Conditions causing acute or sub-acute back pain in adults

Acute mechanical back pain

- Most cases in a 1° care setting are uncomplicated and resolve spontaneously, though be aware of danger signs ('red flags') (see Table 20.1).
- The main differential to musculoskeletal pain is loin pain from the kidney, or, in older patients, vascular pain (aneurysm). If pain is related to posture or movement, especially of the thoracic cage, and local tenderness is felt at the lumbosacral junction then the pain is highly likely to be musculoskeletal.
- It is very important to be seen to take patients' acute back pain seriously to avoid inadvertently triggering or aggravating psychological factors that may lead to chronicity. Reassurance that severity of pain does not necessarily equal severity of cause is important.
- The immediate management is adequate and regular analgesia (not 'as required') such as paracetamol 1 g tds/qds or maximal dose codeine combination analgesics, advising only minimal bed rest, encouraging mobilization and normalization of activities.
- Short courses of diazepam 2 mg bd/tds or nitrazepam 5 mg nocte to ↓muscle spasm and aid rest/sleep should be considered.
- The clinician should explore patient fears and, where appropriate, reassure that serious illness is unlikely, tests are not usually needed, severe pain is often short-lived but milder pain may be present for longer, and that recurrences are common.
- Radiographs are likely to be unhelpful for planning management in most cases and radiologists often advise against getting them, but the role of such investigation in allaying patient anxiety/concern and orienting patients' perception of 'appropriate' management in trying to prevent longer term morbidity is unknown.
- A rehabilitation approach should be considered (see Table 20.2). The strength of evidence for therapies is variable. Adherence may be a problem with rehabilitation programmes but there is some evidence to support the notion that adherence may be augmented by providing patient education literature.

Table 20.1 Warning signs for sinister pathology in back pain

⚠ **'Red flag signs':**

1. First pain age <20 or >55 years

2. Non-mechanical pain (stiffness ± at rest)

3. Thoracic pain

4. Past history of carcinoma

5. On immuno supression (?infection)

6. Unwell/weight loss

7. Abnormal neurology

8. Structural deformity

Table 20.2 Therapies used in facilitating rehabilitation after acute mechanical low back pain

Manipulation	Either done by an osteopath, chiropractor, or physiotherapist. Some controversy as to the size of benefit owing to poor methodological studies. Avoid using in cases of intractable back pain (see Chronic back pain)
McKenzie exercises	Passive extension exercises designed to improve pain and stiffness associated with disc and anterior spinal structure pathology. May aggravate pain from posterior spine structures e.g. facet joints, spinous processes
Hydrotherapy or balneotherapy	Poorly studied but warmth can ease movement and augment land-based exercises. Might be considered after initial painful phase to regain normal movements and mobility. Obviously will only suit a few patients and resources may be limited.
Graded (physio') activity programmes	Useful if patients need a lead and would be unable to gain optimally from home exercise regime. A plan for rehab with milestones is useful for some patients.
Behavioural programmes	Focuses on psychological aspects of pain, involves moderate supervision and planned withdrawal of treatment. Differs from some other approaches in that the therapist takes on the 'control' of the back pain. Limited resources may restrict provision of this approach. Choice of patients for programme important though data scanty on this point.

Back pain and nerve root lesions (see also Chapter 2)

- Root compression occurs most often because of acute or sub-acute disc prolapse or foramenal stenosis. The peak incidence is age 30–50 years. About 70% resolve within 3 months and 90% within 6 months.
- Root compression should be suspected if acute or sub-acute back pain is associated with segmental nerve or sciatic leg pain.
- Acute sciatic pain (outer and posterior leg) is often sharp or burning in nature, most frequently arises from acute disc prolapse of either L4/5 or L5/S1 (>90% cases) and gives distal symptoms in the distribution of L5 and S1 (dorsum and sole of foot) or both.
- 'Straight leg raise' is sensitive for nerve root lesion and positive if pain is felt in the buttock or back at a leg angle of <60°. The test has a low specificity. Eliciting pain in a non-lifted leg could reflect a central (?large) disc prolapse (?cauda equina syndrome—saddle anaesthesia, ↓sphincter control).
- △ A neurological examination is essential: L5 root lesions give ↓strength of the foot and great toe dorsiflexion, standing on heel, and ↓ankle reflex and sensation over great toe. S1 root lesions give ↓strength in plantar foot flexion, difficulty weight-bearing on toes, and ↓ankle reflex and sensation on sole or outer part of foot.

Principles of management

- The natural history is such that 40–50% of patients are free of pain after 1 month.
- Pain relief: consider bed rest (1–2 days) initially and maximal dose paracetamol, NSAIDs, or both or, if severe, codeine combination analgesics with NSAIDs. Avoid under-treatment and giving the perception of not taking the symptoms seriously as this is a risk factor for chronic pain.
- An epidural steroid injection can improve pain in the short-term but data from RCTs does not show better long-term outcome at 3 months or longer compared with controls.
- An 'NNT metanalysis' showed that 1 in 7 patients having a steroid epidural get >75% improvement in pain in the short-term and 1 in 13 get >50% symptom improvement in the long-term.
- Physiotherapy and supervised rehabilitation using lumbar extensor exercise regimes may be of benefit. Efficacy has not been shown in robust RCTs.
- MR can characterize lesions but 25% of asymptomatic people have frank disc protrusions; thus MR gives poor specificity. MR should be used to confirm a diagnosis, not to reach for one.
- The absolute indications for surgery (see Table 20.3) are a cauda equina lesions or progressive muscle weakness and neuropathy causing functional disability.

Table 20.3 Surgical approaches for lumbar disc prolapse

Discectomy	Essential for discs causing cauda equina syndrome and progresssive neurological deficits. Excluding above indications, compared to conservative therapy, in a RCT 66% vs. 33% patients were satisfied following surgery at 1 year, 66% vs. 51% were satisfied at 4 years thus benefit of surgery in the long-term is small. SEs of surgery: mortality <0.2%, dural tears in 4%, permanent nerve root injuries in <1%. About 70% success rate in short term. ↑Risk of failure from surgery relates to ↑hysteria or hypochondriasis scores on MMPI* and presence of litigation claims.
Microdiscectomy	Smaller surgical field results in earlier mobilization and less postoperative disability. Outcomes similar to those of conventional discectomy.
Percutaneous discectomy	Suctioning of central disc material causing disc decompression and relieving nerve root pressure. Associated with low complication rate and rapid rehabilitation. Non-RCT data suggest similar efficacy to discectomy.
Chemonucleolysis	Injection of proteolytic enzyme into disc. RCTs suggest standard discectomy is superior. NICE (UK) suggest efficacy data is not sufficient to support its use. Rare but devastating neurological complications and risk of anaphylaxis (0.3%).
Laser lumbar discectomy	Vaporizing of part of disc by laser introduced through a needle probe. Efficacy possible similar to discectomy. No RCT data. NICE (UK) concluded efficacy and safety data not adequate to support use of procedure.
Prosthetic intervertebral disc replacement	Also indicated for degenerative disc disease, post-laminectomy syndrome and non-specific persistent low back pain. Artificial discs consist of 2 endplates separated by pliable inner core. Anterior approach needed. Good results reported in open series for pooled patient groups. Complication rate may be high (up to 45%). NICE (UK) advise against use owing to lack of long-term efficacy data.

*MMPI = Minnesota Multiphasic Personality Inventory.

Facet joint (FJ) syndromes
- FJ OA of the lumbar spine is common in middle aged/elderly adults, can be part of inflammatory generalized OA, and is associated with spondylolytic spondylolithesis.
- Psoriatic arthritis (see Chapter 8) can also affect FJs and is almost certainly under-recognized as a cause of low back pain.
- It is likely that CPPD arthritis (see Chapter 16) can affect FJs.
- Typical symptoms include pain on extending or rotating the low back, pain referred to the upper buttocks worse on standing still and eased by forward lumbar flexion.
- FJs cannot usually be felt but muscle spasm may accompany flares of FJOA etc. and superficial soft-tissues may be tender.
- Arthritic FJs are best detected using oblique spinal radiographs and bone scintigraphy with SPECT.

Management options for FJ syndromes
- Patients can be treated according to principles applied for all patients with acute mechanical back pain except that extensor exercises are contraindicated as they will aggravate symptoms.
- Short courses of analgesics and/or NSAIDs as for OA (see Chapter 6).
- Generally advise minimal bed rest.
- FJ steroid injections: evidence for efficacy controversial. Bone scan (SPECT) images can inform image-guided steroid injections. However, note injections for any joint OA have limited success and pain from tissues around FJs is almost certain to some degree.
- Radio frequency denervation of medial branches of dorsal rami supplying FJs can help (significantly compared with sham procedure) but the procedure should only be considered if local anaesthetic block works first.

Lumbar canal stenosis
- The diagnosis is frequently missed in the elderly.
- It presents mainly with achy, stiff pains in the legs increasing on walking and eases if the patient stops walking, sits, or leans forward (claudication).
- Symptoms may be aggravated by extension associated with a congenitally narrow spinal canal.
- Bladder involvement is frequently present though often lesions have been long-standing and the consequent sphincter control changes are not regarded as part of the problem by the patient.
- Neurological leg signs can be accentuated after exercise.
- The diagnosis is made using MR imaging the L-spine.
- Surgical decompression should be considered if leg pain rather than low back pain is the major problem, functional incapacity is significantly due to this rather then co-morbidities, the patient has good cardiovascular and respiratory health, and the stenosis is focal not extensive.

Non-traumatic vertebral collapse: work up

- This is usually due to osteoporosis, collapse into an abnormal vertebra (e.g. vertebral haemangioma), or 2° to malignancy or infection.
- The history should therefore focus around such pathologies e.g. ?osteoporosis–post-menopausal ♀, previous fragility fracture, early menopause, steroid use or positive family history of fractures. Also consider alcoholism and in men, hypogonadism. For myeloma or infection—weight loss or systemic symptoms, other bone pains.
- Examine the spine for kyphosis, loss of height (?multiple fractures), neurological compromise (particularly cord compression) and perform a full examination to try to exclude malignancy.
- Investigate with AP and lateral spinal X-rays, MR, bone biochemistry (±PTH), 9 am LH/testosterone, TFTs, serum/urine electrophoresis and tests to disclose 1° malignancy as a cause of metastasis.
- MR is good at discriminating infection and tumours from osteoporosis though biopsy for histology and culture is essential if tumour or infection has not been confidently ruled out by MR.

Non-traumatic vertebral collapse: immediate treatment

- The patient should be assigned to bed rest and there should be monitoring for evolving neurological lesions.
- Pain control often requires bd morphine sulphate with short acting opiate (e.g. oromorph) for breakthrough pain.
- Calcitonin 100–200 IU bd s/c or 200 IU/day by nasal spray has an analgesic effect and reduces bone turnover in osteoporosis. Regular codeine/paracetamol and NSAIDs are unlikely to be sufficiently helpful alone.
- Discuss any pathological malignancy-related fracture with a radiotherapist.
- If conservative measures fail to relieve pain consider vertebroplasty or balloon kyphoplasty.

Post-surgical back pain

- There are numerous causes and no single entity (see Table 20.4).
- Imaging with Gd-enhanced MR may be helpful to delineate inflammatory tissue around the surgical site.
- Persistent pain after surgery may be associated with adverse psychological and social factors and outstanding litigation or insurance claims.
- Nerve root blocks, epidurals, and spinal stimulators may be used.

Sterile discitis

- This is inflammation of the intervertebral disc often associated with annulus enthesitis at the vertebral end-plates and vertebral osteitis.
- The causes include disc degeneration, CPPD disease (probably), AS (Romanus lesions) and other SpAs including SAPHO.
- The lesion should be identified with MR and treatment should include bed rest and aggressive analgesia. In RCTs, steroid disc injections have been shown to be little help overall. IV bisphosphonates (e.g. pamidronate 60–90 mg) has anecdotally been shown to help AS and SAPHO discitis notably.

Table 20.4 Implicated causes of post-surgical back pain

Recurrent disease	e.g. further disc protrusion and radicular features. If re-operation not appropriate consider nerve root block, steroid epidural etc.
Operation for wrong lesion	MR appearances can highlight lesions, which may not be relevant to clinical features. More than 1 or 2 lesions can co-exist. Detailed clinical assessment *prior* to imaging is essential.
Misdiagnosis originally	Many rheumatologists will be familiar with cases of 'failed' surgery undertaken for a structural lesion but where inflammatory disease, typically SpA-related disease, was present and causes on-going symptoms.
Adverse rehabilitation conditions	Resolution of symptoms and regaining functional capacity if slow has been associated with significant psychological and social factors. Poor result of surgery also associated with an outstanding insurance claim or litigation.
Arachnoiditis	Thought to be a direct effect of surgery. Dural tissue becomes inflamed. In nerve root/disc surgery often associated with sensory root symptoms for some months afterwards. Diagnosis with Gd-enhanced MR. Where associated with sensory radicular symptoms, may respond to steroid root block, epidural. If radicular symptoms chronic and disabling consider spinal cord (implanted) stimulator.

Management of chronic back pain

Chronic back pain requires a special approach, quite holistic with emphasis on psychological and social management. Patients are likely to have set beliefs about their problem, the ability of healthcare systems to help them, and are more likely to have developed coping strategies than patients with acute or sub-acute back pain. However, those with chronic back pain who continually seek further and different healthcare options are likely to have less successful coping strategies.

Initial approach to the care of patients with chronic low back pain (see Table 20.5)

- Be confident there is no undiagnosed condition affecting back pain and that no new neurological lesions have evolved. If examination raises concern, use MR to rule out lesions.
- Establish empathy and trust, taking time to get information about the patient's:
  - social situation
  - health and illness beliefs
  - intra-family dynamics
  - true role and perception of their role at work
  - view on conventional and complementary therapies
  - view on what does and doesn't work and on their specific view of exercise therapy.
- With the above information you will be able to plan a more individually-tailored approach to management.
- Plan the management approach with the patient and establish short- to mid-term goals, including whether, and what type of, supervision is required (e.g. graded programme of exercise) and how often a review is needed.
- Consider 'domains' of therapy under the following headings:
  - physical therapy
  - work/life commitments
  - psychological and social support
  - painkillers and medications
  - education (insight and coping strategies)
- Plan to review progress at regular intervals.
- Evaluate patients carefully at baseline if considering long-term opiate use. There may be ↑risk of dependency if the patient currently or previously abused drugs, there's a high level of psychological distress, if short-acting opiates are used, or drugs are prescribed 'as required'.
- Though many strategies, especially those that combine techniques, can be costly, these costs to healthcare are likely to be offset by the saving in 'wages loss cost' in many cases.

Table 20.5 Management options for chronic low back pain

Exercises	RCT evidence supports use. Greater evidence of effect when combined with behavioural methods. Aerobic exercises augment effect of 'back school'. Should be essential part of outpatient physical retraining programme. Less evidence on how much should be supervised, by whom, and how often.
Manipulation	Trials show efficacy on ↓ pain in the long term.
Transcutaneous electric nerve stimulation (TENS)	Disappointing results from 2/3 RCTs in patients with chronic back pain though efficacy for other specific diagnoses unknown.
Posture training	May be more appropriate than corset use and easy to combine training with supervised exercise therapy.
Oral medications	NSAIDs best reserved for acute-on-chronic pain exacerbations. Low-dose tricyclics (e.g. amitriptylene, dothiepin, lofepramine) are useful particularly if chronic neuropathic pain present. Try to avoid long-term opiate drugs though having analgesics to hand that are known to be effective is often useful.
	Chronic opiate use for chronic low back pain is not extensively studied. A mental health evaluation before long-term prescribing is essential to ↓ chance of triggering dependency (see text) and short courses initially for trial period sensible. Best supervised by specialist with experience in pain management.
Back school	Regular programme carrying an educational component. Programmes vary from one to many sessions. May be more effective in occupational setting. Long-term changes in behaviour not extensively studied. Non-compliance and relapse are problems.
Psychologically-oriented rehab programmes	Intensive courses often run by psychologists and 'hands-off' physical therapists can help (highly) selected patients. Focus on learning to cope with pain and ↑ control of effects of pain on functioning and psyche. Not suitable for many patients. Courses few and far between. Cost-effectiveness of courses not proved.
Complementary therapies	Increasingly used (see Chapter 22). By consensus, chiropractic has been shown to be helpful for chronic low back pain. Acupuncture has yet to be proved successful in robust studies. Poor evidence base otherwise.
Intrathecal opiates	Conflicting results from (only) non-controlled studies. Generally results show overall short-term pain ↓ but results on ↑ activity are weaker. Best reserved for patients where all else has failed.
Spinal cord stimulator (SCS)	A number of good studies show that SCS is effective for neuropathic including radicular pain. Technique is relatively safe. Careful patient selection is important. Studies show ↓ pain ≈50% maintained long-term.

Management of back pain in children and adolescents

Children with spinal problems present with deformity, back pain, limping, systemic features, neurological features, or a combination of effects. Back pain in children is common—up to 30%. It is rare in the young <10 years. If severe enough to warrant hospital admission there is frequently an underlying cause. Age determines likelihood of cause, with infection and tumours being more common in young children compared with adolescents.

The principles behind history and examination in children are discussed in Chapter 2.

Non-specific low back pain

- The annual incidence is 10–22% in schoolchildren.
- Adolescent back pain is linked with familial clustering, physical inactivity, sports injuries, ↓muscle strength, psychosocial factors.
- Most children have self-limiting symptoms.
- Management should focus on an explanation of the short natural history, reassurance, addressing predisposing factors (see above) that remain a trigger for recurrence and increasing general health/exercise to improve muscle strength.

Idiopathic scoliosis

- This is often vertebral malalignment in the coronal plane associated with spinal rotation accentuated on spinal flexion.
- It occurs in up to 3% of schoolchildren.
- Most are asymptomatic (≈70%). Progression is more likely in the presence of pain or thoracic curve convex to the left—conditions that should be investigated for more serious underlying spinal pathology.
- Progressive scoliosis (see Fig. 20.1) requires bracing or surgery. Usually curves of 25–45° are braced and those >45° are best considered for surgery.

Congenital (CS) and neuromuscular (NMS) scoliosis

- CS is associated with genitourinary malformations (20%) and, rarely, congenital heart disease. CS is associated with spinal dysraphism (20%), myelodysplasia, and Klippel-Fiel syndrome.
- NMS is associated with cerebral palsy, muscular dystrophy, spinomuscular atrophy, and myelodysplasia.
- To avoid rapid progression and ↑long-term morbidity and disability, refer for prompt correction of progressive curves. Orthotic treatment is an adjunct to, not substitute for, surgery.

Table 20.6 Causes of back pain in children

Developmental

Painful scoliosis

Spondylolysis and spondylolisthesis

Scheuermann disease

Infection

Discitis

Vertebral osteomyelitis

Spinal epidural abscess

Inflammation

Juvenile arthritis

Osteoporosis

Mechanical

Herniated disk

Muscle strain

Fractures

Neoplasms

Benign (osteoid osteomas, osteoblastoma, aneurysmal bone cyst)

Malignant (leukaemia, lymphoma, sacroma)

Visceral

Pyelonephritis, appendictis, retroperitoneal abscess

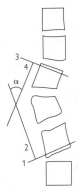

Fig. 20.1 Measurement of the degree of scoliosis by the Cobb method: 1, the lowest vertebra whose bottom tilts to the concavity of curve; 2, the erect perpendicular to line 1; 3, the highest vertebra whose top tilts to the concavity of curve; 4, the drop perpendicular to line 3; α, the intersecting angle. Curves less than 20° are considered to be mild, 20–40° are moderate, and above 40° are severe

Scheuermann's osteochondritis

- This is perhaps the most common cause of spinal deformity and back pain in children and adolescents (3–5% of all adolescents usually 13–17 years). The aetiology is unknown.
- If severe it can form a kyphosis and then frequently becomes symptomatic. Compensatory lumbar lordosis evolves.
- The typical radiographic pattern is one of wedge deformities (<10°) of contiguous thoracic vertebrae with irregular vertebral end-plates.

Management of symptomatic disease

- Avoid repetitive stress-loading activities such as running.
- Extensor exercises for the back and abdominal muscle exercises may improve symptoms but will not correct kyphosis.
- Brace treatment usually prevents progression of kyphosis.
- Surgery is reserved for severe persistent pain, if there are severe or progressive deformities (>70°) or there is great concern about the appearance.

Spondylolysis and spondylolisthesis

- Spondylolysis is a defect in the pars interarticularis, most commonly seen at L5. Alone as a lesion it is common (4% preschool children and 6% at age 18 years).
- Spondylolysis is a risk factor for asymptomatic and symptomatic spondylolisthesis (slippage of one vertebra on another, see Fig. 20.2).
- Progressive slippage is rare in children but can occur during the adolescent growth spurt.

Management

- On serial radiographs if slippage is >25% (Grade II, III, or IV) then advise against contact sports or sports involving lumbar hyperextension.
- Advise should be given on regular abdominal muscle exercises, avoiding gaining centripetal obesity, and consider regular bracing.
- Surgery is considered for *progressive* vertebral slippage or Grade III/IV slip.

Herniated disc

- This is infrequent in children. Most occur after >11 years and are often associated with scoliosis.
- Diagnose disc herniation by MR but be cautious in interpreting normal developmental changes in the growing spine.

Management

- Without nerve root impingement management is conservative: short period of bed rest, adequate analgesics and NSAIDs with early exercise-based rehabilitation regime.
- Over 50% improve with conservative treatment but reported results from surgery for significant nerve root lesion (persistent severe pain ± neurological deficit) are very good.

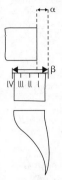

Fig. 20.2 Spondylolisthesis measured as a % slip of L4 on L5 (α/β). Grade I <25%, Grade II 25–50%, Grade III 50–75%, and Grade IV >75%.

Spinal tumours

- ⚠Though rare in children, spinal tumours frequently present with back pain (80% cases).
- It is important to recognize painful scoliosis, radicular pain, night pain, stiffness and effectiveness of NSAIDs which are all (though not specific) features of spinal tumours.

Management

- Urgent radiographs (may be negative in early disease) and MRI are needed to delineate the nature of the problem and the clinician should consider bone scintigraphy (the latter with SPECT) or focal CT to identify posterior element tumours (e.g. osteoid osteoma).
- Adequate analgesia is required: NSAIDs—ibuprofen in recommended doses for weight may not be sufficient, consider naproxen 250 mg qds for adolescents.
- Bed rest is not essential though wise if scans show there is risk of vertebral collapse or cord compression. If the latter is a worry this should be discussed urgently with a paediatric spinal surgeon and radiotherapist.
- Initiate a search for other tumours known to metastasize to spine (see Table 20.7).
- Investigation of adolescents on specific adolescent units is advisable given the specific multidisciplinary input often needed.

Table 20.7 Primary spinal tumours in children and adolescents (see also Table 2.17)

Osteoid osteomas

Benign. Not uncommon. Mainly adolescents. Posterior vertebral bone usually. Pain can be severe. Discriminated from osteoblastomas by size (osteomas are <1.5 cm, osteoblastomas >1.5 cm) as histology is often identical. Lesions are associated with scoliosis (63% cases). Surgical excision is treatment of choice.

Aneurysmal bone cyst

Benign. Symptoms often triggered by vertebral collapse. Care when considering biopsy to discriminate from malignant lesions. Discuss in detail with musculoskeletal radiologist.

Eosinophilic granulomas

Benign—often occurs around age 10 years. Rare. Lytic lesion. May occasionally be multiple/disseminated—staging important. Symptoms often triggered by vertebral collapse. Cord and radicular compression can occur. Biopsy essential to discriminate from malignant lesions. Surgical excision or internal spine fixation not usually needed. Consider radiotherapy if cord compression threatened. Consider external brace fixation in all and monitor for spontaneous resolution. Disseminated lesions can be treated with chemotherapy.

Ewing sarcoma

Overall rarely affects spine (≈10% cases). Can affect any part of spine including sacrum (latter cases often delayed diagnosis). Treat with combination chemotherapy and local radiotherapy. 5-years survival ≈50%. Outcome better for tumour sizes <8 cm or localized disease.

Leukaemia

Consider both ALL and AML in all cases of spinal osteopaenia or single/multiple vertebral collapse. Notorious association with delayed diagnosis. Associated systemic symptoms may not necessarily be present but normal FBC at presentation unlikely (≈10% cases only). Also look for eosinophilia and hypercalcaemia and consider bone marrow aspirate.

Lymphomas

Rarely presents with back pain; however, known cause of persistent back pain. MR is imaging of choice. MR can show vertebral collapse and/or soft tissue paraspinal mass. Biopsy is diagnostic. Case reports of plasmacytomas presenting similarly.

Secondary malignant tumours

Neuroblastoma, rhabdomyosarcoma, Wilms tumour, retinoblastoma and teratoblastoma are know to present with back pain. Usually biopsy evidence for then triggers a search for the underlying primary neoplasm.

Rheumatological emergencies

For vertebral fracture see Chapter 20

Septic arthritis

Infection in a joint can progress rapidly and cause destruction of tissues and permanent deformity and disability. When septic arthritis is suspected investigations should be prompt, appropriate (or appropriate empiric) antibiotics/antifungals should be started without delay, and, where feasible, infected tissue should be removed. The epidemiology of infections is discussed in Chapter 17.

Suspecting infection

- Septic arthritis is uncommon but is more likely to occur in patients with established joint disease, around prosthetic joints, and where patients have co-morbidity such as diabetes or chronic renal disease, or when patients are immunosuppressed. Patients are often not systemically unwell.
- The main differential diagnosis in adults is crystal arthritis (see Chapter 15).
- The commonest causative organisms in children are: *S. aureus* and streps with *H. influenzae* type b only significantly affecting the 7–36 month old age-group though occurring in those up to age 11 years. Gonococci cause almost 30% of cases in children >11 years.

Immediate management of adult joint sepsis
(see Table 21.1)

- Immobilize the joint and provide adequate analgesia.
- Take blood for FBC (CBC), ESR, culture, U/Es Cr, LFTs, CRP, and serology.
- Manage septic shock as appropriate and rule out infective endocarditis (especially in IV drug user (IVDU) or in those with known cardiac valve disease).
- Drain the joint completely (use at least an 18-gauge needle) and send the sample of joint fluid for Gram stain, culture, and for polarized light microscopy (LM). If the polarized LM is positive and cultures negative after 48 hours then consider diagnosis of gout or CPPD.
- Joint fluid with a WCC >50 000/mm^3 (mainly neutrophils) and a glucose < 400 mg/L is highly suggestive of infection.
- Suspect Gonococcus in young, sexually-active adults; where there are pustular skin lesions, tenosynovitis, or migratory arthralgias—further swabs and cultures are required, see below.
- Liaise early with orthopaedics (arthroscopic washout of knee, hip, or shoulder) and with microbiology to arrange a Gram stain of joint fluid and set up cultures/special tests for atypical organisms. See Table 21.1.
- Empiric antibiotic treatment in the absence of a positive Gram stain in adults in a straightforward clinical scenario should be IV vancomycin 1 g bd and cefotaxime 1 g tds to cover staphs, streps, and entero-bacteriaceae. See Table 21.1.
- Consider vancomycin or teicoplanin if Gram positive clusters on LM of joint fluid and patient previously MRSA positive.
- If pseudomonas is suspected (e.g. IVDU) use ceftazidime 2 g IV tds.

Table 21.1 Initial choice of antibiotics for septic arthritis based on Gram stain in adults. All antibiotics are given IV initially

Gram's stain result	Probable pathogen	Antibiotic choice
Gram-positive cocci Clusters	*Staph. aureus* (methicillin resistance suspected)	Nafcillin (2 g every 4 h)
		Vancomycin (1 g every 12 h)
	Staph. epidermis	Vancomycin (1 g every 12 h)
Pairs and chains (urinary, biliary, bowel)	Streptococci	Penicillin G (2.5 million U every 4 h)
	Enterococci	Penicillin G (2.5 million U every 4 h) and gentamycin (1 mg/kg every 8 h)
Gram-negative cocci (haemorrhagic rash, meningitis)	*N. gonorrhoeae* *N. meningitidis*	Ceftriaxone (1–2 g every 12 h)
		Penicillin G (2.5–5 million U every 6 h)
Gram-negative coccobacilli	*H. influenzae* (ampicillin resistance suspected)	Ampicillin (2 g every 6 h)
		Cefotaxime (1 g ever 8 h)
Gram-negative bacilli	Enterobacteriaceae	Cefotaxime (2 g every 8 h)
	Pseudomonas spp.	Ceftazidime (2 g every 8 h)
No organisms seen (healthy young adult)		Ceftriaxone (1–2 g every 12 h)
	N. gonorrhoeae	
(older adult, under-lying disease)	Staphylococci	Vancomycin and cefotaxime
	Streptococci	
	Enterobacteriaceae	
(intravenous drug abuser)	Staphylococci	Vancomycin and ceftazidime
	Pseudomonas spp.	
	Enterobacteriaceae	

Source: Reprinted with modification from Parker, R. H. (1998). Acute bacterial arthritis. In *Orthopedic Infections* (ed. D. Schlossberg), p. 74. New York: Springer-Verlag.

Specific management in children (see Fig. 21.1)

Prompt IV antibiotic therapy is essential. Initially treat according to the most likely organism for age: <3 months cover *S. aureus*, Gram negative enteric organisms and group B strep; for those 3 months to 2 years cover *S. aureus*, *S. pneumoniae* and *K. kingae*. In older children cover staph and strep as for adults.

Post-immediate management of septic arthritis

- Review analgesia regularly.
- Rule out multiple foci of infection.
- Discontinue any immunosupressants but consider an ↑ in steroid dose if systemically unwell and HPA axis suppression likely.
- Adjust antibiotics according to culture sensitivities and in discussion with a microbiologist.
- For affected weight-bearing joints keep non-weight-bearing until improvement obvious from ↓pain, ↓swelling, ↓CRP, ↑passive movement possible on bed and you are confident the patient is on appropriate antimicrobials.
- Physiotherapists should be involved early to help passive mobilization of joint before patient weight-bears.
- The evidence for routine duration of antibiotic course is not strong and the regime should be individualized. Common protocols include IV antibiotics for 1–2 weeks and a further oral course for 2–4 weeks.

Reasons for no/poor improvement

- The wrong diagnosis must be considered: think about crystals, RA (see Chapter 5), and SpA monoarthritis (see Chapter 8).
- Consider that the infection has been successfully treated but that the slow progress is owing to super-added crystal-induced or reactive autoimmune arthritis, foreign body, or background disease (e.g. RA).
- The antimicrobials may not be covering the infection. Consider multiple infecting organisms (re-culture), atypical organisms (re-take history, review evidence from serology/special stains or cultures).

Gonococcal (GC) septic arthritis

- Cultures can be initially negative. If suspected re-culture blood but also urethra, cervix (80–90% positive), rectum, pharynx, pustules, and joint fluid. Send urine for GC nucleic acid detection.
- Use IV ceftriaxone 1–2 g bd for 1 week (as >5% organisms are penicillin-resistant) then, depending on susceptibility, either amoxicillin 500 mg tds or ciprofloxacin 500 mg bd orally for 1–2 weeks.
- Consider empiric therapy for C trachomatis—doxycycline 100 mg.
- All sexual partners should be recommended ceftriaxone 125 mg IM and doxycycline 100 mg orally.
- Consider fluoroquinolone resistance in isolates from men who get infection from homosexual intercourse. Consider HIV testing.
- Discuss with clinical immunologist re: ruling out hereditary complement deficiency (C5–C9) where infection with GC is recurrent.

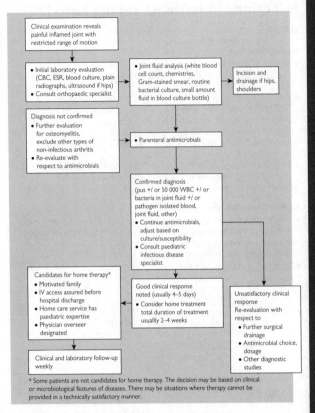

Fig 21.1 Management of suspected septic arthritis in the child.

Reproduced with the permission of Oxford University Press from the *Oxford Textbook of Rheumatology 3e*, edited by Isenberg, David *et al.*

Infections in patients taking anti-TNFα drugs

Background

- Over the last 5 years, immunosupressants, which specifically inhibit the actions of TNFα or IL-1 have become widely used for RA (see Chapter 5).
- Anti-TNFα drugs (infliximab/Remicade®, etanercept/Enbrel® and adalimumab/Humira®) have been/will be increasingly used for Crohn's disease, juvenile idiopathic arthritis (see Chapter 7), psoriasis and psoriatic arthritis (see Chapter 8), AS (see Chapter 8), myositis (see Chapter 13), vasculitis (Chapter 14 and 21) and Behçet's disease (see Chapter 18) for example.
- The risk of infections is ↑ with anti-TNFα use but also the severity and type of infections occurring needs special consideration.
- Deaths from infection have been reported.

Characteristics of infections

- There may be a disassociation of the expected correlation between severity of systemic features and severity of infection in such patients. Patients might actually be sicker and more at risk of severe morbidity than clinical evaluation first concludes.
- Disseminated fungal and viral infections can occur (see Table 21.2).
- Activation of commensal organisms or reactivation of previously contracted infections may be a particular problem. Breakdown in host immunity controlling latent infection may be important.
- The BSR registry (www.rheumatology.org.uk) records details of >7000 patients about adverse effects including infections occurring in anti-TNFα-treated RA patients across UK regions and is a useful repository of information. General conclusions about infections in any single population have not yet been drawn but may be available from analysis of the BSR registry in the near future.
- Numerous reports of TB occurring with anti-TNFα treatment have led to the recommendation of pre-treatment assessment for previous/ present TB, not giving anti-TNFα in high risk TB cases, and either simultaneous TB chemotherapy for a number of months or 6 months chemoprophylaxis in moderate TB risk cases.
- Reactivation of TB should be considered in febrile patients and those not screened for TB before anti-TNFα treatment.
- Infections overall tend to reflect local prevalence of infecting microorganisms rather than a tendency to develop a number of specific infections.
- The risk and severity of infections appears to be ↑ in those also taking other immunosupressants, especially steroids.
- Patients may need a longer than normal course of antibiotics and need careful re-assessment before re-starting anti-TNFα drugs.

Table 21.2 The range of organisms and type of infections reported in the literature or witnessed by authors in association with anti-TNFα treatment. Fatalities have occurred

Organisms		Nature of infection
Bacteria	M. tuberculosis	Disseminated
		Pulmonary
	Atypical mycobacteria	
	Listeriosis	Septicaemia
		Septic arthritis
		Meningitis
	Staph	Septicaemia
		Cavitating pneumonia
	Salmonella	Septicaemia
		Septic arthritis
	Moraxella	Septic arthritis
	Actinobacillus	Septic arthritis
	Nocardia	
Viruses	Varicella	Disseminated 1°
	H. simplex	Severe
	Hepatitis B	Reactivation
	CMV	Disseminated
Fungi/yeasts	Candida	Septicaemia
	Cryptococcus	Pneumonia
	Aspergillosis	Disseminated
	Sporotrichosis	Skin
		Disseminated
	Pneumocystis	Pneumonia
		Disseminated
	Histoplasmosis	Pneumonia
		Disseminated
Parasites	Leishmaniasis	Visceral

Acute SLE

Acute SLE will manifest either in patients with established disease where there is suboptimal disease control or monitoring, or as the first presentation of the disease. Serial measures of C3 (trend ↓) and DNA antibodies (trend ↑) may predict acute disease flares in some patients.

The reader is referred to Chapter 9 for SLE and Chapter 10 for Antiphospholipid syndrome and catastrophic APS.

Diagnosing SLE in an acute medical context

- Consider SLE as a diagnosis in all young and middle-aged ♀ presenting with current/history of joint pain and skin rash, pleuritic chest or abdominal pains (serositis), and unexplained fever or sweats.
- A history of Raynaud's, recurrent mouth ulcers, myoarthralgias and UV-sensitive skin rash, though non-specific, is easy to check for and, if present, a pointer to the diagnosis.
- As labs usually do not test for ANA, C3/C4 and other serology urgently these tests will not help you make the diagnosis initially.
- The CRP is often negative/↓ if acute SLE is not accompanied or preceded by significant infection. Patients with serositis complicating SLE, can have ↑CRP. ↑ESR isn't a reliable sign of SLE activity.

Acute SLE nephritis (adults)

- Check the BP accurately, creatinine, urea, electrolytes, send urine for culture and 24 h urinary protein and US the renal tract to rule out post-renal obstruction.
- Quantification of urinary protein and creatinine grades severity of the renal lesion and guides management approach (see Fig. 21.2).
- Control BP. Often a diuretic, ACEI and β-blocker is required.
- Discuss the need for kidney biopsy with a nephrologist. WHO biopsy activity index can inform treatment decisions (Class III–V is usually treated with steroids + immunosupressant (see below and Fig. 21.2). Steroids alone (0.5 mg/kg/d.) can be used for WHO Class I/II where there is little ↓GFR and proteinuria is mild.
- Steroid-induced osteoporosis and IHD risk should be managed from the outset. Consider getting the following done early: DXA scan and lateral TSp+LSp radiographs (?previous # in women age 50+), ECG, and fasting cholesterol and HDL:LDL.
- If AZA is to be used then consider testing TPMT status early (avoid giving AZA to the 1:300 Caucasians homozygote for no gene activity/low TPMT activity).
- Give weekly bisphosphonate and daily calcium (1000 mg) and vitamin D (800 iu) at the start of steroid therapy in all, and withdraw bisphosphonate if DXA shows the BMD is high (all T scores >−1.5).
- Both oral and pulse IV cyclophosphamide regimes are used. There is a need to counsel patients about infertility, malignancy, and haemorrhagic cystitis risks, the dose schedules (e.g. ±MESNA), monitoring (FBC at day 10 after and prior to IV pulse) and pneumocystis prophylaxis chemotherapy (e.g. cotrimoxazole 460 mg bd every third day). See Fig. 21.2.

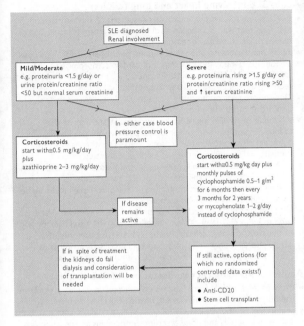

Fig. 21.2 The management of adult renal SLE: treatment algorithm

Reproduced with the permission of Oxford University Press from the *Oxford Textbook of Rheumatology 3e*, edited by Isenberg, David et al.

Acute SLE involving heart and lung (adults)

- Cardiac and isolated pulmonary manifestations of SLE are rare and in many patients with SLE, acute cardiac and pulmonary features may be due to other common conditions.
- ↑CRP may reflect infection or significant pleuropericardial SLE. Lupus pericarditis alone without evidence of cardiac compromise can be treated with NSAIDs and prednisolone 20–40 mg/d for 2–4 weeks reducing dose then over further 2 months.
- Monitor progress of pericarditis treatment closely given the ↑risk of pericardial constriction from steroid therapy.
- If not due to cardiac failure, acute dyspnoea in SLE may be due to intercurrent infection, pneumonitis, pulmonary vasculitis, PE, pulmonary hypertension (more likely 2° to PEs rather than 1°) or ventilatory difficulty from the pain of pleural serositis.
- There is little evidence to favour use of cyclophosphamide over AZA for cardiopulmonary manifestations of SLE even if features severe—assuming acute situation is controlled on steroids though it should be considered for severe ILD/pneumonitis.
- Both oral and pulse IV cyclophosphamide regimes are used. There is a need to counsel patients about infertility, malignancy and haemorrhagic cystitis risks, the dose schedules (e.g. ±MESNA), monitoring (FBC at day 10 after and prior to IV pulse) and pneumocystis prophylaxis chemotherapy (e.g. cotrimoxazole 460 mg bd every third day).

Acute haematological manifestations of SLE (adults)

- Many patients with SLE are Coomb's positive without having significant haemolysis (and do not need treating as such).
- Features of haemolysis include fever, shivers, pyrexia, anaemia, ↑bilirubin in serum and urine, ↓serum haptoglobins and reticulocytosis.
- Acute thrombocytopaenia is a relatively frequent presentation.
- If severe, both haemolytic anaemia (Hb < 7 mg/dL) and thrombo-cytopaenia (platelets < 25 000) require high dose prednisolone 60–80 mg/d. AZA or cyclophosphamide may also be used (see above).

Table 21.3 Important aspects in management of acute cardiopulmonary manifestations of SLE in adults

Initial clinical cardiac assessment should include:	ECG, blood for CK, troponin T, echo
Initial lung assessment should include:	ABGs, CXR, spirometry, HRCT chest, VQ scan
Consider PE	Consider empirical anticoagulation early and check for lupus anticoagulant, APL antibodies, and complete thrombophilia screen.
Pulmonary vasculitis (very rare)	Features: severe dyspnoea, CXR abnormal, ↑KCO. Requires ICU and chest physician support and consider plasma exchange.
Interstitial lung disease	Requires high-dose steroids and either AZA (up to 2.5 mg per kg/d or cyclophosphamide). Cyclo has less chance side-effects as IV regime e.g. 0.5–1 g every 2 weeks x6 then maintenance doses every 3 months reviewed every 6 months.
Antiphospholipid syndrome	PE associated with APL syndrome in SLE requires lifelong anticoagulation.
Specific therapies	
Steroids	Assuming non-viral infections excluded or treated most cardiopulmonary SLE features respond to oral prednisolone 0.5–1 mg/d (max 60 mg/d). Consider initial 3 consecutive days methylprednisolone 500–1000mg IV if clinical situation extreme and IV steroids will not compromise clinical situation.
Mycophenolate	Mycophenolate mofetil (0.5 mg bd initially increasing after 1–2 weeks to 1 g bd) can be considered if AZA or cyclophophamide contraindicated or patient intolerant. It is increasingly being used as an alternative to cyclophosphamide for inducing remission in lupus nephritis. May prove to be as effective as cyclo in inducing remission with less incidence of side-effects.
Anti CD20	Though evidence minimal, rituximab (anti-CD20) 1 g infusion repeated after 2 weeks may be considered if other immunosupressants contraindicated or patient intolerant.
Bone protection	All patients treated with steroids require daily calcium (1 g) and vitamin D (800 IU). Most should also get bisphosphonate initially—withdrawn if DXA scan shows good BMD with all T scores >-1.5

Paediatric SLE—acute nephritis

- The commonest lesion is diffuse proliferative GN (30–45% cases).
- One-third have hypertension which may need aggressive management
- All have microscopic haematuria and proteinuria >3 mg/kg/d. Most have >25 mg/kg/d proteinuria. However up to a third may have serum albumin > 35 g/L and about 50% maintain GFR >100 ml/min/1.73m^2.
- Prognosis and therapy of nephritis is guided by the active WHO-grade pathological lesion and chronicity index; thus biopsy is important.
- Management includes high dose steroids and AZA.
- Cyclophosphamide is reserved for treatment failures or when in renal failure. In acute fulminant renal disease consider plasmapheresis. Mycophenolate is also being increasingly used and MTX can be used to maintain remission (see Fig. 21.3).

Paediatric SLE—acute haematological manifestations

- Overt haemolysis occurs in <10%, thrombocytopaenia in 15–45%.
- Bleeding is uncommon.
- Most with thrombocytopaenia respond to steroids and/or IVIG.
- Thrombotic thrombocytopenia (TTP) is rare but presents with microangiopathic haemolytic anaemia, neurologic and renal disease. In childhood, TTP is commonly associated with SLE unlike in adults where it is rarely associated.
- A high index of suspicion is needed to diagnose catastrophic APLS. It is characterized by multiple organ thromboses and microangiopathic changes.
- All cases require close liaison with haematologists as highly informed interpretation of detailed serial coagulation studies are required.
- The treatment of haematological manifestations of SLE is shown in figure 21.4.

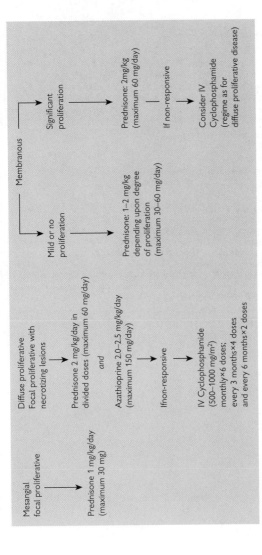

Fig. 21.3 Therapy flow chart for treating paediatric SLE nephritis
Reproduced with the permission of Oxford University Press from the *Oxford Textbook of Rheumatology*, 3e, edited by Isenberg, David et al.

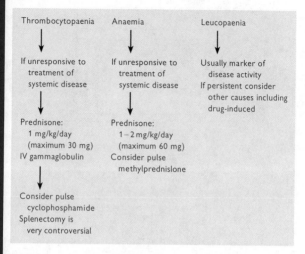

Fig. 21.4 Flow chart for treating paediatric haematological manifestations of SLE
Reproduced with the permission of Oxford University Press from the *Oxford Textbook of Rheumatology 3e*, edited by Isenberg, David et al.

Systemic vasculitis

The management of acute vasculitis is an emergency whether large (giant cell (GCA)) or small (e.g. Wegener's granulomatosis (WG)) vessels are involved because permanent organ damage from ischaemia or infarction can evolve quickly. The specific management of each type of vasculitis is outlined in relevant sections of Chapter 14.

Identifying patients with vasculitis

- Disease presentation ranges from the obvious, with a typical purpuric skin rash, to the difficult because of few specific features (e.g. patient 'unwell', PUO, and ↑ESR).
- The need for treatment varies. HSP, drug-induced, or hypersensitivity skin vasculitis often needs no specific therapy assuming the trigger has been removed. GCA and systemic cANCA positive vasculitis require prompt treatment with high dose steroids and the latter cyclophosphamide or MTX.
- Often a high index of suspicion is required to make a diagnosis and detailed questioning in the history is important. For example, patients with WG may have months/years long history of recurrent stuffy nose with epistaxis, transient recurrent coughs, and previous CXR abnormalities.
- Systemic vasculitis is firmly in the differential diagnosis of causes of non-specific illness associated with ↑CRP/ESR where malignancy and infection are unlikely or have been excluded.
- Be proactive in looking for skin, kidney, lung, neurological, and eye involvement.

Important tests in investigating vasculitis

- Check the ESR, CRP, and complement C3/C4. All are usually ↑ greatly in systemic vasculitis except C3/C4 in SLE-related vasculitis. ↑ Eosinophils are seen in Churg–Strauss.
- Check urinalysis, lightmicroscopy (LM) of urine sediment (?casts), creatinine, and 24-hr creatinine clearance, and if abnormalities arise discuss these with a nephrologist re: a renal biopsy (?WG/MPA).
- Check the ANCA. cANCA pattern with PR3 specificity suggests WG. MPO specificity may be associated with other vasculitides notably microscopic polyangiitis (MPA). The ANA is of less use and is often negative.
- Tissue biopsies: for WG consider nasal, transbronchial or open lung, kidney or skin; for MPA consider kidney; for GCA consider temporal artery; for CSS consider skin/nerve/lung.
- Angiography/MRA or FDG-PET may be of value in investigating Takayasu's arteritis (nonspecifically unwell, ↑ESR/CRP++, absent or diminished pulses). Angiography of coeliac axis and renal artery is valuable in looking for PAN (PET/MRA have too poor resolution to identify small aneurysms).
- Check the hepatitis B status (association with PAN) and hepatitis C serology (associated with cryoglobulinaemia).
- Pulmonary vasculitis/haemorrhage can complicate WG, MPA, and rarely CSS. Prompt diagnosis is important. Check for ↑KCO on lung function and consider broncho-alveolar lavage (BAL).

Table 21.4 Management of systemic vasculitides

GCA	Baseline ESR/TA biopsy/ophthalmology review. Prednisolone: 40-60 mg/d with weekly bisphosphonate, daily calcium 1 g/vitamin D 800 IU and consider PPI in all. Regular aspirin 75–150 mg/d ↓risk of CVAs. If ischaemic ocular lesions may need higher steroid doses—d/w ophthalmologist.
Takayasu's arteritis	Confident angio/MRA or PET scan diagnosis at baseline is important. Treat with prednisolone 1 mg/kg/d initially and taper dose. Disease relapses are frequent. Bone protection as for GCA.
WG and other PR3+ systemic vasculitides	Baseline urine LM, Cr, CrCl/GFR, CXR/PFTs, ANCA, and obtain confident biopsy result. Treat limited (early systemic) disease with either prednisolone 1 mg/kg/d + cyclophosphamide 2 mg/kg/d or MTX 15–25 mg/w. Treat generalized disease with prednisolone 1 mg/kg/d and cyclophosphamide 2 mg/kg/d. After disease remission obtained switch to AZA up to 2.5 mg/kg/d with low-dose prednisolone. Pulsed IV cyclophosphamide is an alternative to oral cyclophosphamide and side effects arguably less, but relapse rates following remission higher. Bone protection as for GCA. Consider initial pulse daily methylprednisolone, plasmapheresis and early dialysis when there is severe renal disease or pulmonary haemorrhage.
Microscopic polyangiitis	Investigate as for WG. Up to 80% have pANCA (MPO). 80–100% have renal involvement. Alveolar haemorrhage is not infrequent (↑KCO, diagnosed on BAL). Treatment approaches are similar to those for WG. Close renal support required including control of BP, dialysis, and considering plasmapheresis. Bone protection as for GCA.
Polyarteritis nodosa	Unless skin (rash/nodules) or nerves involved biopsy material may not be easy to get. Associated with, thus check, hepatitis B. Organ infarction/ischaemia common (e.g. bowel 'angina'). Complete abdominal arterial angiography is usually necessary to make diagnosis in adults. Treat with prednisolone 1 mg/kg/d and either continuous daily cyclophosphamide 2 mg/kg/d or fortnightly IV cyclophosphamide 0.5–1 g x6 to induce remission. Discuss with hepatologist use of vidarabine or zidovudine to treat if hepatitis B positive. Bone protection as for GCA above.
Churg–Strauss vasculitis	Can involve heart, lung, sinus/nose, skin, eye, and nerves. History of previous asthma and ↑eosinophils. Investigate proactively for range of organ involvement. Biopsy lung, nerve or sinus tissue. Treat as for PAN. Bone protection as for GCA.
Henoch–Schönlein purpura	Monitor for gut and kidney involvement. Skin disease alone usually requires no specific drug treatment. NSAIDs for joint pains. Monitor for 2° skin infection. Consider prednisolone 20–40 mg/d if gut involvement. Role of steroids, other immunosupressives and plasmapheresis in adults or children with renal involvement controversial.

Scleroderma (Scl) crises

Renal crisis

- This may manifest as an acute or subacute hypertensive crisis usually in diffuse scleroderma (dcScl) within 5 years of onset (Chapter 12). It can be the presenting feature of Scl.
- Diagnostic criteria include an abrupt ↑BP >160/90 and hypertensive retinopathy grade III or more, with rapid deterioration of renal function and ↑ plasma renin activity.
- Other features include a microangiopathic haemolytic blood film, encephalopathy and convulsions.

Acute Scl renal crisis management

- Control the BP avoiding fast drop with absolute/relative hypovolaemia as perfusion pressures in Scl-affected renal vessels can worsen kidney failure; ⚠ thus avoid labetalol or IV nitroprusside.
- Use ACE-Is and calcium channel blockers aiming to ↓diastolic and systolic BP by 20 mmHg in first 24 h. Maintain the diastolic at 80 mmHg or below.
- Use IV continuous infusion prostacyclin from diagnosis.
- Liaise with the nephrologists about renal replacement therapy: use haemodialysis short-term but PD long-term if required.
- Prompt initial treatment often leads to re-establishment of good renal function and skin Scl can improve.

Pulmonary hypertension (PHT)

- This usually occurs acutely in lcScl patients as a 1° feature. Often patients are anti-centromere positive. It can occur 2° to lung fibrosis often complicated by PE(s).
- It presents acutely/subacutely with SOB, SOA, ↑JVP, normal CXR and lung volumes on spirometry but ↓KCO, normal VQ scan, normal LV function on echo but ↑RV and PA pressures on echo doppler of the heart. The mean PAP is typically >30 mmHg on Doppler.

Management of acute Scl-related 1° PHT

- Stabilize the patient using continuous IV prostacyclin and maintain arterial O_2 >90%.
- Use spironolactone to blunt hyperaldosteronism and consider digoxin for its inotropic effect.
- Rule out a PE with a VQ scan or spiral CT scan of the lung.
- Liaise early with experienced cardiologists (or in UK, regional PHT centre) so that a right heart catheter with vasodilator challenge can be organized ± pulmonary angiogram.
- All patients with PHT need anticoagulation long-term but use heparin prior to heart catheterization.
- For grade III/IV PHT consider bosentan (endothelin-1 receptor antagonist).

Methotrexate-induced pneumonitis

This is rare but it can occur in any patient given methotrexate (MTX). Reports suggest the incidence ranges from <0.5% to 7% of patients (variation due to definition of condition). It is probably much rarer in children/adolescents compared with adults. Life-threatening pneumonitis requiring hospital admission probably occurs in <1% patients taking MTX. It is thought that mild pneumonitis resolves on drug withdrawal alone.

Patients at risk

- Most patients suffering pneumonitis do so within the first few months of starting MTX or after a significant dose ↑.
- In patients on stable-dose MTX, ↑ in blood levels owing to ↓renal function or ↓levels of folate may predispose to MTX-induced toxicity including pneumonitis.
- Consider the diagnosis in all patients on MTX with acute onset of dry cough, dyspnoea, headache, and fever. The differential diagnosis lies between chest infection, acute pulmonary oedema, or acute ILD associated with underlying disease.

Immediate management of severe toxicity

- Admit to a respiratory unit (e.g. ARCU) if possible.
- Check the degree of acidosis and ABGs and arrange urgent respiratory support accordingly.
- Stop MTX and give folinic acid.
- Get a CXR (?bilateral interstitial infiltrates) and consider getting an urgent HRCT chest.
- Take sputum and blood for culture, check the ESR/CRP, urea, electrolytes and creatinine, LFTs, folate (↓levels are a risk for MTX toxicity).
- Check the Hb as anaemia (including haemolysis) may worsen dyspnoea.
- Check procalcitonin (normal level has a high negative predictive value for *bacterial* infection).
- Rehydrate and transfuse as required.
- Discuss with a chest physician: BAL provides no specific information in terms of MTX-induced pneumonitis but can be useful in obtaining material for special stains (?pneumocystis) and culture.
- Investigate as usual for acute cardiac/coronary pathology with acute LVF (ECG, cardiac enzymes, troponin I, TTEcho etc.).

Steroids alone or with cover?

- Early treatment with IV methylprednisolone 250 mg/d (x3 d) then prednisolone 20–40 mg/d and tapering dose over 2–4 weeks is recommended where the diagnosis is likely and condition is severe.
- Co-treatment with appropriate antibiotics, pneumocystis therapy, and anti-fungals depends on the degree of certainty these infections have been ruled out.

Complementary medicine in rheumatology

Introduction

The popularity of alternative and complementary medicine (CM) among people with chronic diseases including arthritis is widely recognized. In some areas up to one third of arthritis sufferers have received CM from CM practitioners[1] and CM use prevalence has been reported at between 30–100% rheumatological patients[2]. Among the most popular are dietary approaches, herbalism and acupuncture. Few interventions, however, have been studied in a robust way.

The prevalence of CM use for chronic arthritis and pain chiefly mirrors that in other chronic diseases and appears to be consistent across Western populations.

CMs appear very popular despite very little evidence for their efficacy. Using 'homeopathy, complementary medicine and arthritis' as prompt words for searching articles on CM and arthritis in a widely recognized search engine for articles written in medical and scientific journals (www.ncbi.nhm.nih.gov/entrez/query.fcgi) revealed 1080 articles (1950–2006); however, using the same words to search the internet with either 'google' or 'yahoo' reveals 321,000 and 212,000 hits respectively (2005).

There may be no universal explanation as to why patients use CMs. Gender, age, income, education, degree of underlying psychological stress, and desire to regain 'greater self control' may all influence use. Published suggestions for CM use also include dissatisfaction with orthodox medicine or the belief that a philosophy associated with a particular CM is desirable and aligns with the patients' own philosophy.

1 Resch KL, Hills, Ernst E. Use of complementary therapies by individuals with 'arthritis'. *Clin Rheumatol* 1997; **16**: 391–5.
2 Ernst E Usage of complementary therapies in rheumatology: a systematic review. *Clin Rheumatol* 1998; **17**: 301–5.
3 Ernst E Musculoskeletal conditions and complementary/alternative medicine. *Best Pract Res Clin Rheumatol* 2004; **18**(4): 539–56.
4 Weiner DK, Ernst E. Complementary and alternative approaches to the treatment of persistent Musculoskeletal pain. *Clin J Pain* 2004; 20(4): 244–55.

Herbal remedies (phytotherapy)[1]

- The likely mechanism of effect of most agents is on eicosanoid metabolism inhibiting either cyclo-oxygenase or lipoxygenase pathways.
- Most efficacy studies illustrate methodological flaws—notably the failure to power studies sufficiently given small differences in outcome vs. placebo. Risk–benefit profiles are generally unknown.
- Adverse reactions similar to those from conventional medicines can occur and include allergy and drug interactions.
- In most countries few legal controls exist to ensure quality of herbal medicine constituents and no legislative 'medicine development' framework exists to reliably ensure safety and efficacy.

Phytodolor

This is a standardized extract of Populus tremula marketed for rheumatic pain. Reviews suggest studies overall show a pain reduction effect in patients with OA (see Chapter 6) compared with placebo.

St John's wort (Hypericum perforatum)

- St John's wort has been shown in relatively robust trials to improve mild depression. This may relate to its effect on inhibiting synaptosomal uptake of 5-HT, dopamine, normetanephrine, glutamate, and GABA.
- Symptom ↓ in patients with arthritis or chronic pain may be 2° to improvements in mood, pain perception or coping strategies.
- There are important interactions with some conventional drugs. Rheumatologists need to be aware of the interaction of Hypericum with ciclosporin—upregulating cytochrome P450 activity and ↓ ciclosporin blood levels. Interference with warfarin levels and elimination of other drugs can also occur.

Gamma (γ) linoleic acid (GLA)

- GLA is a plant seed-oil derived unsaturated fatty acid which suppresses production of Il-1β. It is contained in many different plant seed oils (e.g. blackcurrant seed oil).
- Compared with placebo, 2.8 g/d GLA significantly ↓ symptoms and signs of active RA over 6 months.[2] However, virtually all plant-seed oil preparations that contain GLA are likely to be taken at lower daily doses than those shown to be effective.

Devil's Claw (Harpagophytum procumbens)

- This may work by ↓ cyclo-oxygenase or iNO synthase in joint tissuesor by ultimately ↓ matrix metalloproteinase production from chondrocytes.
- At 60–100 mg/day, harpagophytum extract (harpagoside) has moderate but significant effects on back and joint pain associated with OA.[3]

1 Soeken KL, Miller SA, Ernst E. Herbal medicines for the treatment of Rheumatoid arthritis: a systematic review. *Rheumatology* 2003; **42**(5): 652–9.
2 Zurier RB, Rossetti RG, Jacobson EW et al. Gamma-linolenic acid treatment of rheumatoid arthritis. A randomized placebo-controlled trial. *Arthtis Rheum* 1996; **39**: 1808–17.
3 Gagnier JJ, Chrubasik S, Manheimer E. Harpgophytum procumbens for osteo-carthritis and low back pain: a systematic review. *BMC complement Altern Med* 2004; **4**: 13–23.

Physical and 'hands on' therapies

Acupuncture

- Acupuncture is commonly used to treat neck and back pain and is easily incorporated into primary care consultations.
- Meta-analyses suggest short-term efficacy for low back pain[1] but no overall effect for neck pain.[2]
- Controversy exists among acupuncturists as to adequacy of acupuncture techniques used for back pain in published trials.
- No convincing evidence exists to suggest acupuncture should be advised for mid/long-term relief of symptoms in OA or RA.
- Serious complications of acupuncture exist (e.g. pneumothorax, hepatitis B, spinal cord injury, infection) but are rare. Complications may be under-reported.[3,4]

Tai Chi

- In RA, Tai Chi has been shown to ↑ plantar flexion range and is associated with a higher level of participant enjoyment.
- Trials have shown few benefits in terms of outcome measures. It appears not to exacerbate RA.[5]

Reflexology

- This is one of the most frequently used CMs.
- From the few controlled trials taken together, results do not suggest there is any specific therapeutic effect.

Spinal manipulation

- Of the most rigorous sham-controlled studies of manipulation (for any indication of back pain) none showed benefit compared with placebo.
- Review suggests that about 50% of patients have side-effects though these are chiefly mild or transient.[6,7]
- Reliable estimates of the incidence of serious adverse effects do not exist. Reported effects include vertebral arterial dissection, strokes, disc herniation, spinal fracture, cauda equina syndrome and, possibly under-reported but likely, worsening of undisclosed spinal inflammatory conditions (e.g. AS/SpA, discitis).
- Reports from neurologists suggest serious neurological lesions occurring after neck chiropractic are not infrequent.
- There is concern over excess radiation risk from overuse of radiographs ordered by practitioners.

1 Ernst E, White AR. Acupuncture for backpain: a meta-analysis of randomized controlled trials. *Arch Intern Med* 1998; **158**: 2235–41.

2 White AR, Ernst E. A systematic review of randomized controlled trials of acupuncture for neck pain. *Rheumatology* 1999; **38**: 143–7.

3 Ernst E, White AR. Life-threatening adverse reactions after acupuncture? A systematic review. *Pain* 1998; **71**: 123–6.

4 Ernst E. Acupuncture—a critical appraisal. *J Intern Med* 2006; **259**(2): 125–37.

5 The Cochrane library. Issue 4. 2004.

6 Ernst E. Prospective investigations into the safety of spinal manipulation. *J Pain Symptom Manage* 2001; **21**: 238–42.

7 Ernst E, Canter PH. A Systematic review of systematic reviews of spinal manipulation. *J R Soc Med* 2006; **99**(4): 192–6.

Homeopathy

Homeopathy stems from the belief that tiny quantities of substances have an holistic therapeutic effect. There has been a great publicized debate as to whether homeopathy is genuinely more effective than placebo and whether conventional randomized studies are a relevant way of evaluating its effect. Reports in the medical and scientific literature invariably generate prolonged and sometimes fierce debate in the letters pages for some time afterwards! Nevertheless homeopaths are among the most frequently visited CM practitioners by patients with arthritis.

• Metanalyses of therapeutic trials might suggest the clinical effects of homeopathic remedies cannot be fully explained by placebo effects alone.[1] However, the most robust methodological studies do not show any positive effects compared with placebo.[2,3]

• There is some evidence that short-term improvement in RA symptoms is superior to placebo.[4] A more robust methodological study, however, suggested no symptomatic improvement in RA over 3 months in patients stabilized on DMARDs and NSAIDs.[5]

• Summarizing four RCTs of homeopathy use in OA, there appears to be a positive effect though firm conclusions cannot be reached.[6]

• One of the most frequently used homeopathic remedies is *Arnica montana*. A systematic review of its effects[7] suggests there's no proof of its effect.

• Preparations of *Echinacea* are believed by some to have significant immunomodulatory properties but although historically advocated for pain and arthritis—originally appearing in nineteenth century N.America adapted into 'elixirs' as American Indian people had used the *Echinacea*—containing plant 'purple cornflower' for its 'medicinal properties'—no reliable evidence exists for its efficacy.

1 Linde K, Melchart D. Randomized controlled trials of individualized homeopathy: a state-of-the-art review. *J Altern Complement Med* 1998; **4**: 371–88.

2 Ernst E, Pittler MH. Efficacy of homeopathic arnica: a systematic review of placebo-controlled clinical trials. *Arch Surg* 1998; **133**: 1187–90.

3 Ernst E. Are highly dilute homeopathic remedies placebos? *Perfusion* 1998; **1**: 291–2.

4 Jonas WB, Linde K, Ramirez G. Homeopathy and rheumatic disease. *Rheum Dis Clin* 2000; **26**: 117–23.

5 Fisher P, Scott DL. A randomized controlled trial of homeopathy in rheumatoid arthritis. *Rheumatology* 2001; **40**: 1052–5.

6 Long L, Ernst E. Homeopathic remedies for the treatment of osteoarthritis: a systematic review. *Br Homeopath J* 2001; **90**: 37–43.

7 Ernst E, Pittler MH. Efficacy of homeopathic arnica: a systematic review of placebo-controlled clinical trials. *Arch Surg* 1998; **133**: 1187–90.

Other CMs

Dietary supplements

- Commonly used supplements by patients with arthritis and pain include cod liver oil, fish oil tablets, vitamins and selenium.
- Though there is little available scientific evidence to support any recommendation of any sort of dietary modification, individuals may wish to 'do something for themselves' in the scheme of managing and coping with a chronic disease. Support from the carer is vital. Self-help books may be useful.

Hypnotherapy

- This is of long-standing interest in controlling pain but shown also to improve short-term measures of anxiety and depression.
- There is some evidence for efficacy in fibromyalgia patients.

Relaxation therapy

- Various studies suggest short-term benefit for patients with RA but proof of effects on measures of disease in long are absent.
- Methodological deficiencies in studies and absence of cost-effectiveness data suggests no firm conclusion can be drawn about the role of therapy in specific individuals or disease groups.

Spiritual healing

- A 'therapeutic experience' transmitted by a therapist's touch, non-touch, prayer or 'mental healing'.
- Examples include Therapeutic touch, Reiki and Distance Healing. There's some evidence that 'Therapeutic touch' done by nurses can reduce anxiety in hospital patients. No data exist which compare this to talking to/informing patients about their condition.

Other

- Electrical stimulation ↑ grip strength in RA patients with hand muscle atrophy. Pulsed electrical stimulation can help knee OA symptoms. Data is weaker for an effect on pain from neck OA.
- Thermotherapy for RA—including wax and Faradic baths, hot and ice packs have brief positive effects without causing harm.
- The positive effects and results of trials of balneotherapy in RA and low back pain[1] patients cannot be ignored. Trial methodology has been poor however—trials have generally not studied relevant outcomes.

Further information

- Focus on Alternative and Complementary Therapies (FACT) available from The Pharmaceutical Press (www.pharmpress.com) or website at Peninsula Medical School (fact@exeter.ac.uk).
- Mason S, Tovey P, Long AF. Evaluating complementary medicine: methodological challenges of randomised controlled trials. *BMJ* 2002; **325**: 832–4.(www.bmj.bmjjournals.com).
- If the drugs don't work. *Guardian* 2004; March 2. (www.guardian.co.uk/health/story/0,,1159913,00.html)

---

1 Pittler MH, Karagulle MZ, Karagulle M, Ernst E. Spa therapy and balneotherapy for treating low back pain: meta-analysis of randomized trials. *Rheumatology* 2006 Jan 31; [Epub ahead of print].

Index